Praise for *Niacin: The Re___*

"Dr. Hoffer's early work led to the use of niacin for schizophrenia and as a cholesterol treatment and successfully treated many thousands of patients with high doses of niacin. The authors present some very compelling evidence to support treating most psychotic disorders as a vitamin B$_3$ dependency. Considering it is very inexpensive and has virtually no dangerous side effects, niacin would certainly be worth a consideration for anyone who has a family member with this mental health challenge. I highly recommend picking up this book and learning more about its use."

   —Dr. Joseph Mercola

"*Niacin: The Real Story* is a classic. This book should be read and even studied by everyone. It will help keep readers healthy and save many lives. More people will benefit from the teachings of Drs. Hoffer, Saul, and Foster."

   —Richard Passwater, PhD

"This new edition of *Niacin: The Real Story* clarifies and describes the latest scientific evidence on supplementing with this important vitamin. Niacin (vitamin B$_3$) is inexpensive and comes in several forms that the body incorporates through slightly different pathways. As shown many decades ago by Dr. Abram Hoffer, when taken in safe and appropriate doses, it can enhance brain function—reducing the risk of mental illness. Saul's clear writing style explains how niacin can also reverse kidney disease and the risk of several types of cancer, and contribute to health body-wide."

   —Robert G. Smith, PhD, Research Associate Professor,
   Perelman School of Medicine

"Niacin is the real thing! It is anti-inflammatory and neuroprotective. Research also shows positive results for coronavirus as well as some other viral and bacterial diseases."

   —Bo H. Jonsson, MD, PhD, Karolinska Institutet, Stockholm

"Dr. Hoffer worked with well over 2,000 children under the age of four using nutrient therapy including an adequate amount of niacin/niacinamide and saw great responses to it. What a boon it would be for children with ADHD, along with their parents, to have that critical choice as opposed to drug treatment only. Dr. Hoffer's research on niacin proved to be lifesaving for many thousands of patients with schizophrenia, bipolar, and other mental health conditions, as well as many other conditions, such as high cholesterol, arthritis, and more. His work continues to be a gift to the world."

—**Rosalie Moscoe**, author of *Frazzled Hurried Woman*

"Dr. Hoffer's writings changed my son's life. His schizophrenia was cured with niacin treatments. My son, fully recovered, went on to become CEO of a marketing company ten years later."

—**Atsuo Yanagisawa, MD, PhD,** President of the International Society for Orthomolecular Medicine

"*Niacin: The Real Story*, Abram Hoffer's final book, has a wealth of information about Dr. Hoffer's favorite vitamin, which he recommended optimal doses of to many of his patients and tens of thousands of readers. Abram Hoffer even advised his mother to take niacin and it helped her. Everyone who reads Abram Hoffer's writing will find it interesting and helpful. Books such as *Niacin: The Real Story* will continue to give readers the chance to learn the facts so they can use that information to support safe, effective, and restorative care for a wide range of patients. Each copy sold could save a life!"

—**Robert Sealey**, author of *Finding Care for Depression, Mental Episodes & Brain Disorders*

"I found this book to be a real treasure. It made me love dietary supplements, especially vitamin B_3, in view of the very positive effects that it offers to our body. Everyone should have this book as a health support."

—**Tahar Naili, MD**

"*Niacin: The Real Story* is a great book. It shows patients their path to health, and it shows doctors who didn't learn about niacin in medical school how to make their patients healthy."

—**Bernhard Welker, MD**

Also by Andrew W. Saul, PhD

AS AUTHOR

Doctor Yourself: Natural Healing That Works

Fire Your Doctor!: How to Be Independently Healthy

AS COAUTHOR

The Vitamin Cure for Alcoholism

Vitamin C: The Real Story

Orthomolecular Medicine for Everyone:
Megavitamin Therapeutics for Families and Physicians

I Have Cancer: What Should I Do?:
Your Orthomolecular Guide for Cancer Management

Hospitals and Health:
Your Orthomolecular Guide to a Shorter, Safer Hospital Stay

The Vitamin Cure for Children's Health Problems

The Vitamin Cure for Depression

Vegetable Juicing for Everyone:
How to Get Your Family Healthier and Happier, Faster

The Vitamin Cure for Infant and Toddler Health Problems

AS EDITOR

The Vitamin Cure for Women's Health Problems

The Vitamin Cure for Eye Disease

The Vitamin Cure for Chronic Fatigue Syndrome

The Vitamin Cure for Digestive Disease

The Vitamin Cure for Arthritis

The Orthomolecular Treatment of Chronic Disease:
65 Experts on Therapeutic and Preventive Nutrition

The Vitamin Cure for Heart Disease

The Vitamin Cure for Diabetes

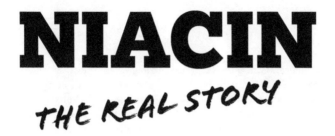

NIACIN
THE REAL STORY

SECOND EDITION, REVISED, UPDATED, AND EXPANDED
BY ANDREW SAUL

Abram Hoffer, MD, PhD,
Andrew W. Saul, PhD,
and Harold D. Foster, PhD

FOREWORD BY
W. Todd Penberthy, PhD

Basic Health Publications, Inc.

BASIC HEALTH PUBLICATIONS, INC.
AN IMPRINT OF TURNER PUBLISHING COMPANY
Nashville, Tennessee
www.turnerpublishing.com

Niacin: The Real Story 2nd Edition

Cover design by William Ruoto
Book design by Tim Holtz

Library of Congress Cataloging-in-Publication Data

Names: Saul, Andrew W., author. | Hoffer, Abram, 1917-2009, author. | Foster, Harold D., author. | Penberthy, W. Todd., writer of foreword.
Title: Niacin : the real story / Abram Hoffer, MD, PhD, Andrew W. Saul, PhD, and Harold D. Foster, PhD; foreword by W. Todd Penberthy, PhD
Description: Second edition. | Nashville, Tennessee : Turner Publishing Company, [2023] | Includes bibliographical references and index.
Identifiers: LCCN 2022026765 (print) | LCCN 2022026766 (ebook) | ISBN 9781684429028 (paperback) | ISBN 9781684429035 (hardcover) | ISBN 9781684429042 (epub)
Subjects: LCSH: Niacin—Therapeutic use—Popular works. | Vitamin therapy—Popular works.
Classification: LCC QP772.N55 H64 2023 (print) | LCC QP772.N55 (ebook) | DDC 615.3/28—dc23/eng/20220720
LC record available at https://lccn.loc.gov/2022026765
LC ebook record available at https://lccn.loc.gov/2022026766

Printed in the United States of America

Contents

To all the physicians who have demonstrated that niacin cures disease, with particular honor to Joseph Goldberger,
William Kaufman,
Rudolf Altschul,
Edmond Boyle,
William B. Parsons,
Humphry Osmond, and Abram Hoffer.

Acknowledgments

We would like to thank Steven Carter, Director of the International Society for kind permission to use material that originally appeared in the *Journal of Orthomolecular Medicine*. We are indebted to the late Charlotte Schnee Kaufman for gracious encouragement and permission to extensively reprint text from her husband's privately printed book *The Common Form of Joint Dysfunction* and also to publish correspondence, notes, and other writings of her husband, Dr. William Kaufman, thus making his important work widely available to the public. We greatly value the specialized input of Dr. Robert G. Smith, Stephen D. McConnell, Nick Fortino, and all other valued contributors to the *Orthomolecular Medicine News Service*, many articles of which are incorporated in this book. A very special thanks to Dr. W. Todd Penberthy for providing the foreword and for many important additions to the text. The Brattleboro (Vermont) Historical Society kindly provided background information on Dr. Kaufman's printed work, and *WholeFoods* magazine graciously granted permission to use the Dr. Passwater interview series.

Foreword

BY W. TODD PENBERTHY, PHD

Niacin raises high-density lipoprotein (HDL), or good cholesterol, more than any known pharmaceutical, while simultaneously lowering total cholesterol, triglycerides, and the most pathogenic form of cholesterol-associated lipoprotein, very low-density lipoprotein (VLDL). This wide array of generally clinically desirable chemical adjustments is undeniable based on precise biochemical measures. Niacin (extended-release formula, Niaspan) has been shown to reduce disease progression in four other clinical trials as well.[1] Medical doctors with proper knowledge of niacin will prescribe it for reducing cardiovascular disease risk and provide a description of how to use it. Niacin is frequently the gold standard control used for basic research experiments using animal models of atherosclerosis. In clinical trials, when niacin has been compared to other marketed drugs it has led to most undesirable effects for business, but most therapeutically beneficial effects for the fortunate patients. Cardiovascular disease (CVD) kills more individuals than any other disease. Accordingly, there is tremendous drive in the pharmaceutical industry to produce drugs to combat CVD. Merck and Schering-Plough convinced doctors to spend 21 billion dollars over seven years selling Zetia (ezetimibe). Ultimately, however, clinical trials revealed that Zetia actually increases cardiovascular events, making mean arterial walls thicker![2] Thus, it is no longer a good business idea for the pharmaceutical industry to compare drugs to niacin head-to-head. Immediate release (IR) niacin works just as well as prescription extended release (ER) niacin, but it costs approximately fifteen dollars a day to obtain 3 grams, while IR niacin costs just fifty cents. ER niacin causes less of a flush response initially, but with regular usage, IR niacin results in little to no flush at all, while all of the benefits are still reaped.

While the benefits of niacin for treating CVD are undeniable, given the rigorously precise biochemical measures, there has been more controversy over the benefits of niacin for treating schizophrenia and behavioral disorders. Seventy years ago, Dr. Abram Hoffer entered this scene at the all-time height of psychiatry equivocation when he first proposed with Dr. Humphry Osmond to try much higher doses of vitamin B3 for treating what resembled the dementias seen in the pellagra epidemics of the 1940s. Sigmund Freudian-based psychotherapy was all the rage in the early 1950s. "Refrigerator moms" (emotionally unresponsive mothers) were given as the causal explanation for schizophrenia. Hoffer and Osmond's results were stunningly effective in the cure rate for schizophrenia, and were more effective than today's best medicine used for treating schizophrenia. Nonetheless, poorly understood drugs are repeatedly marketed to suffering schizophrenics, while an ever-increasing variety of newly defined mental and behavioral disorders are identified. This book, *Niacin: The Real Story*, relates niacin to descriptions of the three main psychotic disorders: bipolar disorder (characterized by dramatic mood swings), schizophrenias (characterized by perceptual hallucinations and delusions), and schizoaffective disorders (characterized by periods of dramatic mood swings and also hallucinations and delusions).

As illustrated above with the Zetia example, it is rare that anyone addresses the question "What works best?" It is such a simple question. Instead, too much research today proceeds primarily from a for-profit motive. It is also so rare to have someone who was around to witness the historical transformation of medical motives from a "health-and-improvement motive" to a "much-increased-profit motive," as Abram Hoffer and Harold Foster did. The profit machine ultimately consumed the spirit or focus of many a well-intentioned doctor, but Abram persisted in weathering the storm, risking his stature among his peers to maintain the premise of his work, always addressing the question: "What works best?" With an open mind and an incredible work ethic, Abram continued following the most recent research right up until the end.

There is so much more to the story of niacin than its success in treating CVD. Firstly, there are other distinct molecular versions of nicotinamide adenine dinucleotide (NAD) precursor besides niacin. They are also covered in this book. Secondly, there are many observations that would remain hidden from modern medical education if it were not for the work of the author of this book, Dr. Andrew Saul. Abram Hoffer's experiences treating patients with high doses of niacin or niacinamide were almost too numerous to tell.

Even today, niacin, functioning as a precursor to NAD, perennially excites and stimulates modern discovery in molecular biology and pharmacology research. One of the most amazing mice used by scientists for twenty-plus years has been the Slow Wallerian Degeneration (WldS) mouse.[3] Wallerian degeneration is the process of neuronal degeneration that occurs after physical insult to the neuron via razor excision or crushing of axons, all occurring in a petri dish. Normal neurons completely degenerate within twenty-four hours of damage; however, the Wlds mouse resists degeneration. Amazingly, WldS neurons survive for over two weeks, all without a nucleus, while still being able to be excited for at least a week![4] Eventually the gene was mapped and determined to involve triplication of the NAD-synthesizing enzyme encoded by Nicotinamide mononucleotide adenylyl transferase 1 (NMNAT1), where NAD itself could in part substitute for the neuroprotective activity conferred by this fortunate genetic mutation.[5] Further research realized a role for the NAD-dependent pathways frequently involving histone deacetylase enzyme Sirt1 in Wallerian degeneration, multiple sclerosis, diabetes, Alzheimer's disease, and others in the best animal models available for studying human disease.[6] This same Sirt1 enzyme was previously identified as being critical to conferring caloric restriction (CR) dependent increases in lifespan,[7] where CR is the only proven approach shown to consistently extend lifespan in all animal models.

However, with the genome(s) sequenced at the end of the shining day of the molecular biology revolution, the most important question remains: "What works best?" To this day, niacin ranks among the best answers. Based on sheer historical observation, pellagra was the most devastating nutritional deficiency epidemic ever reported in the United States of America. This epidemic deficiency was in large part the result of modern developments in food refining, when technological advancements enabled mass milling and the production and introduction of white rice and white flour to large populations of people. The pellagra epidemics followed, and then the golden age of vitamin discovery began. We realize from this history that modern human beings are most susceptible to niacin (and vitamin B_1/ beriberi) deficiencies. Thus, it simply makes sense that we would most likely benefit from higher dose application of niacin during stress or disease situations, which are well known to actively deplete NAD. Once niacin is transformed to NAD inside the cell, it is used in more biochemical reactions than any other vitamin-derived cofactor (over 450).[8] This surely factors into the molecular basis for its varied physiological activities. Does it not therefore come as little surprise that niacin works to provide relief for so many conditions? Unfortunately, as Abram Hoffer once said, "Niacin works so good that nobody believes it." Reality is what one wants to believe, but sometimes it is hard to believe. The fact is, there are so many situations where increased NAD is what we need to allow our body's endogenous chemistry to catch up to the insults inflicted on it—whether it is consumption of too much sugar or alcohol, too much stress, too much fat, and ad infinitum.

There have been many amazing developments in niacin-related clinical research since the 2012 edition of *Niacin: The Real Story*, beginning with Alzheimer's disease. More than 99 percent of 200 clinical trials designed to develop effective treatments for Alzheimer's disease have failed. It wasn't until 2022 that investigators began to examine the use of high-dose niacin therapy for treating Alzheimer's disease in clinical trials.[9] Research published in 2022 revealed that the niacin flush is key and uniquely important in this regard as well.[10,11] Similarly, only recently have clinical trials begun to examine the use of niacin in the context of brain tumors, owing to promising results stemming from prior research in multiple sclerosis-related myelination research led by Dr. Wee Yong, Chairman of Neuroimmunology at the University of Calgary and with 320 published peer-reviewed manuscripts.[12,13] It is increasingly clear that we need to fix human health problems using the parts that the human body machine divine instead of the come-and-go, routinely failing xenobiotic molecules that are pushed to clinical trials by the patentable-profit motive while all too often tragically failing the Alzheimer's disease-afflicted patients and families.

Also, since the 2012 edition *Niacin: The Real Story*, the myth of niacin-related hepatotoxicity (alleged liver damage) that arose from sustained release forms of niacin in the early 1960s has been thrown on its head.[14] It has since been learned that the immediate release least expensive form of niacin is in fact so healthy for the liver that it commonly reduces fatty liver by 50 percent and is now being pursued for drug development to treat nonalcoholic fatty liver disease.[15,16] Researchers recently published a study entitled "Niacin Cures Systemic NAD+ Deficiency and Improves Muscle Performance in Adult-Onset Mitochondrial Myopathy" in *Cell Metabolism*, one of the highest-impact biomedical scientific journals.[15] To date adult-onset mitochondrial myopathy has been a condition for which there has been no successful consensus treatment. Even in the control groups there was increased muscle strength and decreased fatty liver after simply taking 1g of niacin daily for over one month. Finally, it is now known that niacin can correct congenital malformations arising from defects in the conversion of tryptophan to NAD.[17] The full range of niacin's benefits in the context of early development remains poorly understood.

Clinical trial research has routinely proceeded at a glacial pace with respect to consideration of orthomolecular medical approaches involving niacin, but as the mountain of supporting basic and genomic research accumulates it becomes undeniable that we must examine high-dose niacin in a much wider range of contexts to explore how many indications can respond favorably. The future looks bright, but physician/specialist education will be key to getting to implement its use in practice when an individual is not learned and confident in doctoring oneself.

In basic scientific research, there are many experiments that obviously can never be performed on human beings. We must learn the tragic way. This involves simple observational analysis, with the most medically significant lessons arising in urgent response to wars rather than through the standard biomedical scientific method. Abram and Harold lived through such wars and worked with the victims and reported with Andrew Saul on many of these most important examples of treatment with high-dose niacin. Their lessons are veritable timeless treasures. Aside from their research, reports of high-dose niacin treatment do not exist in the standard medical education literature. In this book, you will observe firsthand examples of the results of clinical niacin use as it has never been told before. It is an invaluable resource for everyone interested in maintaining optimal health.

Preface

Many people have no idea how many illnesses are caused by too little niacin, and practically no one realizes just how many illnesses can be cured with megadoses of niacin. It is the authors' intent to change that. Our objective is to provide a reader-friendly, problem-solving book. This book is not nearly so much about the niacin molecule as it is about what can be done with a lot of niacin molecules. Therefore, this book concentrates on niacin's clinical benefits in a number of health conditions. These conditions, successfully treated by pioneering niacin researcher Abram Hoffer, MD, PhD, are based on his more than fifty years of medical practice. Dr. Hoffer, whose capacity for work continually astounded me, began this book at the age of ninety-one. Unfortunately, he died before it was completed. Medical geographer, professor, coauthor, and longtime collaborator Harold D. Foster also suffered untimely death during the early stages of writing this work. So, if you wonder why this book is not thicker and more comprehensive, there you have your main reasons. This is most certainly not a textbook. However, standing on the shoulders of these two giants of nutritional science, I have endeavored to add to and complete the existing manuscript without altering Abram's and Harry's voices: Harry, the medical theorist and scholar; Abram, the experienced and courageous physician and researcher. (You often will find Dr. Hoffer's voice in this book, in first person, with the initials AH following in parentheses.) The other voice is mine (AWS), that of teacher, raconteur, and parent.

I am honored beyond measure to have worked for years with Dr. Hoffer and Dr. Foster. I think they were, and will ever be, regarded as two of the great medical innovators of the modern era. Dr. Hoffer was the world authority on niacin. This constitutes his final work, of which he said, simply:

"This book is designed primarily for clinicians and the public who want to learn more and more about niacin and its wonderful properties."

I hope this handbook may prove to be a significant part of his legacy, and of real help to all readers.

Andrew W. Saul

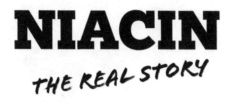

CHAPTER 1

Why Should You Read This Book?

In theory, there is no difference between theory
and practice. In practice there is.
—Attributed to Yogi Berra

In *The Structure of Scientific Revolutions,* Thomas Kuhn says that advances in science do not occur in an evolutionary or straight-line manner.[1] Instead, such steps take place in a series of violent revolutions separated by long periods of relative peace. During dramatic uprisings, "one conceptual world view replaces another." These intellectual revolts are not random events. They are promoted by the discovery of significant anomalies: emergent facts that the ruling dominant theory and its supporters fail to adequately explain. These "exceptions to the rule" are the termites of scientific theory. As they multiply, they become more and more difficult to ignore. The newly infected ruling theory weakens until it eventually collapses. A paradigm shift occurs as another takes its place.

While the drug-based pharmaceutical industry continues to control conventional medicine, its support structure is increasingly termite riddled. Weaknesses are being illustrated by new highly critical books, with titles such as *Deadly Medicine,*[2] *Overdo$ed America,*[3] and *Death by Modern Medicine.*[4] Of course, the drug-based approach to health will not be abandoned any time soon unless society has a viable alternative, waiting, like an understudy, in the wings. There it must be quietly attracting its own, more open-minded supporters.

The authors of this book are members of one such group: advocates of orthomolecular (nutrition-based) medicine. They support an approach to human wellness that does not involve the use of drugs, but instead

1

encourages the use of substances that naturally occur in the human body.[5] Niacin is one of these, and as such, seems destined to eventually play a significant role in the upcoming, inevitable medical paradigm shift. It is impossible to here make note of all the advantages society will gain by switching to nutrition-based medicine. However, this initial chapter provides a variety of examples, drawn from several specific categories of wellness. The remainder of the book seeks to examine, in much more detail, the case that can be made for the far more widespread use of one such nutrient, niacin, for the prevention and treatment of health issues.

"Orthomolecular" means the right or the correct molecule. Conventional pharmaceuticals tend to be "toximolecular." Vitamins and insulin are examples of orthomolecular therapeutic substances. Chemotherapy is an example of a toximolecular therapy.

By eating diets that are deficient in essential nutrients, many individuals trigger their own chronic degenerative diseases later in life. It has been known for millennia that the basis for health is good nutrition. Orthomolecular medicine, a description coined in 1968 by Linus Pauling,[6] goes further. Pauling describes a medical modality that uses nutrients and normal (that is, "ortho") constituents of the body in specific optimum quantities as the dominant treatment. Such health-nutritional relationships have been comprehensively explored most recently by Hoffer and Saul in *Orthomolecular Medicine for Everyone: Megavitamin Therapeutics for Families and Physicians*.[7]

It has been further recognized that individuals are unique in their daily requirements for vitamins, minerals, or protein.[8] For *each* nutrient, at least 2.5 percent will need higher levels than the rest of the population. There are about three dozen nutrients. When one does the math, it becomes apparent that most people are deficient in something—even if they consume USRDA (United States Recommended Dietary Allowance) nutrient levels every day.

"Orthomolecular" means the right or the correct molecule. The name was coined by Linus Pauling in 1968. Conventional pharmaceuticals tend to be "toximolecular." Vitamins and insulin are examples of orthomolecular therapeutic substances. Chemotherapy is an example of a toximolecular therapy.

We are all different, and you are a bit different every day. Illness, medications, age, variations in diet, fatigue, and stress are among the many factors that today can make you different from the you of yesterday. It has been said that you are what you eat. This very orthomolecular concept is true. But, in a deeper way, you are what you absorb. To illustrate, as Hoffer and Saul point out:

> In regard to nutrients, there may be a problem with absorption in the intestine. Thus, with pernicious anemia, specific areas in the gut that normally absorb vitamin B_{12} are lacking, or after the vitamin is absorbed, it may not be combined effectively into its coenzyme, or it may be wasted or held too tenaciously by some organ system, thus depriving other parts of the body.[9]

We need all the nutrients all the time, in the same way that an aircraft needs all its wheels and wings. Roger Williams[10] has described a basic concept called the "orchestra principle." Just as it is impossible to claim that one instrument in an orchestra is more important than another, to maintain health, all the nutrients required by the body must be available to ensure well-being. Though impossible to outline the enormous number of illnesses that can develop as a result of nutritional imbalance, it is possible to illustrate the principle. It seems likely that calcium and selenium deficiencies promote many cancers,[11] excess aluminum and inadequate magnesium and calcium are linked to Alzheimer's disease,[12] and a lack of sulfur is associated with osteoarthritis.[13] Certainly there are many other well-known nutrition-illness connections as well.

As will be seen from the remainder of this book, niacin plays an especially significant role in orthomolecular medicine. Inevitably, its use will increase as the medical paradigm shift occurs. Orthomolecular treatments are typically far less expensive than drug-based conventional protocols. Embracing orthomolecular treatments will make prevention and treatment available to the poor. If this statement might seem overly ambitious, consider this: a single orange may cost one dollar. It would provide about 50 milligrams of vitamin C. A bottle of 100 tablets of vitamin C, 500 milligrams each, costs about five dollars. In terms of vitamin content, the orange gives you 50 milligrams per dollar. The supplement gives you 10,000 milligrams per dollar. There are of course other nutritional factors and advantages to eating oranges, such as sugars, taste, bioflavonoids, and fiber. However, one cannot easily deny, at least in terms of vitamin C, that the supplement is 200 times cheaper, costing about half a cent for the amount of vitamin C in a one-dollar orange. Even if your oranges could cost only one-tenth as much, an impossible ten cents each, the supplement is still twenty times less expensive.

The same is true for niacin. Niacin supplements cost approximately five dollars for 100 tablets of 250 milligrams each. That works out to be about 5,000 milligrams niacin per dollar. Healthy foods naturally containing significant amounts of niacin cost far more. Once again, the many nutritional advantages of eating kidneys, liver, whole-grain bread, nuts, and green leafy vegetables are considerable and undeniable. In terms of niacin content, however, there is no competition. Several dollars' worth of these foods provides only tens of milligrams of niacin. Niacin-fortified foods such as breakfast cereals, white bread, and pasta are slightly less expensive niacin sources, but not by much. Interestingly, the fact that milled grains have any niacin at all is due to niacin being added to them in the manufacturing process. Adding niacin to foods is a common form of low-dose supplementation.

The U.S. Recommended Dietary Allowance (RDA) for niacin is less than 18 milligrams per day, which is far too low. Yet bodily need for niacin varies with activity, body size, and illness.[14] About half of all Americans will not get even the RDA amount of niacin from their diets. Niacin's special importance is indicated in that the RDA for niacin, which we again say is too low, is actually twenty or more times higher than the RDA for other B vitamins. Twenty teaspoons will not clean up after a hurricane much faster than one teaspoon will. We think that a lack of sufficient niacin is a real and continuing public health problem.

CHAPTER 2

What Is Niacin?

For every drug that benefits a patient, there is a natural
substance that can achieve the same effect.
—Carl C. Pfeiffer, MD, PhD

Niacin is a small molecule, smaller than the simplest sugar, glucose. Niacin is made of only fourteen atoms—$C_6H_5NO_2$. How can just one molecule have such profound effects on health?

Niacin is a member of a family of substances involved in the pyridine nucleotide cycle. It plays a role in over 500 reactions in the body. Interfering with any of these vital reactions will cause disease and, conversely, improving and restoring these reactions will be therapeutic.

Why, then, is the medical profession so ignorant of this vitamin and its vast importance? After all, in 2022, a Google search will hit (find a match on) "niacin" nearly 50 million times. Antipsychotic drugs have been promoted with multimillion-dollar budgets, while niacin has not been promoted at all, except by physicians who found its properties so valuable. There are few advertisements in medical journals from niacin manufacturers. Niacin is still advocated by word of mouth. Drugs are heavily advertised in both the medical journals and in the popular press. They have to be; it takes a lot of public persuasion to promote

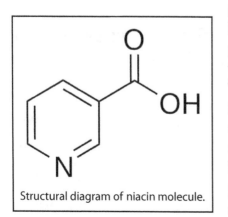
Structural diagram of niacin molecule.

products that are rarely effective and carry with them dangerous side effects, including death. The major side effect of niacin is longer life.

It is not possible to document and describe everything that is known about niacin to date. Instead, the contents of this book will concentrate on its clinical aspects and on conditions that one of us, Abram Hoffer (AH), found were benefited by niacin, during over fifty years of psychiatric practice.

Niacin's original chemical name was nicotinic acid. The name was changed to niacin to remove confusion with nicotine. Niacin was also known early on as vitamin B3 since it was the third water-soluble vitamin to be identified. Normally, this term would have been eliminated once its chemical structure had been determined, but it was brought back by Bill Wilson, cofounder of Alcoholics Anonymous (AA), who wanted a catchy name he could use to inform members of AA about its immense value for the treatment of alcohol addicts. There is a question whether niacin was misclassified when it was classed with the vitamins because it can be made in the body from tryptophan, and is used by the body in quantities more appropriate to amino acids. It has instead been suggested that it should be classed as an amino acid.

Gutierrez outlined a study at the University of California at Irvine which showed that liver cells in vitro treated with niacin did not take up as much HDL, which could explain why it increased HDL in blood.[1] This may be the first explanation of why niacin is so effective. But it also shows that niacin is not toxic to liver cells. We are making this point straight away to help quell the delusion held by so many doctors that niacin is liver toxic.

FORMS OF NIACIN AND HOW THEY DIFFER IN ACTION

Derivatives of niacin (nicotinic acid) have been examined for their ability to alter lipid levels as well as niacin does. It would be advantageous to many if the niacin vasodilatation (flush) were eliminated or removed.

Niacin lowers cholesterol, elevates high-density lipoprotein (HDL) cholesterol, and reduces the ravages of heart disease, but causes flushing when it is first taken. The flushing reaction dissipates in time, and in most cases is gone or is only very minor, within a matter of weeks. Niacinamide, which is not a vasodilator, does not produce a flush, but it has no effect on

	Niacin	Niacinamide	Inositol Hexaniacinate	Sustained Release (Hard Tablet)	Extended/Time Release
Blood Lipid Benefits	Yes	No	Yes	Yes	Yes
Psychiatric Benefits	Yes	Yes	Yes	Yes	Yes
Flush	Yes	No	No	Sometimes	No
Nausea at Several Thousand mg/day	No	Yes	No	No	No
Highest Degree of Liver Safety	Yes	Yes	Yes	No	No
Complete Tablet Dissolution	Yes	Yes	Yes	No	Yes

blood fats (lipids). Inositol hexaniacinate will lower cholesterol without the flushing side effect, but does not do so as well as plain niacin.

Niacin

Both niacin and niacinamide are effective against mental illness. Both will prevent and treat simple nutritional deficiency. Niacin (but not niacinamide) taken in high doses will produce a skin flush in most people. This is why niacinamide is the much more common form used in multiple vitamins and other dietary supplements. Unlike many other vitamins, all forms of niacin are exceptionally stable, and each has a long shelf life. The vitamin is not harmed by heat.

Several formulations are available to decrease the intensity of the niacin vasodilatation or flush. The best known is called "no-flush" niacin and is available over the counter. It is an inositol derivative with six niacin molecules attached to each benzene ring. There are other flushless forms available by prescription only, but they are much more expensive. Billions of dollars have been spent trying to find something as good as niacin that can be patented. This is a major waste of money and time, since the best anti-flush preparation is niacin itself. Most people stop flushing with continued use. The best antidote to the flush is an informed patient and doctor. As Dr. William Parsons Jr. wrote, "A doctor must know niacin in order to use it."

Another major difference between niacin and niacinamide is that niacin normalizes blood lipid values. It lowers low-density lipoprotein cholesterol ("bad" cholesterol), elevates high-density cholesterol ("good" cholesterol), lowers triglycerides, lowers lipoprotein(a) [Lp(a) is considered a risk factor for heart disease], and lowers the anti-inflammatory factor C-reactive protein. It therefore is the best substance known for these important therapeutic effects. Niacinamide has none of these properties.

Niacinamide

The other common form of niacin is nicotinamide, known more commonly as niacinamide. Both niacin and niacinamide forms are precursors to the active anti-pellagra factor NAD (nicotinamide adenine dinucleotide). A third form of vitamin B_3, nicotinamide riboside, was discovered in 2004, and little is known about it. Your body uses NAD (with a hydrogen, it is NADH) in over 450 biochemical reactions, most of which are involved in anabolic and catabolic reactions. Most people tend to associate NAD with glycolysis (sugar breakdown) and adenosine triphosphate (energy production). However, NAD is involved with many other reactions as a cofactor, including either the synthesis (anabolism) or the breakdown (catabolism) of just about every molecule our cells make: steroids, prostaglandins, and enzymes. NAD is also involved in cell signaling and assists in ongoing repair of DNA. There are several important reactions where it functions as a substrate for the enzymes PARP, Sirtuin, and IDO.[2,3,4]

Niacin and niacinamide have different properties. The most commonly observed difference is that when niacin is first taken, it causes a flush that starts in the forehead and travels down the body with varying intensities. Niacinamide does this very rarely. If there is a flush from niacinamide, it is very unpleasant.

Niacinamide is more likely to cause nausea at long-term, medium-high dosages (several thousand milligrams per day) than are the other forms of B_3. Niacin and inositol hexaniacinate generally do not cause nausea unless the dose is extremely high, on the order of tens of thousands of milligrams per day. Nausea is indicative of overdose. No one would need to take that excessive amount of B_3, and no one should. On the other hand, niacinamide has been successfully used at maintained doses of several thousand milligrams per day by Dr. William Kaufman to treat arthritis (see chapter 8). He reported virtually zero side effects.

Inositol Hexaniacinate

For those who cannot tolerate niacin, there is the option of using inositol hexaniacinate. This preparation has most of the therapeutic advantages of niacin and none of the side effects. It is available in health food stores as "no-flush niacin." It costs perhaps three times as much as "regular" niacin, but this is still much better than the cheapest statins (the most expensive of which costs a small fortune). Drug coverage plans should cover inositol hexaniacinate as they now cover niacin to achieve some of this savings and, even more important, improve the health of their patients.[5,6]

Inositol hexaniacinate is an ester of inositol and nicotinic acid. It is sometimes called inositol hexanicotinate. Each inositol molecule contains six nicotinic acid molecules. This ester is broken down slowly in the body. It is about as effective as nicotinic acid and is almost free of side effects. There is very little flushing, gastrointestinal distress, or other side effects. Inositol, considered one of the lesser-important B vitamins, does have a function in the body as a messenger molecule and may add something to the therapeutic properties of the nicotinic acid. The name "nicotinic" is often confusing. Remember that niacin (nicotinic acid) and nicotine have no physiological properties in common.

I (AH) used this compound for thirty years for patients who cannot or will not tolerate the flush. It is very gentle, effective, and can be tolerated by almost every person who uses it.

Extended-Release, Sustained-Release, or Time-Release Niacin?

Get ready to be confused a bit: these terms are often used interchangeably. Sometimes "sustained release," "time release," or "extended release" niacin is simply inositol hexaniacinate. Sustained-release, time-release, and extended-release niacin may also refer to physical or chemical tableting variations of regular niacin, generally either a hard-matrix tablet or coated little pellets in a tablet or capsule. If a vitamin tablet physically dissolves slowly, there is a sustained-release effect. Extended-release and time-release are very similar: release is chemically delayed. The goal of all these preparations is a reduced niacin "flush." (We further discuss the niacin flush in chapter 4.)

Sensitive persons sometimes report that the harder matrix of some sustained-release tablets can be felt in the stomach. Taking sustained-release tablets with a meal or snack may help reduce this sensation. Hard-matrix sustained-release tablets are the most likely to fail to break down in the digestive tract of elderly people. In other words, one may not be getting what the label claims, not because it isn't in the tablet, but because the tablet never breaks down completely enough to release it.

Sustained-, extended-, and time-release niacin are often advertised as not causing a flush at all. This claim may not be completely true; sometimes the flush is just postponed. It may be difficult to determine your optimum level with an extended-, sustained-, or time-release product. All three are also more costly. But the biggest reason to avoid sustained-release niacin is that relatively more reports of side effects stem from use of that form.[7] A 2007 review by Guyton and Bays of many niacin therapy studies reveals that regular ("immediate release," or IR) niacin is quite safe; extended- or time-release are safe, but unnecessarily pricey, and sustained-release (SR) has the most side effects. They write:

> Shortly after Altschul and colleagues described cholesterol lowering by niacin in 1955, sustained-release (SR) formulations were developed in an attempt to reduce flushing. However, these were quickly found to be hepatotoxic in some patients. . . . Henkin et al.[8] found 8 cases of hepatitis in 15 patients using SR niacin, compared with none in 67 patients using regular niacin. Three patients who had experienced hepatitis with SR niacin were subsequently able to tolerate equal or higher doses of regular niacin.[9] McKenney et al.[10] directly compared IR and SR niacin in a randomized clinical trial with dosage escalation from 500 to 3,000 milligrams per day over a period of 30 weeks. None of the 23 patients taking IR niacin developed hepatotoxic effects, whereas 12 of 23 patients (52 percent) taking SR niacin did. The increase in liver toxicity with SR niacin mainly occurred with doses of 1,500 milligrams per day.[11]

We therefore prefer and recommend manual, divided, doses of regular, immediate-release niacin, not sustained-release niacin. For those who simply must avoid the flush, the alternative forms of niacin are acceptable.

NADH Supplements

NADH (nicotinamide adenine dinucleotide, plus hydrogen) is an antioxidant coenzyme, an activated form of niacin, and is involved in cellular energy production. While NADH research is promising, but not definitive, it has been available in a stabilized form as a dietary supplement since the mid-1990s. NADH is extremely costly per milligram, but only a few milligrams are normally taken. It is claimed to help with chronic fatigue and other energy-related disorders, and is possibly beneficial for treatment of Alzheimer's disease, Parkinson's disease, and depression. Niacinamide also increases the body's production of NADH, but since NADH is naturally and continually made in the body from niacin, we think taking a lot of niacin is a far cheaper therapy. Niacin has a longer, and stronger, track record of effectiveness. We also think that, generally speaking, vitamin C is a much cheaper way to get antioxidant benefits.

Tryptophan

All forms of vitamin B_3 are anti-pellagra, all are precursors of NAD, are available commercially, and all have major therapeutic properties beyond what most people expect from their nutritional, anti-pellagra properties. Tryptophan is also a precursor to NAD. However, at high doses, tryptophan may have health concerns. Tryptophan has been connected with eosinophilia-myalgia syndrome, characterized by elevated white blood cell levels and muscle pain. The connection may be primarily due to manufacturing error with genetically-engineered materials. However, limited plasma tryptophan plays key roles in limiting a potentially hyperactive immune system. Thus, tryptophan is not generally taken as a precursor to NAD.

Other "Niacins"

One may occasionally come across what may be described as other forms of niacin. These include xanthinol niacinate (or xanthinol nicotinate), nicotinyl alcohol, ciclonicate, and etofylline nicotinate. All are vasodilators, which means they cause blood vessels to expand slightly. Nicotinyl alcohol also lowers cholesterol. Are these "designer niacins" worth seeking out and paying for? Maybe, maybe not. When niacin and xanthinol nicotinate were compared in a double-blind experiment, it was found that niacin "treatment resulted in improvement of sensory register and short-term memory, while xanthinol nicotinate improved sensory register, short-term memory, and long-term memory. In comparison with placebo, both active compounds yielded improvements of 10 to 40 percent."[12] Xanthinol niacinate seemed to work better in elderly subjects.

However, xanthinol is a derivative of theophylline, a molecule that resembles caffeine, and is present in tea and cocoa leaves. Theophylline is a central nervous system stimulant with properties similar to caffeine. It is therefore questionable whether the active part is the niacin or the xanthinol. Ciclonicate is a drug that was abandoned in the mid-1980s. It is still available outside the United States, but nothing has been published about it in well over twenty years, and it would not be considered as a form of niacin, regardless what may be claimed by promoters.

Chromium polynicotinate (or chromium polyniacinate) is a chromium supplement that contains niacin. It is also known as "niacin-bound chromium." There have been several studies that have shown niacin-bound chromium may be more effective in increasing insulin sensitivity, improving glucose tolerance, and reducing excess body fat than other forms of chromium. Niacin-bound chromium has also been reported to help lower cholesterol and systolic blood pressure.[13-16] It may be that some of chromium's claims to fame are not so much due to niacin enhancing the biochemical delivery of chromium but are actually due to chromium enhancing the delivery of niacin. (Niacin in cardiovascular disease will be discussed in chapter 11.)

WHAT ABOUT NIACIN IN FOODS?

Many foods contain a little niacin. None contain therapeutic quantities. Foods relatively high in niacin include lean meat, fish, organ meats (kidney, liver), clams, shrimp, pork, dairy products, nuts and seeds, wheat germ, whole wheat products, beans, and green leafy vegetables. So, is it enough to just eat more of them? Unfortunately, no. Even an ideal diet, very heavy in all of these nutritious foods, will not come close to even a 100 milligrams niacin supplement. We need extra niacin.

CHAPTER 3

How Niacin Therapy Began

*People's minds are changed through observation
and not through argument.*
—Will Rogers

$\mathbf{D}$eficiency is present when the very small amounts of nutrients that are needed to keep one going in the usual common state of poor health are not present in the diet. Most of the people living in North America cannot get enough vitamins and trace minerals from their food and therefore are suffering from various degrees of micronutrient deficiency. The daily recommended doses established by government are grounded in deficiency. They are derived from the old vitamins-as-prevention paradigm, now 100 years old, and ignore the modern vitamins-as-treatment paradigm. The classical deficiency diseases are beriberi, pellagra, scurvy, rickets, and pernicious anemia.

PELLAGRA (VITAMIN B₃ DEFICIENCY) AND SCHIZOPHRENIA (VITAMIN B₃ DEPENDENCY)

After Dr. Joseph Goldberger discovered the cause of pellagra, a deficiency disease, and Dr. Conrad Elvehjem discovered that niacin and niacinamide were the anti-pellagra vitamins, pellagra was vanquished. The timely mandatory fortification of white flour in 1942 by the United States government during the Second World War saved humanity incalculable numbers of lives and disability, and trillions of dollars in costs. This brilliant decision may have even influenced the outcome of the war.

Joseph Goldberger, MD (1874–1929)

Goldberger is my model of a brilliant scientist.
—ABRAM HOFFER, MD, PHD

Joseph Goldberger was born in 1874 and studied medicine at Bellevue Hospital Medical School in New York, graduating with honors in 1895. After an internship at Bellevue Hospital College, he engaged in private practice for two years and then joined the Public Health Service Corps in 1899. During routine work as a quarantine officer on Ellis Island, Goldberger rapidly acquired a reputation for outstanding investigative studies of various infectious diseases, including yellow fever, dengue fever, and typhus. Goldberger devoted the latter part of his career to studying pellagra. After quickly contradicting the contemporary general belief that pellagra was an infectious disease, he spent the last fifteen years of his life trying to prove that its cause was a dietary deficiency. During the first half of the twentieth century, an epidemic of pellagra produced roughly 3 million cases in the United States, about 100,000 of which were fatal.[1]

Abram Hoffer adds:

> In the early 1940s, the United States government mandated the addition of niacinamide to flour. This eradicated the terrible pandemic of pellagra in just two years, and ought to be recognized as the most successful public health measure for the elimination of a major disease in psychiatry, the pellagra psychoses. The reaction of contemporary physicians was predictable. Indeed, at the time, Canada rejected the idea and declared the addition of vitamins to flour to be an adulteration. The United States has long been the leading nation in nutrition research.

Knowledge comes at a cost: Goldberger had yellow fever, dengue, and very nearly died of typhus. According to the U.S. National Institutes of Health, he "stepped on Southern pride when he linked the poverty of Southern sharecroppers, tenant farmers, and mill workers to the deficient diet that caused pellagra."[2]

In the end, Goldberger was nominated for the Nobel Prize. Had he not died earlier in the year, he might well have shared it with vitamin researchers Christiaan Eijkman and Frederick G. Hopkins in 1929.

Alan Kraut's prize-winning book, *Goldberger's War: The Life and Work of a Public Health Crusader*, is an excellent source on this outstanding pioneer.

In 1930, 30,000 Americans died from pellagra in the southeast United States. Pellagra is characterized by the four D's: dermatitis, diarrhea, dementia, and death. The dementia or psychosis associated with pellagra cannot be differentiated on clinical grounds alone. It can be readily distinguished by the nutritional history and the use of vitamin B_3 as a diagnostic test. If patients given niacin recovered in a few days or weeks, they were diagnosed as having pellagra. If it took a lot longer or did not occur because too little was given, they were diagnosed as schizophrenic. This was the style of diagnosis by pellagrologists in the United States in the mid-1930s once niacin/niacinamide was identified as the anti-pellagra vitamin.

The major difference is that pellagra is caused by total malnutrition generated by a diet high in corn and non-nutritious food, while in schizophrenia, the major deficiency is vitamin B_3 in most cases where starvation is not endemic. The skin lesions in pellagra are responsive to tryptophan. Like pellagrins, schizophrenic patients exposed to the sun suffered skin pigment changes. The pellagrologists in the 1930s and 1940s were very good observers. How could they miss this obvious similarity between schizophrenia and pellagra? They did not miss it. But they were so indoctrinated by the vitamins-as-prevention paradigm that they were blinded by theory rather than guided by what they observed. They knew pellagra was a deficiency disease and that only small amounts were needed to cure and to prevent further relapses in most cases. They knew schizophrenia was a major intractable chronic mental disease. Because they were blinded by the old vitamin paradigm, they insisted the two were different conditions. When niacin became available, they gave it to both pellagrins and schizophrenic patients. According to their definition, they were pellagrins if they responded in a short period of time, even if it took 1,000 milligrams daily. They remained schizophrenic if they did not respond at these doses. The pellagrologists were unable to make the differential diagnosis on clinical grounds alone. And because these experts were so certain the diseases were not the same, investigators thereafter would no longer examine the issue.

HOW DR. HOFFER BECAME INVOLVED WITH NIACIN

I (AH) looked on niacin as a drug, as did the FDA, and not as a vitamin. Only much later did I realize what we were dealing with. The vitamin-as-prevention paradigm was enshrined around the following beliefs: (1) Vitamins are needed only to prevent the classical well-known deficiency diseases; and (2) Only very small doses, the usual vitamin doses, are needed. It followed that one should not give vitamins unless deficiency diseases were present, and large doses were not needed and were forbidden. Giving large doses of niacin to schizophrenic patients broke every rule of the vitamin-as-prevention paradigm. Had the pellagrologists properly determined the optimum dosage for the B vitamins on a large scale, and not been blinded by the vitamin-as-prevention paradigm, we might have had a treatment for schizophrenia much earlier.

The adrenochrome (oxidized adrenaline) hypothesis of Hoffer, Osmond, and Smythies in 1954 suggested that any decrease in the production of adrenaline would be therapeutic for schizophrenic patients, as this would decrease the amount of catechol that could be converted into adrenochrome. Niacin is one of the major methyl acceptors in the body, and it was possible that by depleting methyl groups, less noradrenalin would be converted into adrenalin. Niacin was safe, could be taken forever, and protected against pellagra, a recent scourge of mankind. It had remarkable antipsychotic effects with the pellagra psychosis, so it became reasonable to test its effect on schizophrenic patients. In 1952 I did not realize that the pellagra psychosis was identical with the schizophrenic psychosis. Our first pilot trials were very successful. We followed these with a small series of double-blind, randomized, placebo-controlled, prospective studies on nonchronic patients,

COMPARISON OF SCHIZOPHRENIC AND PELLAGRA PSYCHOSIS		
	SCHIZOPHRENIA	PELLAGRA
Perceptual		
Visual	Yes	Yes
Auditory	Yes	Yes
Others	Yes	Yes
Thought disorder	Yes	Yes
Mood disorder	Yes	Yes
Behavior changes	Yes	Yes
Skin pigmentation	Yes-minor	Yes-major
Gastrointestinal	Yes-minor	Yes-major
Deaths increased	Yes	Yes
Reasons	Heart; Malnutrition	Suicide
Treatment	Diet	Diet
	Niacin 3,000 mg and up	Niacin 100 to 1,000 mg
Time required	Months to years	Months

the first in psychiatric history. We doubled the two-year recovery rate to 75 percent compared to 35 percent for the placebo. Once you have seen schizophrenic patients become normal, it remains unforgettable. These controlled studies have been confirmed by a large number of clinical open studies, through my own experience in treating well over 5,000 patients since 1952, and in one NIMH-sponsored double-blind controlled trial by Wittenborn in 1974.[3]

CHAPTER 4

How Niacin Works,
and Why We Need More of It

Half of what we will teach you is wrong.
The problem is, we don't know which half.
—DR. ABRAM HOFFER, QUOTING ONE OF HIS MEDICAL
SCHOOL PROFESSORS ON THE FIRST DAY OF CLASS

For many biological variables, if one charts the number of individuals having a characteristic against its frequency in the population, the curve on the chart follows a so-called normal distribution form. For example, if one measures the height of men, there will be a range between a low figure to a high figure, but the majority of men will be somewhere in the middle. More men will be five foot ten than five feet tall, and fewer will be six foot ten than five foot ten. Almost all biological variables have this variation. The curve is a bell-shaped curve, and most of the values will lie within two standard deviations from the mean. The same distribution applies to our need for nutrients.

Roger J. Williams made it very clear in his writing about biochemical individuality that we are not alike and we do differ in this way. We have different needs for calories, for example, and of course for nutrients, which are so essential. But the *optimum* needs for vitamins have not been determined. For example, I do not know of any study where the optimum needs for vitamin C have been determined. The vitamin-as-prevention paradigm has been the major obstruction to conducting such research. It forced everyone to accept that vitamins were needed only in very small amounts. It limited examination of needs to individuals who required lower amounts than the average by excluding the needs of those who required much more. The vitamin-as-treatment paradigm broke this rule and forced serious examination of the population who required much more no matter what the reasons were. It is known that disease, stress, and many other factors determine how much of a nutrient is needed, and this is not a static figure.

Let us assume that the most reasonable hypothesis is, if one measured the optimum nutrient requirements of a large population, it would follow the same bell-shaped curve as most other biological variables. The individuals in this population would not be well unless they received whatever was their own optimum requirement. The current Recommended Dietary Allowances (RDAs) are based on very little good research done so many years ago and enforced by legal action that did not take this important hypothesis into account.

Once the mean optimum value had been determined, one would expect that people consuming values on the low side of the value would not be as healthy as people taking the mean value. The further from the mean these individuals were, the sicker they would be. If they were two standard deviations away from the mean, they would develop pellagra, the niacin deficiency disease. The closer they were to the mean optimum intake (MOI), the healthier they would be.

If one could depend only upon the natural amount of the vitamin in food, it would be easier to meet one's nutritional requirements, and much less attention would have to be paid to the quality of the diet. However, that isn't typically possible, so supplements are used or prescribed. The optimum dose of vitamin supplements is that which meets the physiological needs of a particular person, without experiencing side effects. Ingesting more than the optimum requirement is not typically harmful unless enormous doses are taken. This is in striking contrast with pharmaceutical drugs, where taking too much is much more harmful than taking too little.

Just the opposite is true with vitamins. Taking too little is more harmful than taking too much—again within reason. Any substance—no matter how safe—will have side effects if the amount is much too great. Thus, if vitamin C is taken in large doses, it will cause diarrhea in some people. This is not necessarily toxic, but if the diarrhea is excessive it might be. Therefore, the onset of loose stool is used as an indicator that the person has reached the upper end point of how much vitamin C he or she should take. This is known as the sublaxative level.

Ideally, we should talk about the relative deficiency of a nutrient in a particular person. If a person needs 1,000 milligrams of vitamin C each day and eats only 100 milligrams, their intake will be 10 percent of optimum need. If they require 100 milligrams daily and ingest only 30 milligrams, that person is getting only 30 percent of their optimum need. Taking more than the optimum is of little value, but as it is not dangerous, it is typically better to err on the side of a bit too much, rather than risk deficiency. The only waste will be in the cost of the vitamin and fortunately, as they are not patented, their costs have not jetted into the stratosphere.

WHY DO WE NEED MORE NIACIN?

Subjects who do not get enough vitamin B3 because of their diet will develop pellagra. Patients whose vitamin B3 requirements are in the upper range will never get enough through their diet, and they will have to use supplements. They are the vitamin dependent group. The range of vitamin B3 requirements varies from the left end of the bell-shaped curve to the group who need a lot more at the right end of the requirement distribution. We believe that half or more of the population needs vitamin B3 supplementation.

FETAL DEVELOPMENT AND FUTURE DISEASES

A woman's diet during pregnancy has very significant ramifications on her fetus.[1] This, of course, has been known for millennia. Much more recently, however, it has been demonstrated that nutrition is the number-one intra-uterine environmental variable that alters expression of the fetal genome.[2] As a result of its impact on the genes of the fetus, what a mother eats has lifelong consequences for her child. To illustrate, her diet can greatly alter the risk of her offspring for developing specific diseases in adulthood, a phenomenon known as "fetal programming." Optimal maternal nutrition, therefore, can both promote healthy fetal growth and lower the risk of her child experiencing various chronic diseases in adulthood.[3]

In some regions, soils and potable water are so deficient in a specific mineral(s) that certain infant abnormalities are commonplace and said to be endemic. Iodine deficiency, for example, which interferes with the normal production and regulation of thyroid hormones, is associated with a spectrum of deficits ranging from cretinism, hypothyroidism, and dwarfishness to deafness.[4] Endemic abnormalities triggered by maternal iodine deficiency occur in 1,550 Chinese regions.[5] Extreme selenium deficiency is also experienced in parts of China, resulting in endemic diseases such as Keshan disease, an endemic cardiomyopathy, and Kaschin-Beck disease, an endemic osteoarthropathy.[6]

Intrauterine environmental nutritional deficiencies can alter the expression [development] of the fetal genome with specific lifelong consequences.[7] It has been suggested, for example, that fetal iodine deficiency may result in an abnormally high requirement of dopamine, which, in adulthood, increases the risk of illnesses such as Parkinson's disease and multiple sclerosis.[8,9] This phenomenon is termed "fetal programming" and has led to the belief that there are often "fetal origins of adult disease."[10]

NUTRITION AND GENETIC INDIVIDUALITY

Consider that chimpanzees' protein-coding DNA is at least 94 percent genetically identical to humans. What a difference that other 6 percent makes!

Genes are blueprints that permit the production of proteins. These in turn are needed to create, among other things, enzymes. Nevertheless, slight differences in specific genes, called alleles, occur from one person to the next. As a result, many genes carry two, several, or even many variants of the same genetic information. Accordingly, even members of the same family may have distinct genetic information in specific genes. While some of these minor genetic differences cause almost insignificant variations in information and do not significantly affect well-being, others can have profound negative impacts.[11]

A study published by Dr. Robert Ames and coworkers in the *American Journal of Clinical Nutrition* points out that "The proportion of mutations in a disease gene that is responsive to high concentrations of a vitamin or substrate may be one-third or greater."[12] Roughly one-third of such genetic mutations appear to create enzymes that have very decreased binding activities for their coenzymes. This results in an enzyme that is less reactive than normal, making the human carrier of this polymorphism more susceptible to health problems associated with an inadequacy in the enzyme involved.

Genes are not destiny, however. As Ames and colleagues explain:

About 50 human genetic diseases due to defective enzymes can be remedied or ameliorated by the administration of high doses of the vitamin component of the corresponding coenzyme, which at least partially restores enzymatic activity. Several single-nucleotide polymorphisms, in which the variant amino acid reduces coenzyme binding and thus enzymatic activity, are likely to be remediable by raising cellular concentrations of the cofactor through high-dose vitamin therapy.[13]

Simply put, there are numerous people who carry genetic mutations that mean they must eat diets that are unusually elevated in a particular nutrient. If they eat a typical diet, they cannot produce effective levels of the enzyme activity required for health. As a result, they will inevitably begin to develop the associated deficiency disease. For people carrying certain alleles, very high intakes of vitamin or mineral supplements are not a health threat or a fad—they are the only way they can remain healthy. In some cases, they require as much as one thousand or more times the Recommended Dietary Allowance of a particular nutrient.

Ames and colleagues provided details of many of such coenzyme-decreased binding affinity disorders and the nutrients that are likely to ameliorate them.[14] One example is the enzyme cystathionine b-synthase, which catalyzes homocysteine and serine, creating cystalthionine. People who have a defective form of this enzyme cannot do this and, as a consequence, have abnormally high blood and urine homocysteine levels. These are known to be associated with numerous health problems including mental retardation, vascular and skeletal defects, and optic lens dislocation. In approximately 50 percent of cystalthionine b-synthase deficient patients, very high doses of vitamin B_6 can provide significant improvement by lowering the homocysteine and serine concentrations to normal levels.[15]

NUTRIENTS AND INFECTIOUS DISEASES

Humans have evolved very complex immune systems to protect themselves against infection by a wide variety of pathogens. Conversely, pathogens possess a diverse genetic versatility that permits them to mutate and so escape such population immunity.[16] These conflicting host-pathogen objectives have led to an evolutionary "arms race." In this battle for supremacy, pathogens typically seek to deplete their hosts of specific nutrients that are necessary for the functioning of the human immune system. Once infection occurs, the pathogen continues to rob its host of the same nutrient(s), often causing many of the disease symptoms and sequela [negative aftereffects].[17]

This means that specific diets and supplements can greatly reduce the risk of infection by a particular pathogen. Even after this "invasion" has occurred, the same nutrients may help to hasten disease recovery and reduce its severity. Numerous examples of these relationships are apparent in the literature.

- In malaria, Plasmodium falciparum competes with its host for vitamin A.[18] In some cases, an extreme deficiency of this vitamin leads to blindness. Plasmodium falciparum also abstracts zinc[19] from its host. Interestingly, 200,000 International Units of vitamin A, given to children four times a year, can greatly lower susceptibility to malaria.[20] So, vitamin A is both a promising preventive and treatment for the disease.

- In contrast, infection by the Coxsackie B virus seems to result in a selenium deficiency because this pathogen encodes for an analogue of glutathione peroxidase. This trace mineral deficiency-viral infection has been associated with both myocardial infarction[21] and Keshan disease. As suggested here, selenium supplementation can cause dramatic drops in the incidence of Keshan disease.[22] It also lowers heart attack risk, reducing reinfarction rates.[23]

- HIV-1 depletes its host of the four nutrients required to make the selenoenzyme glutathione peroxidase. As a result, those infected slowly become deficient in selenium and three amino acids: cysteine, glutamine, and tryptophan. These deficiencies cause major symptoms that together are referred to as Acquired Immunodeficiency Syndrome

(AIDS).[24] Open and closed African trials involving high doses of these four nutrients have shown that the correct nutritional supplements can reverse the symptoms of AIDS and prevent HIV-positive patients from developing the disease.[25]

It is apparent, therefore, that the supplementation of diet with specific nutrients, including vitamins, minerals, and amino acids, can reduce infection by numerous pathogens. Beyond this, when infection occurs, the use of such nutrients to treat the resulting illness may prevent or reverse many of the symptoms and sequela commonly associated with diseases as different as malaria, myocardial infarction, Keshan disease, and HIV/AIDS.

SUPPLEMENTS AND LONGEVITY

Research has shown that there may be an important link between life expectancy and the use of vitamins. The June 2009 issue of the *American Journal of Clinical Nutrition* includes evidence that multivitamin supplements may prolong lifespan by reducing the speed with which telomeres shorten.[26] The Sisters Study analyzed data collected from 586 women, some of whom had developed breast cancer, and their cancer-free siblings. As part of this research project, blood samples were taken for DNA analysis and information was collected from participants on their use of vitamins during the previous twelve years.

According to lead researcher Dr. Honglei Chen, head of the Aging and Neuroepidemiology Group at the U.S. National Institute of Environmental Health Sciences, it was discovered during the Sister Study that "multivitamin use was associated with longer leukocyte telomeres." Telomeres, the end portion of chromosomes, protect against damage, but shorten each time cells divide. It is generally believed that this process sets limits to the number of possible cell divisions and, as a result, to lifespan.[27] The Sister Study showed that telomeres were, on average, 5.1 percent longer in women that had taken multivitamins. This greater length corresponds to about 9.8 years less age-related telomere shortening. While this evidence is not conclusive, it is highly suggestive that taking multivitamin supplements increases life expectancy. This is not surprising. In their book *Feel Better, Live Longer with Vitamin B₃*,[28] two of the current authors pointed out that doctors inducted into the Orthomolecular Hall of Fame had lived an average of eighty-three years. This is greater than the normal lifespan for both men (76 years) and women (81 years). While this is not conclusive, it is highly suggestive, especially since many of these inductees were born in the nineteenth century, when general life expectancy was lower than it is today.

While adverse side effects are the hallmark of conventional drug-based medicine, they are exceptionally uncommon in the practice of orthomolecular treatments. Once the new paradigm is widely adopted, treatments will go into areas untouched by conventional medicine. Nutritional mixtures are already available that can mitigate serious surgical and genetic brain damage, significantly improve antisocial behavior, and enormously reduce the incidence of both infectious and chronic degenerative diseases. As will now be demonstrated, niacin will be highly involved in the coming orthomolecular revolution.

Niacin's Biochemical Pathways

by W. Todd Penberthy

There are two distinct niacin biochemical pathways. This is important when comparing against the other popular NAD precursors: nicotinamide riboside/Niagen, NMN, niacinamide/nicotinamide. One is niacin as a building block precursor to NAD synthesis. The other is niacin as an activator of GPR109a receptor. The latter pathway is the flush pathway, and it is the one that corrects lipodystrophy (disorder of blood lipids).

NAD categorically functions in basic bioenergetics (glycolysis and respiration to generate adenosine triphosphate), substrate reactions (poly ADP-ribose polymerases, sirtuins, etc.), and redox reactions. Ultimately, NAD is required for over 400 gene functions.

Niacin activation of GPR109a signaling pathway leads to a massive transient release of prostaglandins that work through other g-protein coupled receptors to elicit the flush with associated distinct therapeutically beneficial effects including correction of lipodystrophy and increased mitochondrial biogenesis (PGD2>PPARgamma>

PGCɪalpha) at the most basic level. This pathway should not be persistently activated; rather it appears to be best to activate this pathway transiently perhaps three times a day.

No other NAD booster to date has been able to correct lipodystrophy nearly as well as niacin because this niacin activity works not through NAD, rather it works through the prostaglandin pathways. Niacin has been studied for over 50 years and running in clinical trial after clinical trial that has focused on the most common cause of death, which is cardiovascular disease; niacin's activities are unparalleled in their ability to safely reduce cardiovascular disease risk.

Niacin increases HDL (the good cholesterol), reduces triglycerides, and can either increase or reduce total cholesterol depending on the individual. Overall, cholesterol deficiency is a more serious concern than elevated total cholesterol.

A GENETIC HYPOTHESIS TO ACCOUNT FOR THE NEED FOR VITAMIN B₃ BY SO MANY

The synthesis of niacin from tryptophan is a very inefficient process, and 60 milligrams of the amino acid are necessary to provide 1 milligram of niacin. This process also involves vitamins B_1, B_2, and B_6. It also requires vitamin C for the first reaction catalyzed by indoleamine 2,3-dioxygenase. If these vitamins are in short supply, the synthesis of vitamin B_3 will be even less efficient. It must also be remembered that tryptophan is not usually very readily available in diet, especially if that diet contains a high level of corn. So humans have the ability to synthesize niacin, but this process is ineffective and is likely in evolutionary decline. Of course, vitamin B_3 is also available from many foods. If diet contained enough of this vitamin to supply bodily requirements, there would be no need to convert tryptophan to niacin. This would liberate energy for other uses and free up tryptophan for the production of serotonin, a major neurotransmitter. Humanity has been depending more and more on vitamin B_3 derived from diet, but niacin has become less available from food. As a result, subclinical pellagra and other niacin deficiency disorders are becoming widespread.

According to Miller,[29] tuberculosis (TB) is one such example of niacin deficiency and an important factor in the evolution of schizophrenia. In a thorough study of the relationship between schizophrenia and tuberculosis, Miller formulated the reasonable hypothesis that the rapid spread of tuberculosis, which began with the dawn of industrialization, was due to the evolution of the bacteria and it becoming more persistent in the human body, thus making it more easily transferred to others.

Many years ago, a surgeon called me (AH) and told me that he had tuberculosis of the pericardium and that none of the drugs used had stopped the infection. He was so weak he could barely dress, look after himself, concentrate, or read. In my tuberculosis reprint file, I had several papers published many years ago showing that niacin inhibited the growth of the bacterium. I gave him the references and suggested that he take 1,000 milligrams niacin, three times daily, after meals, along with the same amount of ascorbic acid (vitamin C). Two weeks later, he called back. He was now able to concentrate and read, and had a lot more energy. A couple of years later, I suddenly remembered him and called him at his hospital. To my surprise, he was not able to come to the phone because he was busy in the operating room.

I sent this case history to Miller, who replied, "What I envision is this—that in the TB-infected tissue, the bacterium is pumping out niacin by depleting NAD (nicotinamide adenine dinucleotide) and furthermore, must somehow inhibit the recycling of niacin into NAD by producing an inhibitor of the host NAPRT1 enzyme. However, dietary niacin (as you provided the TB patient) would allow their non-TB-infected tissue to generate NAD and thereby save the host from the huge NAD sink that TB represents. Obviously, low NAD in all tissues equals death."

Unless their diet is high in niacin or tryptophan, schizophrenics may still not have optimal NAD (though not anywhere close to the near-death levels in TB patients) because the deficiency of the niacin receptor causes a compensatory shift toward niacin conservation. The prediction is that these patients should be more resistant to TB than their ethnically matched counterparts, because the niacin receptor deficiency keeps the kynurenine pathway activated.

NAD is central to the model presented here for the intersection of two diseases, poised in the balance between disease susceptibility and disease resistance. The sheer magnitude of the importance of NAD to bioenergetic homeostasis provides the driving force for the compromise of related pathways. Thus, the architects of new pharmaceuticals for schizophrenia and for TB would do well to incorporate an in-depth understanding of the many nuances of the pathways to NAD.

Some 50 percent of the population of the developed world seems to suffer from disorders or diseases that respond beneficially to niacin or niacinamide supplementation. This figure is probably an underestimate. Sufferers from arthritis (20 percent), addictions (10 percent), children with learning and/or behavioral disorders (5 percent), cardiovascular disease, coronary disease and stroke (30 percent), cancer (50 percent), schizophrenia, or severe stress (unknown) would very likely improve if given more niacin.

This brings us back to diseases associated with niacin deficiency. Hoffer and Foster have shown there are numerous dangerous diseases and disorders associated with our inability to synthesize adequate vitamin B_3. Any genetic aberration promoting such a deficiency state, if it was to widely diffuse in the human population, must have carried with it some enormous counterbalancing advantage(s). If it did not, it would soon have disappeared from the human gene pool. What then are the advantages of the apparent inadequate synthesis of niacin?

Schizophrenic genes are actually good genes. Dr. David Horrobin[30] was convinced that the introduction of schizophrenic genes into our genetic configuration was largely responsible for the creation of modern society. He surmised schizophrenic genes could not have survived millions of years of evolution unless they conferred some evolutionary advantage[31]—and they do—but only for the healthy relatives of patients. For the patient, there is no advantage in being sick, and society usually treated affected patients so badly that they could not possibly have had any evolutionary advantage. Horrobin posited that if a person became schizophrenic at age forty-five, and until then had been normally productive and creative, it surely meant there was not much wrong with their genes, but instead some long-term environmental trigger factors were responsible. It means that these genes, which have been normal for forty-five years, are no longer able to obtain the nutrients from their environment that they must have in order to remain well.

THE EVOLUTIONARY ADVANTAGES OF HAVING SCHIZOPHRENIC GENES

Schizophrenic patients, before they become sick and after they recover, have many physical and psychological advantages over the population lacking these genes. Physically they are more attractive and they age more gracefully. Their hair does not gray as quickly. They can withstand severe pain better. They become arthritic less often, and they have cancer much less frequently. If they do get cancer, they recover when treated by standard and orthomolecular methods. Out of over 5,000 schizophrenic patients, and over 1,500 cancer cases that I (AH) have treated since 1955, only eleven had both diseases.[32] All but one recovered with orthomolecular treatment combined with standard treatment for their cancer.

Schizophrenic patients' first-order relatives (parents, siblings, and children) are also protected against cancer, but not to the same degree. I have seen many families with many cases of cancer and very few schizophrenics, and families with many schizophrenic members and hardly any cases of cancer. The following table records what I had observed.

	NUMBER OF RELATIVES	NUMBER WITH SCHIZOPHRENIA	NUMBER WITH CANCER	NUMBER OF INDEX CASES
Cancer	785	3	89	114
Schizophrenia	437	20	26	95

This natural antagonism between these two major diseases also applies to first-order families (parents, siblings, and children)—there is a striking difference in incidence.

The best explanation I have been able to come up with for this correlation is that both schizophrenia and cancer are adrenochrome diseases. One of the major causes of schizophrenia is too much adrenochrome, and one of the major causes of cancer is too little. Adrenochrome is a hallucinogen and also has antimitotic properties because it inhibits cell division, and cancer, of course, is cell division that has gone rampant. Since all the schizophrenic patients were treated with vitamin B$_3$ (niacin or niacinamide) and ascorbic acid, this suggests that the clear differences I observed were also related to these two vitamins. The conclusion is that schizophrenic patients on niacin and vitamin C will get cancer less frequently than either the same patients not on these vitamins or the nonschizophrenic population.

Professor Diona Damian's finding that niacinamide protects the skin against UVA and UVB rays and was more effective than sunscreens in protecting against skin cancer and protects the immune function of the skin was reported by *The Sydney Morning Herald* on November 19, 2008. Perhaps it has the same effect in protecting against all cancers. Niacin will be as effective as niacinamide as they are interconvertible in the body. Niacin might even be better than niacinamide, as it tends to increase pigmentation of the skin. This has led to the erroneous idea that niacin causes acanthosis nigricans, a skin disorder, which it does not (see chapter 6).

People with the beneficial schizophrenic genes have an evolutionary advantage, but they have to be fed properly. They need vitamin B$_3$, and relief from excessive oxidation in the body. It is as if schizophrenic episodes use, deplete, and ultimately demand more vitamin B$_3$. This requirement must be met with supplementation as it cannot be met by the normal diet.

Psychologically, schizophrenics are more creative and enterprising than the nonschizophrenic population. They tend to see relationships in the world that others do not see. Many brilliant writers, poets, artists, and even Nobel Laureates had these good genes.

SCHIZOPHRENIA: THE CLINICAL PICTURE

Schizophrenia is characterized by a combination of perceptual changes and thought disorder, which may lead to strange or psychotic behavior. When schizophrenic patients are well, however—either before they become sick or after they have recovered—they do possess several physical and psychological advantages. If schizophrenia is caused by hyperoxidation of the catecholamines, leading to increased production of adrenochrome and similar chrome indoles, then it should be possible to predict what the syndrome will be like as an intellectual exercise, simply by knowing the properties of adrenalin and adrenochrome.

Adrenochrome has the following properties, and each should lead to the described consequences in schizophrenic patients:

1. A neurotransmitter inhibitor: perceptual changes and thought disorder.
2. A mitotic inhibitor: interference with growth if first occurs in childhood; decreased incidence of cancer; better response of the cancer to treatment.
3. Toxic to heart muscle: increased incidence of cardiac disease.
4. Formation of melanin pigments: skin changes in pellagra and in some schizophrenic patients.
5. Patients made worse by oxidative stress.
6. Antioxidants are therapeutic.

Schizophrenia can be triggered by factors that increase oxidative stress. Conversely, antioxidants and decreased stress will be therapeutic. Schizophrenia is characterized by changes due to sensory misinterpretations of stimuli and an inability to judge that these changes are not true. Psychotic behavior is comprehensible if one determines the perceptual distortions.

EVOLUTION AND NIACIN DEPENDENCY

Adrenochrome and similar compounds, in common with the hallucinogens, cause perceptual changes. Vitamin B_3 is required to prevent excessive oxidation of adrenalin to adrenochrome in the brain. Factors which facilitate formation of NAD from tryptophan and B_3 supplements will be therapeutic.

There is an evolutionary advantage conferred by vitamin B_3-dependent genes. The energy needed to transform tryptophan to NAD becomes available for other uses. The increased oxidation to adrenochrome and similar oxidized catecholamines provides protection against cancer and arthritis and perhaps many more diseases except heart disease. The decreased prevalence of cancer in these patients and their families will lead to a spread of these genes into the total population given enough time. Ideally only a little adrenochrome would be made, as may be the case with first-order relatives. But whether a little or too much is made, the individual is protected by taking optimum amounts of vitamin B3. This will protect against the effect of adrenochrome on the brain and will also protect the heart by keeping cholesterol levels normal. In time, due to evolutionary pressure, we will all have these schizophrenic genes but no one will be sick because we will be adding enough B3 to our food to replace what our bodies no longer can make and need.

In 1960, Dr. Osmond and I (AH) suggested the following criteria for a good hypothesis. First: It must account both inclusively and economically for what is known already; a hypothesis that fails to do this would be automatically disqualified. Second: It must do this better than any previous hypothesis. Third: It must be testable in a way that will readily lead to its refutation should it be false, using methods available to science under scrutiny. It should also be useful in directing research into productive areas. Is there any reason why psychiatry should require anything different from the rest of science?

I think our adrenochrome hypothesis meets all these criteria. It does take into account most of the clinical findings in schizophrenic patients, but of course cannot account for the large number of biochemical findings that are being discovered. It takes into account clinical findings but cannot be compared to any previous hypothesis, as none have been as inclusive and comprehensive. The purely psychological hypotheses of schizophrenia have been dismal failures and have hurt many patients and their families. Biochemical hypotheses have been crude and have not led anywhere. Infection hypotheses may play a minor role, as any serious brain pathology can produce the schizophrenic syndrome. The adrenochrome hypothesis is testable and has been tested to a limited degree but unfortunately, psychiatry has been too preoccupied with drugs and the minutia of how they work to look comprehensively in this direction. It has finally led to the treatment of schizophrenia using orthomolecular methods, which are much more successful than using only drugs. Thousands of schizophrenic patients are able to live a more normalized life as a result of orthomolecular therapy.

DEFICIENCY AND DEPENDENCY

A deficiency is present when the amount of any nutrient in the diet is below what the average person needs. Classically it applies to the well-known deficiency diseases such as scurvy, beriberi, pellagra, and rickets. Scurvy is caused by deficiency of ascorbic acid. This deficiency alone has killed millions of people. Pellagra is caused by too little vitamin B_3 in the diet. Supplementation with these vitamins prevented these diseases. This was the basis of the old vitamins-as-prevention paradigm developed about 100 years ago and reluctantly accepted by the medical profession about 50 years ago. Since then, it has become so solidly established, it is as if it is written in stone, even though it is totally out of date, wrong, and harmful to so many patients. It is inadequate because it assumes that everyone has the same nutritional needs. That is like assuming that everyone has the same fingerprints. A large number of people have much higher vitamin requirements than modern diets can provide, and if they depend upon their diet alone, they will never achieve optimum health. For these people, the correct term is dependency.

A deficiency will become a dependency if the deficiency is chronic. The rapidity with which this occurs depends on several factors including severity of the stress, severity of the malnutrition, and iatrogenic (physician-induced) causes. These are trigger factors. The European concentration camps and prisoner of war camps in the Far East were ideal for throwing people into the dependency state if they lived long enough. In Japan's prison camps, Canadian soldiers were incarcerated for forty-four months. There they suffered severe malnutrition, from a diet of about 800 calories daily, which caused several deficiency diseases. This was combined with severe physical and psychological stress. One-quarter of the prisoners died in camp. The soldiers who lived remained sick for the rest of their lives, with the exception of a few who were given niacin, three grams daily, after their release.

The risk of becoming dependent varies with the duration and intensity of malnutrition, with the presence of disease such as infection of the gastrointestinal tract, food allergies, the duration and intensity of systemic infections, and with the level and duration of stress. When all three factors are operating at high levels, the time needed to become dependent will be shortened. Cleave[33] found that it took twenty years before saccharine disease developed on a high-sugar, highly refined carbohydrate, and low-fiber diet without abnormal stress. The Canadian soldiers in Japan's Hong Kong camps became dependent in four years. But their malnutrition, presence of disease, and stress were much more severe.

Miller[34] suggests that tuberculosis increased susceptibility toward schizophrenia and that this has been a major factor in driving the evolutionary development of the disease. This bacterium depletes the body of its NAD by forcing an increased production of niacin, which is made from NAD. This ensures the survival of this infectious disease and its ready spread. It is uncommon in developed countries but is still a major pandemic in Africa, associated with the HIV virus. Tuberculosis is a trigger factor which converts a deficiency into a dependency.

Vitamin B$_3$-deficient and -dependent patients will share many symptoms but they will not be identical since the reason for the relative deficiency is different. The vitamin-deficient person is also lacking many other nutrients because their diet is so poor in quality. But the vitamin dependents may be dependent on only one vitamin and may be getting enough of the others from their diet.

CAUSES OF THE DEPENDENCY

The causes of B$_3$ dependency have not been studied because the concept has not been examined seriously. No doubt there are many reasons. The cause may be genetic and present from birth due to the absence of genes or the presence of defective enzymes. In the majority of cases, they start to work after birth and may develop at an early age, but they also may come on toward the end of one's life. There are two major factors 1.) A long-term deficiency will become a dependency if the condition is not treated. 2.) Prolonged stress of any type, including malnutrition, chronic disease, and psychosocial stress including war and brutality, will lead to deficiency and dependency.

Long-Term Deficiency

Pellagrologists in the 1930s observed that when dealing with well-recognized cases of pellagra, there were a few patients who did not become well until the amount of B$_3$ was increased to 1,000 milligrams daily, although most would recover on much less. They could not understand the reason for this.

It was also shown that the canine equivalent of pellagra, called black tongue, showed the same variable responses. If dogs were maintained on a diet deficient in B$_3$ for a few months and then given the vitamin again, they would quickly recover on the usual small doses. But if the dogs were deprived for more than six months, they would need much larger doses to recover. Being kept deficient eventually made these animals dependent. The same occurred with pellagra patients.

I think the same thing is happening today on a much wider scale. People who appear to be well for many years, on a diet only mildly deficient, will eventually become dependent. This accounts for the fact that so many of the modern diseases of affluent society develop in middle age and later, although there is evidence that these conditions are beginning to appear much earlier than they used to. For example, if patients with early-onset arthritis with very little joint degradation but with pain and stiffness are given B$_3$, they recover very quickly. My (AH) mother, who at age sixty-six was developing typical arthritis with Heberden's nodes, was well after only one month on niacin, 1 gram three times daily after meals. She lived another twenty years and wrote two books during that time.

Prolonged Stress

The second major cause is prolonged stress of any type, including malnutrition, chronic disease, and psychosocial stress including war and brutality. Post-traumatic stress disorder (PTSD) is a very common diagnosis. An example of severe stress was the experience of the above-mentioned Canadian soldiers in World War II, when they were incarcerated in Japanese prison camps for forty-four months. Other examples were the Holocaust camps, which killed most of the prisoners. A current example is the enormous stress of unrest, malnutrition and starvation, disease, and war in Africa. These victims suffer from a combination of all three forms of stress. The adverse impacts of combined psychosocial stress, starvation, and malnutrition peaked in the concentration camps of Europe and the prisoner of war camps in the Far East.

If the condition is allowed to damage the person for a longer period of time, it will require more vitamin and more time to recover. The time required on a deficiency diet to convert into dependency depends upon the degree of deficiency. If it is mild, it will take much longer to show up. If it is severe, as it was in Japanese war camps, it will take only a few years. I think that with the average North American diet it may take twenty years. If the nutrients are replaced at any time during the development phase, the process can be interrupted; if the deficiency is slight, small amounts of vitamins will cure. These are found in the standard B-complex preparations, which contain almost all of the B-complex vitamins. If the deficiency has been prolonged and severe, taking multiple-vitamin preparations in the usual small doses will be of little help in counteracting the dependency. It would be like giving too little antibiotic for a disease when a large dose is needed. This will be disappointing to many who have heard from their friends how well they became on the small dose preparations, because they did not know their own needs were so much greater.

Niacin and Prisoners of War

The link between niacin deficiencies and diet have been noted through research conducted on prisoners of war, in multiple settings, and by a number of researchers. Hoffer and Foster have previously described the impact of severe niacin deprivation, in their publication *Feel Better, Live Longer with Niacin*:

> The effects of this stress-malnutrition combination did not end upon release. Its subsequent impacts were obvious on the aging process. Over two thousand untrained Canadian soldiers were sent to Hong Kong to defend it from invasion from the east. But the Japanese attacked from the west and soon all these Canadian soldiers were in prison camps. Forty-four months later, one-quarter of them had died and the rest were left permanently impaired. On their way home in hospital ships, they were fed the strongest vitamin preparation then available, rice bran extracts, and they rapidly began to regain their health. Those that had survived had lost up to one-third of their body weight [and now] began to replace some of this loss. Although they appeared to become well again, they did not. A survey conducted by the federal government established that they were much sicker than Canadian soldiers who had fought in Europe, and, as a result, they were given special pensions. After the war, they suffered to an exaggerated degree from all the diseases of

aging, including arthritis, blindness, heart disease, neurological deterioration, and depression. Dr. Hoffer estimated that one year in a Far Eastern prisoner of war camp aged these soldiers about five years, as compared to a normal year living at home. A soldier imprisoned in such a camp at chronological age thirty-five would come out four years later with a biological age of fifty-five.

One of these former Hong Kong veterans, GP, was the administrator of a retirement home for many elderly men and women. GP had been depressed, experienced severe arthritis, was fearful, was heat and cold intolerant, and had spent some time on a psychiatric ward for veterans. He had been diagnosed as having a personality disorder. Much to his surprise, after two weeks on niacin he became normal. All these symptoms had disappeared, and he remained well until he died years later as Lieutenant Governor for the Province of Saskatchewan. Through his intercession, some 20 more Hong Kong veterans, as they were called, and American former prisoners of war came to see Dr. Hoffer. Given niacin treatment, they all recovered. It was concluded that the high-dose niacin had reversed the health deterioration caused by the extraordinarily severe stress of these camps.[35]

Life was hell for these men. They were treated with extreme brutality, were starved of calories, vitamins, and minerals, and they suffered from many deficiency diseases including scurvy, pellagra, beriberi, and infections.

Hans Selye tried to develop a measure for the severity of stress. He defined severe stress as a set of circumstances that would kill 10 percent of the exposed animals. As these prisoners died at a rate two and a half times greater than that, it is clear that they had been exposed to terrible stress indeed. When the soldiers were freed, shortly after the atomic bomb was dropped, the doctors in charge knew what was wrong. The men were fed the crude vitamin preparations then available on the hospital ships that brought them back to Victoria (see quotation above). The soldiers appeared to recover, but in fact they had not. Their subsequent loss due to disability and death has been enormous, yet little attention was given to the plight of these veterans.

In response to continuous complaints from the Hong Kong Veterans Association, Dr. H.J. Richardson (who conducted a special study from 1964 to 1965 on the problems and disabilities of Hong Kong veterans) compared the health of a sample of the veterans against their brothers in arms who had served in Europe. The Hong Kong veterans were found to be, as a group, much sicker. The death rate from heart disease was greater, and incidence of crippling arthritis, nervousness, tension, weakness, blindness, and depression was much higher. In recognition of these findings, Hong Kong veterans received higher pensions. It became clear that these men had been deteriorating both physically and mentally at a rate much higher than normal, and higher than that of soldiers who were not exposed to severe stress and malnutrition. William Allister was one of the Canadians held in these camps. He died at eighty-nine. His obituary describes the severe stress they suffered.[36]

However, the history for one small sample of veterans was much different, because post-captivity, they had been prescribed 3 grams of niacin per day. The twelve veterans recovered from their deficiencies, and remained well as long as they continued to take the quantity of niacin prescribed to them, on a regular basis. One of the last three survivors died in Victoria in July 2006. He was over eighty years old and had been on niacin for several decades and getting on well. He died of a coronary heart attack, but his last few weeks were marred by the hospital not allowing him to stay on his niacin. He felt terrible over this, as did his wife. This is another example of cruelty to patients for absolutely no reason whatever aside from rigid nutritional ignorance.

One of the survivors of the Hong Kong POW camp was Mr. GP, who was sick from the time he returned to Canada in 1944. His Veterans Administration file—all five pounds of it—got thicker, but he did not get any better. Most of his file contained results of frequent medical examinations and investigations. Throughout the documented period, GP was heavily medicated with amphetamines, to keep him alert during the day, and barbiturates, to allow him to sleep at night. He did not get well on this regimen. In fact, on one occasion, he was investigated in a psychiatric ward, which made him worse.

GP suffered from arthritis so incapacitating that he and his wife had to work up to one hour each morning to mobilize him so he could go to work. He also suffered from chronic anxiety and fear, for which he received psychotherapy. For example, he would not sit in any room with his back to the door. On his way to Hong Kong, he was a healthy young physical instructor, approximately six feet tall, weighing around 190 pounds. When he returned to Canada, his weight was approximately 120 pounds. Even though he was able to regain his weight, he was not well. Eventually he was treated in a Veterans Administration hospital, where he was diagnosed as suffering from anxiety. In fact he was suffering because he could not function properly.

In 1960 I started a project to study the effect of niacin on aging patients. GP was the director of the institution housing the patients, so I described the effects of niacin and the associated flush. A few months later he asked me whether he could also take the vitamin. I wondered why he would want to, and he told me that it would be easier for him to explain the flush to the elderly men living there if he experienced it. At that time I knew nothing about his wartime background.

A few months later he told me that he was "okay"—but I did not know what he meant. Then he told me about his forty-four months in the prisoner of war camp. Two weeks after starting the niacin, his arthritis was gone, he was able to lift both arms high over his shoulders, he was no longer heat and cold intolerant, and he was no longer anxious. He suffered a relapse several years later when he forgot to take his niacin on a trip to the mountains with his son. Two weeks later he was well into a relapse, and he never forgot again. A medical health officer who had been in the same camp with GP could not believe that the niacin had been of any value and accused GP of having had a placebo response. Later GP—George Porteous—became Lieutenant Governor of Saskatchewan. He was very proud of his recovery and told as many people as would listen to him about it. And because he described his recovery so freely, he helped many Hong Kong Veterans and United States ex–POWs.

THE DEFICIENCY DEPENDENCY CONTINUUM: FROM PELLAGRA TO SCHIZOPHRENIA

Vitamin B3 deficiency produces a large variety of psychiatric syndromes. Green and Kaufman, independently, described these quite well through their various publications.[37,38,39] It appears that a good deal of modern psychiatry depends on patients suffering from unidentified pellagra for its bread and butter. They would do a much better job if the basic treatment instead restored the insufficient vitamin. At the extreme end of the optimum-need continuum, the syndrome is much more likely to be even more severe and chronic. This includes the psychoses of aging, bipolar disease, and schizophrenic psychoses. Therefore, it is logical to drop the word "schizophrenia," and to use the correct term, pellagra, which would be described as "light to severe" or as "brief" or "prolonged." The pellagra caused by a deficient diet could be called deficiency pellagra and the pellagra caused by an increased requirement would be called dependency pellagra.

Clinically, schizophrenia and the pellagra psychosis could not be distinguished from each other in the southern mental hospitals, where they had the most experience in dealing with these syndromes. The differential was made on the basis of what the patients ate and the typical skin color of the condition. When niacin became available as a treatment it was used—and the schizophrenic patients who recovered with small doses of niacin were re-diagnosed as pellagra sufferers, while the schizophrenic patients who did not recover on the small dose continued to be diagnosed as schizophrenic. Schizophrenics did not have the same degree of skin discoloration because they were not exposed to the sun as much as the pellagrins.

The major clinical analysis accepted by the pellagrologists was that only pellagrins would respond to better diets and small amounts of niacin. They did try up to 1,000 milligrams daily, and were surprised that a few pellagrins needed the higher doses, which was considered enormous in those days.

Since schizophrenia and the pellagra psychosis are almost identical, and since the differences can be readily accounted for by the fact that they represent extreme ends of the B_3-requirement continuum, why do we not use the correct name? The development of a dependency is related to the severity of the initial deficiency and its duration. People with a minor deficiency will present symptoms for brief periods of time, say months rather than years, and will respond more quickly to smaller doses of the vitamin. They are like the pellagrins who responded so quickly to "vitamin" (small) doses of B_3, and like the dogs with black tongue that were not kept deficient too long. Schizophrenic patients have been on a deficient diet for years rather than months and they need large doses of B_3. They will also respond more slowly to treatment, as did the chronic pellagrins and the black tongue dogs that were maintained on a deficient diet too long.

In "High-affinity Niacin Receptor HM74A is Decreased in the Anterior Cingulate," Miller and Dulay's last paragraph states:

In conclusion, one important implication of the data we present here is that the early clinical studies by Abram Hoffer reported in a notable degree of success through treatment of unmedicated patients with niacin, but inconsistently replicated in follow-up work by others, should now be re-evaluated in the context of the limitation imposed by a deficient receptor, . . . The possibility that a deficiency in the high-affinity receptor is a core feature of many individuals with schizophrenia provides a basis for research into more potent receptor agonists and therapies that might significantly increase expression of the fully-functional protein.[40]

Miller and Dulay's research provides us for the first time with a clear indication of one of the causes of schizophrenia. The nicotinic acid receptors are not functioning properly, either because there are too few, or because they are malformed, or because they are less responsive to the presence of the vitamin in the fluid external to the cells. Using the lock and key analogy, either the lock or the key is not right for the other, or there are too few pathways into the cell. This can be overcome by increasing the head of pressure into the cell by using large doses.

If it quacks like a duck, walks like a duck, looks like a duck, and flies like a duck, then surely it must be a duck. Pellagra is that duck.

Schizophrenia and pellagra are clinically the same, and often one cannot be distinguished from the other unless the niacin therapeutic test is given. They are both nutritional diseases with major social and economic implications, and they both respond to proper treatment with optimum doses of niacin. Pellagra is a B_3 deficiency condition: there is not enough in food to meet the patient's requirements. Pellagra is also a dependency disease because there is not enough niacin in even the best of diets, and it must be supplemented. The word *schizophrenia* is therefore redundant. Even more, it is damaging to patients, to their families, and to society. The correct word should be *pellagra*, which can be qualified by the term *dependency pellagra* to distinguish it from deficiency pellagra. Deficiency pellagra is, of course, also complicated by deficiencies of other vitamins, protein, and essential fatty acids. I hope Cato the Elder will not mind: *Schizophrenia delenda est.* (Schizophrenia must be eliminated.)

Niacin Treatment of Schizophrenia

Recent Research Confirms Abram Hoffer's Original Work

by Robert G. Smith, PhD

Schizophrenia is a devastating and complex disease that can include a variety of specific clinical conditions. Drugs to treat schizophrenia have not advanced much beyond the 1960s; in many cases they are not very effective, and they have severe side effects. The problem is that the cause of schizophrenia is unknown, and precisely how the drugs affect brain circuitry is also unknown. Schizophrenia is thought to have a substantial environmental component (toxins, culture, upbringing, lifestyle, diet, etc.), but its onset is likely to be predisposed by genetic factors.[41] Genetic analysis has recently made great progress in identifying genes that cause diseases. Many diseases that strike young adults, as schizophrenia often does, have been shown to be caused by one or just a few specific mutations. For example, some diseases that cause blindness are now known to be caused by a mutation in one or more of the genes that code for molecules in the brain essential for sight. In one recent case, gene therapy approved by the FDA to correct the mutation has restored sight in blind people.[42]

Pessimism about Schizophrenia

Research into the possible genetic cause of schizophrenia has not found any obvious candidate gene mutations. Part of the problem is that schizophrenia is not just one disease; it comprises a family of interrelated conditions and is diagnosed by several criteria, which implies that a variety of causes may contribute. Apparently, many gene mutations may contribute to schizophrenia, but none yet found have an influence strong enough to be the exclusive cause.

A recent presentation on solving the puzzle of schizophrenia at the Society for Neuroscience (SfN) conference in Washington, D.C. had a pessimistic tone, explaining that there are no easy answers in the search for better treatment. No helpful novel drug treatments for schizophrenia have been found in recent years, and the lack of obvious genetic markers that are correlated with the disease presents a severe challenge. The SfN presentation, however, did not mention recent research into dietary causes and treatments for schizophrenia.

Niacin Cures Many Schizophrenics

In the early 1960s, Hoffer and Osmond published studies showing that niacin (also known as nicotinic acid or vitamin B_3) given at sufficiently high doses could effectively treat some schizophrenia patients.[43-47] Although Hoffer and Osmond's theories about how niacin could treat schizophrenia were never sufficiently proven to convince the rest of the field, their results in treating thousands of patients with niacin therapy and curing many were striking. The term "orthomolecular" was coined by Linus Pauling for the use of essential nutrients such as niacin in preventing disease, and in particular, schizophrenia.[48] A recent search conducted on PubMed of the terms "schizophrenia niacin" returned several dozen articles. One of them asserts that some schizophrenics can be well treated with niacin, and refers to Hoffer and Osmond's early studies, reviewing several theories about likely mechanisms.[49]

> "Abram Hoffer backed up his treatment with clearly
> explained biochemistry, as he had a degree in biochemistry
> before obtaining his MD. I personally found his
> presentation fascinating as well as convincing."
> —Ralph Campbell, MD

Niacin Skin Test

Most people get a "niacin flush" on their skin for a few minutes when a large dose of niacin is taken orally. This is a normal consequence of niacin activating prostaglandin pathways that cause vasodilation in the skin and is not harmful. Niacin is utilized by several hundred metabolic pathways in the body, so oral niacin is taken by many to treat illness and maintain good health. To avoid the skin flush, one starts with small doses (typically 25 milligrams per day)

and gradually increases the dose over several days to achieve a therapeutic effect. However, some schizophrenics don't get a niacin flush
with the normal doses, suggesting that they have a deficiency of niacin and likely other essential nutrients. Therefore, niacin applied to
the skin or taken orally has been used as a test for predisposition to
schizophrenia. Hoffer noted that in some cases where schizophrenics
recovered, they reverted to a normal skin flush.[50] A flurry of recent
studies show that about one third of schizophrenics have a blunted
niacin skin flush, suggesting that this test can be used as a diagnostic
tool.[51–60] Several recent studies attempted to determine what aspect
of the metabolic disturbance might cause problems for the brain.
Although most of the studies don't explicitly discuss the use of niacin
as a treatment, the underlying theme is that niacin treatment can
help many schizophrenics.

> "Dr. Abram Hoffer observed a recovery to a normal niacin-
> flush response in an otherwise previously flush-resistant
> schizophrenic. Dr. Hoffer used either niacinamide or niacin,
> although he favored the lipodystrophy-correcting/flush-causing
> niacin form more. He also recommended essential fatty acids."
> —W. Todd Penberthy, PhD

Nutrient Dependencies

Many schizophrenic patients have severe nutrient *dependencies* that
can be treated with niacin and other vitamins and nutrients. Several
recent studies review the evidence for a benefit from good nutrition
(niacin, other B vitamins, vitamin C and D, omega-3 fatty acids,
etc.) on brain function.[61–68]

The use of niacin therapy for testing and treatment of schizophrenia and many other conditions appears to be rapidly expanding.
It is inexpensive and widely used for health, but can also help those
in desperate need of treatment. For a therapeutic effect, Hoffer recommended gradually increasing doses up to 3,000 milligrams per
day of niacin in divided doses, along with 2,000 milligrams per day
or more of vitamin C and other essential nutrients. For some people, high doses can cause temporary side effects, so many people take

niacin for its health benefit at lower doses (500 to 1,000 milligrams per day). Niacinamide has similar benefits but does not cause the skin flush.

Conclusion

It is straightforward to understand the historical bias against niacin therapy for schizophrenia. Niacin is inexpensive and can't be patented. It is known to be effective at preventing heart disease.[69] One can imagine that the drug industry is working to make a form of niacin or a niacin-like drug that can produce profits.[69-70]

CHAPTER 5

How to Take Niacin

*There is a principle which is a bar against all information,
which is proof against all argument, and which cannot
fail to keep man in everlasting ignorance. That principle
is condemnation without investigation.*
—WILLIAM PALEY (1743–1805), OFTEN ATTRIBUTED
TO HERBERT SPENCER (1820–1903)

The keys to taking niacin therapy are *quantity, frequency*, and *duration*. You need to take enough, take it frequently, and take it long enough to see benefit.

TAKE ENOUGH

Adequately high supplement doses need to be employed to get the job done. As there is a certain, large amount of fuel needed to launch an aircraft or a spacecraft, there is a certain, large amount of a nutrient needed to cure a sick body. With vitamin therapy, speed of recovery is proportional to dosage used. Dr. Hoffer's standard prescription was 3,000 milligrams per day.

Much less is needed for prevention and daily good health maintenance. The Recommended Dietary Allowance (RDA) for niacin is under 18 milligrams per day. That is outdated guidance and far too low. In 2007, an independent review panel of twenty-two researchers and physicians issued their recommendation for niacin intake for an adult as 300 milligrams per day.[1]

Vitamins

How Much to Take?

In his classic health book, *Supernutrition*,[2] Richard A. Passwater suggests a simple and utterly nontechnical method to determine what amounts of vitamins you personally need to take for optimum health. Wisely, no one prescriptive list is given; no "one size fits all" approach is offered. Rather, Dr. Passwater builds a careful and well-documented case for megavitamin therapy, and then shows how to increase your own vitamin doses in two-week intervals until peak health has been achieved. Essentially, you take the smallest amounts of supplements that give the greatest results. If you go over and beyond that level, your health benefits will stay the same or decline. That would be the point of diminishing returns, the point of wasting money, and/or a potentially harmful overdose. If this seems like common sense, perhaps that's because it is. Interestingly, when doctors use this very same approach with drugs, it is called a "therapeutic trial." With drugs, it is trial and error. With nutrients, it is trial and much, much less risk of error.

TAKE FREQUENTLY

Niacin is a water-soluble vitamin. This means that it is lost from the body easily during the course of a day or even a few hours. Therefore, divide the daily niacin dose and take a third of it with every meal. Taking niacin with meals improves absorption.

Dr. William Kaufman and other experienced physicians have advocated for the importance of the frequency of doses. With the water-soluble vitamins, at any given quantity, frequently-divided doses are invariably more effective. (There is more about Dr. Kaufman's treatment for arthritis in chapter 7.)

TAKE IT LONG ENOUGH

Some persons will notice benefits right away. Blood lipid benefits take more time. Long-standing mental illness may respond slowly, over a period of weeks or even months. Every patient is different, and this is why we recommend that you work in close cooperation with your personal physician.

HOW DO I KNOW IF NIACIN IS HELPING?

There are two ways to tell if your niacin supplementation is working for you: subjectively and objectively.

SUBJECTIVE PROOF

If you are fighting mental illness, you will know full well when you feel better. It is just that simple. Friends and family may comment positively. Dr. Hoffer's standard measure of recovery was this: recovered, truly well patients pay income tax. It sounds odd, but a person must be successfully holding a job in order to do so. Placebos rarely achieve that result. Critics of Hoffer's work have claimed that it was his pleasant, positive bedside manner that resulted in cured patients. Dr. Hoffer replied, "I am nice to all my patients. However, only the ones getting niacin get better."

Common Sense Caution:

Work with your doctor. Persons who are pregnant or have a history of heavy alcohol use, liver disorders, or diabetes will especially want to have their physician monitor their use of niacin in quantity.

OBJECTIVE PROOF

Ask your physician to check and see. For example, laboratory tests can easily verify if your blood lipids are benefiting from niacin. Watch especially for lower triglycerides and higher "good" HDL.

HOW MUCH IS TOO MUCH?

A person's absolute upper limit for niacin is the amount that causes nausea, and, if not reduced, vomiting. The dose should never be allowed to remain at this upper limit. Dr. Hoffer's usual therapeutic dose range was 3,000 milligrams daily, divided into three doses of 1,000 milligrams each. Sometimes some patients need more. The toxic dose for dogs is about 5,000 milligrams per 2.2 pounds (1 kilogram) of body weight. It is not known what the toxic dose for humans is since niacin has never been shown to have killed anyone.

Monitoring long-term use of niacin is a good idea for anyone. It consists of having your doctor periodically (perhaps once or twice a year) check your liver function with a simple blood test. Correct interpretation of these monitoring tests is important.

Niacin is not liver toxic, but niacin therapy does increase liver enzyme test results. This elevation means that the liver is active—it does not indicate an underlying liver pathology.

SO-CALLED "SAFE UPPER LIMITS"

In spite of all this, there is now a government-sponsored "Safe Upper Limit" (or "tolerable upper intake level") for niacin consumption. It is 35 milligrams per day.[3] We offer this book as a charge-leading rebuttal against the arbitrariness and absurdity of that figure. Among many reasons why it is preposterous is that the so-called Safe Upper Limit is only about twice the RDA! There is no clinical or laboratory evidence that proves that niacin, or any other vitamin for that matter, is dangerous at double the RDA.

Instead, authoritative-sounding speculation is offered to the public in the form of statements like this:

Supplement users at risk from ignorance of tolerable upper limits
. . . Consuming too many nutrients can lead to harmful side effects,

a fact many users were worryingly unaware of, said researchers . . . (T)he tolerable upper level of one B vitamin, niacin, was exceeded by nearly 50 percent of all the participants in their study who reported taking supplements . . . (D)ietary supplements exceeding the tolerable upper limits were fairly common in the U.S., as the supplement industry is not regulated in the same way as the pharmaceutical industry.[4]

The authors of this paper claim that side-effect symptoms will likely occur in half of those persons taking 100 milligrams of supplemental niacin, and that it is impossible to identify those who are at greatest risk.[5] We consider such statements to be scaremongering and sensationalism.

In his fifty-five years of experience with thousands of patients, Dr. Hoffer found that even 40,000 milligrams of niacin daily is not toxic. He estimated that over 200,000 milligrams per day is fatal. In fact, there is a built-in safety valve with niacin: vomiting. Nausea will occur far in advance of any risk of fatality. Most people would never exceed a few thousand milligrams daily, an amount that orthodox physicians frequently give patients to raise HDL. The safety margin is very large. For more than twenty-five years, data collected by the American Association of Poison Control Centers (AAPCC) confirms that there is not even one niacin-related death per year. (You may download Annual Reports of the American Association of Poison Control Centers free of charge at http://www.aapcc.org/. The "Vitamin" category is usually near the end of the report.)

THE NIACIN FLUSH AND VASODILATATION (VASODILATION)

Niacin usually causes a flush a few minutes after it is taken. A few people will flush with 25 milligrams, more people with 50 milligrams, and most people with 100 milligrams. The flush begins in the forehead and works its way down the body, rarely affecting the toes. The higher the initial dose the greater the initial flush, but if any dose causes a maximum flush, a larger dose taken later will not cause a greater flush. The capillaries are dilated and the blood flow through the organs is increased. There is an internal increase in blood flow as well as in the skin, which may last up to several hours.

Patients must be warned that flushing will happen. If not, they may be very surprised or even shocked by the onset of the flush, and believe that they are experiencing an allergic reaction, or worse. Patients can be started on lower doses until they have adjusted to the decreased intensity of the flush. Then the doses may be increased gradually.

> With large initial doses, the niacin flush is more pronounced and lasts longer. But with each additional dose, the intensity of the flush decreases, and in most patients becomes a minor nuisance rather than an irritant. To minimize flushing, niacin should be taken right after eating.

Each time niacin is taken, the flush is repeated, but to a much lesser degree. In most cases it is almost entirely absent after a week or so, and is a minor nuisance at worst. However, some patients do not tolerate the flush and will have to discontinue the niacin. Non-flush preparations are available for these individuals (see chapter 2). If the routine is interrupted for several days and then resumed, the same sequence of flushing will occur, but the initial flush usually will not be as strong as the original one. The intensity of the flush is minimized by taking the pills after meals and by taking them regularly, three times daily. I (AH) have been taking niacin for fifty-five years and at most have very minor flushes. It is a drier flush, not like the wet menopausal flush, or the flush suffered by male hormone blockers used in treating prostate cancer. Niacinamide does not cause flushing in the majority of patients. In perhaps 1 percent of patients, it will cause a very unpleasant flush, in which case it cannot be used. Probably their bodies convert the niacinamide into niacin too rapidly. This is unlikely to be you.

Vasodilatation (often called vasodilation) is sometimes very helpful. Many patients, particularly arthritics, have reported that they feel much better when their joints are warmed up by the flush, and some will stop taking niacin for a few days in order to experience the flush once more. But for most patients, the sensation is not pleasant. It is tolerable if patients know what to expect and are properly prepared by the physician. William Parsons Jr. writes that only physicians who understand niacin should use it. No-flush and slow-release preparations, which are also no-flush, are available. The best-known no-flush product is inositol hexaniacinate, which is an ester of inositol, a vitamin, and niacin. Doubling the niacin dose may be necessary, but only trial and error will determine which is best for some patients.

SOME HISTAMINE HISTORY

Back in 1962, with only about a decade of niacin research behind me, I (AH) wrote:

> Little is known about the physiology of the nicotinic acid vaso-dilatation; it resembles histamine flushing in its mode of onset, unpleasantness, and bodily distribution but in contrast to the histamine-induced flush, there is no fall in blood pressure. Possibly it releases a histamine-like substance, either histamine itself or serotonin.

Edmond Boyle, then director of research at the Miami Heart Institute, believed the dilatation was caused by the histamine released. He had examined the mast cells [found in skin and connective tissue, and the mucous linings of the nose, mouth, lungs, and digestive tract] before and after taking niacin and had seen that the mast cell vesicles containing histamine were empty after the flush. It is believed that niacin causes a flush by a complicated mechanism which releases histamine, interferes in prostaglandin metabolism, may be related to serotonin mechanism, and may involve the cholinergic system.[6]

Histamine is clearly involved. The typical niacin flush is identical with the flush produced by an injection of histamine. It is dampened down, if not prevented entirely, by antihistamines and by some of the original tranquilizers such as chlorpromazine. The adaptation to niacin is readily explained by the reduction in histamine in the storage sites such as the mast cells. When these are examined after a dose of histamine, these cells contain empty vesicles, which contained the histamine and also heparinoids. If the next dose is spaced closely enough, there will have been no time for the storage sites to be refilled, and therefore less histamine will be available to be released. After there is complete adaptation to niacin, a rest of several days will start the flushing cycle again. This decrease in histamine has some advantage in reducing the effects of rapidly released histamine. Dr. Edmond Boyle found that guinea pigs treated with niacin were not harmed by anaphylactic shock. Because the flush is relatively transient, it cannot be involved in the lowering of cholesterol, which remains in effect as long as niacin is continued. Prostaglandins appear to be involved. Thus, aspirin[7] and indomethacin[8] reduce the intensity of the flush.[9]

Boyle found that niacin increased basophil leukocyte count. These white blood cells store histamine and heparin, and protect the body against microorganisms causing disease. We earlier implicated a histamine-glycosaminoglycan histaminase system as well as histamine in lipid absorption and redistribution. Boyle suggested that the improvement caused by niacin is much greater than can be explained by its effect on cholesterol. He thought it might be due to the release of histamine and to the eventual reduction in the intravascular "sludging" of blood cells."[10] Cheng et al. presented evidence that prostaglandins are involved in the niacin flush, but they admit "the flushing is not completely understood."[11] I am sorry the histamine idea was shelved, as I think there is powerful evidence that it too is involved in the flushing process. Probably all the systems are interrelated.

When histamine is injected subcutaneously (under the skin) there is almost an immediate flush, which is indistinguishable from the niacin flush in distribution and intensity. However, when niacin is taken along with histamine, the flush is not immediate. It may come on much more slowly unless histamine is injected intravenously, in which case the flush is immediate. The flush that occurs following injection of niacin alone is identical to the flush observed when histamine is injected subcutaneously. The niacin flush, however, typically is not associated with a decrease in blood pressure as it is with the histamine flush.

FACTORS IN FLUSHING

The rapidity with which the flush appears depends upon the concentration of niacin achieved. When taken by mouth with a meal or snack, the rate of absorption largely depends on the amount of food in the stomach: more food means slower absorption and less flushing. Another variable would be taking niacin with either a hot or cold beverage: more flushing is likely with a hot drink. Medication is another factor. You can look up any prescription or over-the-counter drug that you are taking in the *Physicians' Desk Reference*, or any of the many drug facts/side effects/interactions websites that are available online. If the niacin is absorbed rapidly, the flush will come on more quickly. Lower doses induce the flush after a time period that varies enormously from person to person. The flush also depends on unknown resistance factors. There are some people who cannot tolerate even a small dose of niacin, say 50 milligrams, before they flush, and have such severe flushes that they cannot take any niacin except no-flush preparations (discussed in chapter 2). A very few cannot even tolerate the no-flush preparations. Their histamine storage sites may be too sensitive and release histamine too quickly. Oddly enough, the best "no-flush preparation" is uninterrupted use of niacin. The flush returns if the niacin is not taken for a day or more, but when it is resumed, the original flush is not as intense. Also, elderly patients and children do not flush as heavily as adults.

Schizophrenic patients are usually less disturbed by the flush. Many schizophrenic patients do not flush until after several months and for as long as up to several years after starting to take 3 grams of niacin daily. This inability to flush may be related to their disease, for an appreciable number of schizophrenic patients begin to flush after several years of medication. This is a good prognostic sign and usually coincides with complete recovery.

These observations suggest that there may be a two-phase process occurring. The first involves the prostaglandins, which become activated and stimulate the release of histamine. If the prostaglandin reaction is primary, this would explain why the time to flush is variable, as it would depend upon the amount of histamine released. If the histamine release came first, the flush should be almost immediate. The way to test this hypothesis would be to check histamine blood levels as a kind of histamine tolerance test. I would expect that after niacin, there would not be an immediate release with little histamine in the blood, and later it would build up in concordance with the intensity of the flush. This two-phase reaction would account for the anti-flush effect of some of the antihistamines and the older antipsychotic drugs, which act on the histamine system. It would also explain the effect of aspirin, which acts on the prostaglandin system. (By the way, Kunin, who was the first to observe that aspirin is a partial antidote to the niacin flush, is hardly ever given any credit.)

NIACIN REDUCES ANAPHYLACTIC SHOCK

While he was working at Henry Wellcome Laboratories, Nobel Laureate Sir Henry Dale discovered that histamine was released during anaphylaxis, a life-threatening allergic reaction. This is a very complex, severe reaction, and apparently acetyl choline and heparin are also involved. Guinea pigs are very sensitive to anaphylactic shock. Boyle found that if guinea pigs were pretreated for a week with niacin, they did not die after a second dose of protein—a procedure that killed all the animals not pretreated.

Common Sense Caution:

Anaphylactic shock is life-threatening. Work closely with your doctor if you have any history of this or other severe reactions. It is generally safe for your doctor to try a supervised therapeutic trial of niacin. It is unwise for you to do it alone.

I have used this technique to protect patients against anaphylactic shock. In 1996 I saw a patient who was very fearful for his life. He was peanut sensitive and avoided all traces of peanuts, but over a six-month period he had five major reactions and nearly died from the last one. I advised him to start with ascorbic acid, 1 gram taken after each of three meals. Ascorbic acid destroys histamine, which is why scorbutic patients who are deficient in this vitamin have high blood histamine levels. I wanted to build up his blood ascorbic acid levels. After one week he was to take 100 milligrams of niacin three times daily after meals. This was designed to release a small amount of histamine with a gentle flush. My hypothesis was that the histamine would be destroyed by the ascorbic acid and would therefore be neutralized to a degree. The niacin dose was increased to 250 milligrams twice a day. This was his maintenance dose. He came back ten years later for an unrelated problem. He had not taken any niacin the previous two years after his doctor told him to stop. (This is an example of a totally illogical fear of niacin, when the same doctor would, with no hesitation, prescribe any and all of the toxic drugs that are available.) I advised him to resume the niacin and to increase the dose until he was on 1 gram after each of three meals. As a result, he had no more reactions, but was advised to be as careful as before.

I have also used the combination of niacin and ascorbic acid to protect patients against the hives induced by insect bites. And I found it very helpful in decreasing the intensity of the allergic reactions, no matter what type of substance the patient is reacting to, although it will not completely prevent these reactions.

OTHER CLINICAL USES OF NIACIN

Some additional and interesting therapeutic uses of niacin include treatment of Meniere's syndrome (ringing in the ears and associated nausea) and high-tone deafness. In long-term therapy, improvement was obtained with only 150 to 250 milligrams daily.[12] Resistance to x-radiation was greatly improved at around 500 to 600 milligrams daily. Radiation-induced nausea was also reduced. Supplemental niacin could therefore be of great value for cancer patients undergoing radiation therapy. Even healing after surgical shock and other trauma including burns, hemorrhage, and infection is more rapid with niacin administration. More clinical uses of niacin are discussed in chapter 11.

TO FLUSH OR NOT TO FLUSH?
THE NIACIN FLUSH AS DOSAGE INDICATOR

I (AWS) have found that the best way to accurately control the flushing sensation is to start with small amounts of niacin and gradually increase the dosage until the first flush is noticed. If you are new to all of this, one very gentle method is to start with a mere 25 milligrams three times a day, most likely with each meal. The next day, try 50 milligrams at breakfast, 25 milligrams at lunch, and 25 milligrams at supper. The following day, increase the dose to 50 milligrams at breakfast, 50 milligrams at lunch, and 25 milligrams at supper, and the next day take 50 milligrams at each of the three meals. Continue increasing the dosage by taking 75 milligrams, 50 milligrams, and 50 milligrams the next day, then 75 milligrams, 75 milligrams, and 50 milligrams, and so on. In this way you have increased at the easy rate of only 25 milligrams per day. You would continue to increase the dosage by 25 milligrams per day until the flush occurs.

It may take quite a while. It is difficult to predict your personal optimum level for niacin because each person is different. As a general rule, the more you can hold without flushing, the more you need. If you flush early, you don't need much niacin. If flushing doesn't happen until a high level, then your body is utilizing (and needs) the higher amount of the vitamin.

Now that you've had your first flush, what's next? Since a flush often indicates temporary saturation of niacin, it is desirable to continue to repeat the flushing, just very slightly, to continue the saturation. This could be done three or more times a day. Niacin can be taken to saturation at bedtime too, to get to sleep sooner at night. You might be asleep before you even notice the flush.

An important point here is that niacin is a vitamin, not a drug. It may relax you (a good thing) but it does not "put you to sleep" or anything like it. Niacin is not a hypnotic (sleeping pill). It is not habit forming. Niacin does not require a prescription because it is that safe. It is a nutrient that everyone needs each day. Different people in different circumstances require different amounts of niacin.

People in fairly good health often choose to increase their doses gradually in order to minimize flushing. If they do increase the dose slowly, what I describe is pretty accurate. For instance, I have been taking niacin for many years, in daily but varying doses depending on my stress level or dietary intake. I know by the flush when I've had enough for the moment. It is like turning off the hot water when the tub is full enough for a nice bath.

When you flush, you can literally see and feel that you've taken enough niacin, at least for now. The idea is to initially take just enough niacin to have a slight flush. This means a pinkness about the cheeks, ears, neck, forearms, and perhaps elsewhere. A slight niacin flush should end in about ten minutes or so. If you take too much niacin, the flush may be more pronounced and longer lasting. If you flush beet red for an hour, well, you took too much. Large doses of niacin on an empty stomach are certain to cause profound flushing.

Most people flush when they start niacin supplementation and gradually get adapted to it unless they stop for a few days and then resume. A few never get used to it, and they take the no-flush preparations. But the intensity of the flush is very variable. *Generally, people who need niacin the most flush the least.* That includes arthritics, schizophrenics, and people with cardiovascular problems. Some schizophrenics do not flush until they get well and *then* they begin to flush. *But the presence of the flush or its intensity cannot be uniquely used to measure the need for niacin,* as there are too many variables such as food in the stomach, whether the drink taken with it is hot or cold, the kind of food taken with it, and other medications the patient takes. Antipsychotics reduce the intensity of the flush as do aspirin and antihistamines.

Plain niacin may be purchased in tablets at many pharmacies, discount stores, health food stores, or online. Tablets typically are available in 50 milligrams, 100 milligrams, 250 milligrams, or 500 milligrams dosages. The tablets are usually scored down the middle so you can more easily break them in half. You can break the halves in half too, to get the exact amount you want. An inexpensive pill-cutter may be useful for this purpose.

Remember, if a niacin tablet is taken on an empty stomach, a flush will occur (if it is going to occur at all) within about thirty minutes, usually sooner. If niacin is taken right after a meal, a flush may be delayed. In fact, the flush may occur long enough afterward that you forgot that you took the niacin. Don't let the flush surprise you. Remember that niacin does this, and you can monitor it easily.

You can powder the niacin tablet if you want a flush right away. This is easily done by crushing it between two spoons. Powdered niacin on an empty stomach can result in a flush within minutes. Take it with a hot beverage and the flush will occur even sooner. Niacin is heat-stable, so the temperature of food will not affect it at all.

Dr. Hoffer reported that side effects that may occur with really high doses of niacin are partly or largely offset by taking large doses of vitamin C. Hoffer had his patients take at least as much vitamin C as niacin. More vitamin C works even better. We have already mentioned the most common side effects: the flush, of course, and possibly nausea if you take way too much. Side effects tend to be more common in people with a history of liver disease and/or substantial alcohol use, commonly believed to be indicated by elevation of liver function tests. We will discuss this and other niacin side effects in the next chapter.

It is a good idea to take all the other B-complex vitamins in a separate supplement, in addition to the niacin. The B vitamins, like professional baseball players, work best as a team. Still, the body seems to need proportionally more niacin than the other B vitamins. Even the U.S. Recommended Dietary Allowance (RDA) for niacin is much more than for any other B vitamin. Orthomolecular (nutritional) physicians consider the current RDA for niacin of only 18 milligrams or less to be far too low for optimum health. While the powers that be continue to discuss this, it is possible to decide for yourself based on the success of doctors who use niacin for their patients every day.

Does Niacin Cause Macular Edema?

Rarely. Niacin can sometimes cause cystoid macular edema (spaces of fluid that form within the retina). This condition is unusual and completely reversible. Such changes are obvious in a standard retinal fundus exam when the patient reports symptoms of a visual deficit.[13]

This maculopathy is not associated with the characteristic leakage from retinal arterioles caused by diabetic retinopathy, as it goes away when niacin is discontinued or the dosage is reduced. There is a threshold dose.[14] Some case reports show that going from 3,000 milligrams per day down to 1,000 to 1,500 milligrams reverses the cystoid maculopathy.[13] The critical dose is likely to be related to the body weight, so that smaller people would have a lower threshold and larger people a higher figure. The reversibility and ease of detection factors are very important to niacin users. Persons taking niacin should note any changes in their vision, especially in reading, which uses the fovea and macula. Of those people taking niacin at high doses, only those that report visual symptoms need to be evaluated by an ophthalmologist.[15] The rate is very low, less than 1 percent of those taking high doses of niacin for reducing cholesterol.[13]

Some papers on this topic[16] offer authors' assessments of ocular side effects from herbals and nutritional supplements which seem a little alarmist, potentially leading the reader to generalize from the specific problems described in the article to an overall conclusion that nutrients and herbal supplements will inevitably lead to problems with toxicity. That is not the case. It is important that people understand that the side effects of niacin are specific to the patient's prior conditions and to the dose.

Cataract surgery is a common and necessary procedure for many elderly persons. One possible side effect of cataract surgery is retinal detachment. It is then possible that surgery for retinal detachment may increase the risk that high doses of niacin could lead to cystoid macular edema (CME). Either decreasing the dose of niacin, or switching to niacinamide, may help conventional anti-inflammatory medication via eye drops. Niacinamide, since it doesn't increase prostaglandins like niacin does, is unlikely to be a factor in causing CME. You should work closely with your ophthalmologist in addressing this, or any, eye concern.

People will notice if they develop eye problems. Because the side effects of niacin are reversible and easy to detect, this is a small and manageable problem. If those people taking supplements know that niacin has been reported in rare cases to cause eye problems, and that the problems are reversible, this will point them and their medical professionals in the right direction.

CHAPTER 6

Safety of Niacin

The physician must know niacin in order to use it.
—WILLIAM PARSONS, JR., MD

*P*harmakon is an ancient Greek word that means both a remedy and a poison. It aptly describes drugs, but not orthomolecular substances like vitamins. Vitamins have established an excellent safety record, and this allows a very large margin for error. Still, there is a right way and a wrong way to do anything. In this chapter we will address the safety of vitamin B$_3$ therapy.

DOES NIACIN RAISE BLOOD SUGAR?

Sometimes it does. Many decades ago I (AH) began giving niacin to all my diabetic patients to keep their cholesterol levels normal and to decrease the serious vascular side effects of diabetes that lead to blindness and loss of legs. I did not see that many, but none of my diabetic patients on niacin suffered from those side effects. Their eyes remained normal as did their circulatory system. Many physicians had the idea that because niacin increased blood glucose levels in some patients that this was contraindication. However, that increase was usually minor, and the patients did not suffer from those slight elevations. I found that one-third of my diabetic patients had to increase insulin levels a little, one-third had to *decrease* it, and the rest did not need to make any change.

No Deaths from Niacin (or Any Other Vitamin)

Safety Confirmed by America's Largest Database

The 38th annual report (2020) from the American Association of Poison Control Centers (AAPCC) revealed **zero deaths from vitamins**. Supporting data is from the most recent information collected by the U.S. National Poison Data System (in Table 22B, p 1476–1478), at the very end of the full report published in *Clinical Toxicology*.[1] It is interesting that it is so quietly placed way back there where nary a news reporter is likely to see it. The AAPCC reports zero deaths from multiple vitamins. And, there were no deaths whatsoever from vitamin A, niacin, pyridoxine (B6), or any other B-vitamin. There were no deaths from vitamin C, vitamin D, vitamin E, **or from any vitamin at all**.

On page 1,477 there is an allegation of a single death attributed to an unspecified, unknown "Miscellaneous Vitamin." If the substance cannot even be specified, it cannot be used to blame a category. The obvious uncertainty of such a listing eliminates it as a valid claim.

Additionally, there were no fatalities from amino acids, creatine, blue-green algae, glucosamine, or chondroitin. There were no deaths from any homeopathic remedy, Asian medicine, Hispanic medicine, or Ayurvedic medicine. None.

Fifty-five poison centers provide coast-to-coast data for the U.S. National Poison Data System, "one of the few real-time national surveillance systems in existence, providing a model public health surveillance system for all types of exposures, public health event identification, resilience response and situational awareness tracking."

Zero deaths from vitamins. Want to bet this will never be on the evening news? Well, have you seen it there? And why not? Well over half of the U.S. population takes daily nutritional supplements. Indeed, a Harris Poll showed that for American adults, the number is 86 percent.[2] But let's just use the low number. Should each of those people take only one single tablet daily, that still makes close to 170 million individual doses per day, for a total of well over

60 billion doses annually. Since many persons take far more than just a single vitamin tablet daily, actual consumption is considerably higher, and the safety of vitamin supplements is all the more remarkable.

Throughout the entire year, coast to coast across the entire USA, there was not one single death from a vitamin. If vitamin supplements are allegedly so "dangerous," as the FDA, the news media, and even some physicians still claim, then *where are the bodies*?

STUDIES ON NIACIN AND BLOOD SUGAR

In a 1987 study by Vague et al., juvenile diabetics were given three grams (3,000 milligrams) of niacin per day. That dosage produced remissions in a large proportion of these young patients. The report on this study concluded, "Our results and those from animal experiments indicate that, in Type I diabetes, nicotinamide slows down the destruction of B cells and enhances their regeneration, thus extending remission time."[3]

In 2006, Canner et al. reported that niacin was valuable in treating post-infarction patients, whether or not they had the sugar metabolic syndrome. They did not find that niacin was contraindicated.[4] Similarly, Dube et al. reported that extended-release niacin "in doses up to 2,000 milligrams daily was safe, well-tolerated, and efficacious in HIV-infected subjects with atherogenic dyslipidemia. Increases in glycaemia and insulin resistance tended to be transient."[5]

Kirkey reported the results of a study, published in *The Lancet* in 2008, that concluded that most people with diabetes should be taking statins. Kirkey writes, "Diabetics should take cholesterol-lowering drugs,"[6] which of course would include niacin. You can visualize how much more therapeutic niacin will be if the statins, which are only a very poor distant cousin in effectiveness to niacin, were helpful. The statins only lower total cholesterol, do not elevate HDL, do not lower triglycerides, and do not lower lipoprotein(a). The statins decrease the least important metabolic factor, which has little relationship to heart disease, and which does not extend life as niacin does. Abnormality in blood lipid levels are main components of this cardiovascular syndrome, which is also associated with decreased sugar tolerance and obesity. Since the main pathological side effects are changes in blood lipids and arteriosclerosis, niacin, which normalizes blood cholesterol levels, should theoretically be an important constituent of any treatment program for this condition and for type 1 and type 2 diabetes. Giving people niacin must be a most important treatment if we are to decrease the major pathology that both of these serious diseases generate.

But not everyone knows this. Here is an example of just how far irrationality seeps into medicine. In one study by Zhou et al.,[7] the authors claim that a mere 100 milligrams of niacinamide raises blood sugar. This is contrary to common sense, as well as contrary to Dr. Hoffer's extensive clinical experience. Hoffer found that several thousand milligrams daily, long-term, raised blood sugar only slightly if at all. Another study by Li et al.[8] borders on the comical. After looking at blood glucose levels in exactly five people, the authors conclude that niacin . . . contained in fortified foods! . . . is a cause of childhood obesity. How so? The authors claim that niacin stimulates appetite. How much niacin? This is the funniest part: in this case, the authors are talking single-digit RDA-levels—far, far less than even 100 milligrams. Might it be more likely that, just possibly, the cause of childhood obesity is overconsumption of fat and sugar? Perhaps the McNothing meals kids eat, or their huge consumption of soda, or lack of exercise? We think that observations on the blood glucose levels of five people are hardly the basis for reconsideration of niacin levels for a whole country. Research like this does not pass the straight-faced test.

DOES NIACIN CAUSE LOW BLOOD PRESSURE?

Somewhat, but with qualifications. Generally speaking, supplemental niacin does not lower blood pressure very much if at all, and it is probably not a first-line therapy for essential hypertension. Dr. Hoffer's standard niacin prescription for his psychiatric patients was 3,000 milligrams per day, in divided doses. People requiring more were gradually acclimated to an increase. He reported no hypotension in the thousands and thousands of patients he treated during more than half a century of medical practice.

STUDIES ON THE RELATIONSHIP BETWEEN NIACIN AND BLOOD PRESSURE

It is possible that a sudden, excessively large (over 5,000 milligrams at one time) dose may sometimes cause an abrupt drop in blood pressure. This is another good reason why self-administration of irrationally huge amounts of niacin is inappropriate. We again state that persons should obtain their physician's participation when using high doses.[9]

It is precisely because of this dramatic acute effect that niacin has been considered as a long-term blood-pressure-lowering agent. A 2009 placebo-controlled study of 1,613 men and women showed that extended-release niacin was associated with significant reductions in systolic blood pressure (SBP) and diastolic blood pressure (DBP) after twenty-four weeks. Reductions were not large: only about 2 to 3 millimeters mercury (Hg) for either SBP or DBP.[10]

Another published paper said the following:

> Small clinical trials of acute niacin administration have shown significant BP-lowering effects of niacin in patients with hypertension but not necessarily in normotensive individuals.... Most large, prospective, randomized clinical trials involving niacin and niacin-containing regimens showed either no clear significant effects of niacin or slightly lower mean BP among some niacin treatment groups compared with placebo.... Larger studies, such as the Coronary Drug Project, suggest that niacin may lower BP when administered over a longer period of time.[11]

Common-sense caution applies: use niacin in cooperation with your doctor. In order to obtain and maximize such cooperation, be sure your doctor reads the following section.

TOXICOLOGY

Vitamins are not toxic. Xenobiotics (drugs) are toxic. There is therefore no toxicology for vitamins. When taken in enormous amounts (as is even true with water), they can have undesirable side effects, but there have been no deaths from vitamins. However, in spite of all the evidence that vitamins are safe and nontoxic, and in spite of the fact there is no evidence that they are toxic, most physicians still believe that niacin especially is toxic—simply because of its vasodilatory effect, the flush that occurs when it is first taken. This has been a bonanza for the drug companies, who are spending barrels of money trying to find a compound that they can patent that works as well as niacin for cholesterol management. They are looking for substances that will moderate the niacin flush. This is unnecessary, since the best anti-flush product is niacin itself. *With continued use, very few patients continue to experience flush.* I have been taking 3,000 mg and more niacin daily for over fifty years and will, on occasion, have a mild flush (which I can feel but no one can see) if I have missed one dose.

It May Be Some Kind of Record, But Don't Do It

A young female teen-aged schizophrenic patient was given a month's supply of niacin, 200 tablets, each 500 milligrams. She became angry at her mother and the next day swallowed the whole bottle. For three days afterward, she had a sore abdomen but experienced no additional side effects. Another teen schizophrenic, after reading a paperback book on megavitamins and schizophrenia, could not find any physician to monitor her. So, she began to increase niacin dosage on her own, and when she reached 60 grams (60,000 milligrams) niacin daily, the voices she was hearing stopped. Two years later her maintenance dose was 3 grams (3,000 milligrams) per day. However, these are very extreme situations from Dr. Hoffer's 55 years of psychiatric practice. Most people would have flushed severely, or would have been very nauseous, long before they got near such exorbitant doses. The take-home lesson is this: Even though niacin is safer than almost all over-the-counter drugs, you need to use good judgment. Be informed. Work out your personal dose in cooperation with your doctor. And, whenever you notice a reaction that is unpleasant or worrying, contact your physician.

NIACIN DOES NOT CAUSE LIVER DAMAGE

One reader wrote to us: "I am megadosing on niacin and my liver function tests are elevated. So now, my doctor has told me to stop taking niacin. Just how significant are these liver function changes, anyway?"

The myth that niacin causes liver damage was thoroughly debunked by Dr. William B. Parsons Jr. in his book on niacin and cholesterol, *Cholesterol Control Without Diet! The Niacin Solution.*[12] The book discusses this problem extremely well.[13] We consider Dr. Parsons to have been the most knowledgeable physician when it comes to treating patients with lipid problems using drugs and niacin. From his publication, it is clear that he favors the use of niacin, not drugs, when treating patients experiencing lipid problems. In fact, he was the first physician outside of Saskatchewan, Canada, to use niacin. He instigated the first niacin cholesterol studies and with his associates corroborated the claims that niacin lowered cholesterol made by Dr. Altshul, Dr. Stephen, and me (AH) in 1955. This discovery might have languished and never been rediscovered had we not gotten this corroboration from the prestigious Mayo Clinic, where Dr. Parsons was chief resident.

Dr. Parsons provides the evidence, based upon his own studies and the vast literature available, that using niacin to lower elevated cholesterol levels is the only practical, effective, safe, and cost-effective method for restoring lipid levels to normal. Niacin does more than decrease levels of low-density cholesterol. It elevates HDL, decreases lipoprotein(a) [Lp(a)], and lowers triglycerides. In comparison with the statins, it is the clear winner. And it decreases mortality and extends life even after patients have already suffered their first coronary.

Niacin is a vitamin, not a drug. In addition to its effect on the lipid blood profile, it has the usual positive vitamin properties of megadose vitamin B_3. Most physicians do not really know niacin since it is not patented, has no solicitous parent corporation to promote it, and is not advertised. It is difficult to pick up a medical journal without seeing some statin ads. There are none extolling the virtues of niacin. Since many physicians do not know niacin, they are suspicious of it. I find exasperating the total ignorance of niacin and the fear it generates. The medical profession is afraid that niacin is liver hepatotoxic, which it is not. Dr. Parsons points out that increases in liver enzyme tests, unless they are very substantial, such as more than threefold, usually does not indicate liver pathology. There are many compounds that elevate liver enzymes—all the statins do, as do acetaminophen (Tylenol) and ibuprofen (Advil).

A second acceptance problem is the flush that accompanies niacin when one first starts to use it. Physicians who understand this and know how to work with it seldom have a problem, and their patients get along well with it. However, physicians who do not know anything about it tend to impart their lack of knowledge to their patients, who soon stop using it. According to Parsons, inositol hexaniacinate, the usual no-flush niacin in health food stores, is not nearly as good for lowering cholesterol, although it is as good for other conditions in which niacin is helpful, including psychoses, schizophrenia, and anxiety.

Since I (AH) began using megadoses of vitamin B3 in 1952, I have seen a few cases of obstructive-type jaundice that cleared up when the niacin was stopped. In one case I had to resume the use of niacin because the patient's schizophrenia recurred. He recovered and the jaundice did not recur. I have seen so few cases of jaundice that there is little evidence that the jaundice arose from the use of the niacin. Jaundice has a natural occurrence rate, and within any series of patients, a few will get jaundice from other factors. In rare cases, too much niacin causes nausea and vomiting, and if this persists because the niacin is not decreased or stopped, then dehydration might become a factor. The main danger from taking niacin is not jaundice—it is that people will live longer.

Understanding Niacin Side Effects

by Robert G. Smith and Andrew W. Saul

Niacin (vitamin B$_3$) famously produces a warm body flush in most persons taking any substantial dose for the first time. Abram Hoffer, MD, PhD, the world's foremost expert on niacin therapy, would tell his patients to expect it, and put up with it, for the first two weeks. Then, with continual intake, the flush would gradually go away. Persons wishing to avoid the flush entirely may choose sustained-release niacin, niacinamide or inositol hexaniacinate. Sustained-release niacin is known to have the most side effects. Niacinamide does not affect blood lipids. Inositol hexaniacinate is slightly less effective, milligram for milligram, than niacin.

Elevation of Liver Enzymes

A side effect of high-dose niacin therapy includes possible elevation of liver enzymes. This is one of the most physician-invoked cautions against niacin. The level of concern is somewhat overblown. William B. Parsons Jr., of the Mayo Clinic, has clearly shown that slight to moderate elevation of liver enzymes is a sign of liver activity, not liver pathology. An increase in liver activity is to be expected with higher levels of niacin, as it is a precursor for NAD, which is a cofactor in hundreds of essential biochemical reactions, utilized in many organs throughout the body and especially in the liver.[14]

"The physician must understand niacin in order to use it."
—William Parsons Jr., MD

Retinal Edema

A rare and reversible side effect of niacin may be retinal or cystoid macular edema. Periodic media allegations of niacin causing eye problems center on this issue. The side effect has been known for decades,[15,16] but has been reported as a new and dreadful conse-quence of megavitamin therapy. That is misleading at best, as niacin in multi-gram quantities has been used to successfully lower choles-terol for decades, with remarkably few reported problems other than the flushes and liver enzyme elevations described above.

The mechanism by which niacin can cause cystoid macular edema is still unknown. In this condition, the retinal layers are thickened and distorted by buildup of fluid, which can be seen with a mod-ern visualization technique called Optical Coherence Tomography (OCT) that scans the retina with light to produce a cross-sectional view of the retinal layers. An OCT image of retinal cystoid macular edema shows that within the affected region (the macula—near the center of vision) the retina has separated from the photoreceptor layer, creating a "cystoid space." This condition is unrelated to leakage from blood vessels in diabetic retinopathy because it is reversible. One hypothesis about this rare effect of niacin speculates that niacin can cause some type of inflammatory mechanism, which then triggers fluid leakage from blood that filters through capillary walls, and an accumulation of extracellular fluid into cystoid spaces within the retina. Although leakage of blood is not seen in this condition using standard fluorescent angiography, a selective filtration from capillaries might prevent the relatively large fluorescent tracer molecules from leaking out. Another hypothesis suggests that one of the retinal cell types, Mueller cells, become engorged with fluid due to some type of toxicity derived from niacin.[17] A similar hypothesis was suggested by a recent report that when tested with electroretinography (ERG) the retinal b-wave, known to reflect the function of the Mueller cells, is significantly attenuated.[18] However, as the b-wave reflects electric current flow through several pathways, it is possible that any distortion of electric current flow in the outer retina could cause a similar effect, even without engorgement of the Mueller cells. Further, since this condition is quite rate, the affected individuals may have a genetic predisposition where some cells in the retina have a toxic reaction to high levels of niacin.

Threshold Effect

Although the exact cause is still unknown, retinal cystoid macular edema is known to rapidly reverse without permanent damage upon lowering the niacin dose, so that it exhibits a "threshold effect." Doses below the threshold (approximately 1,000 milligrams per day, in divided doses) don't cause retinal macular edema.[19] For the rare affected individuals, it is not necessary to completely stop taking niacin. Very likely the threshold dose is related to body weight, i.e., for those individuals who are affected, the threshold dose for larger individuals is higher. This means that even for individuals who may get the cystoid macular edema, they can lower the dose, allowing the retina to recover its normal function, while still receiving a benefit from niacin.[20]

Dosage

For those who plan to take high-dose niacin, the best advice appears to be to start a very low dose, e.g., 25 milligrams per day. This may cause a skin flush (30 to 60 minutes of warm skin) at first, but over several days the body gradually adapts to this dose and does not cause the skin flush. Then, slowly increase the dose over several weeks, taking the niacin in divided doses throughout the day, building up to 500 milligrams per day, and over several months up to 1,000 milligrams per day or higher, in consultation with your physician. You can start by breaking up 100 milligrams tablets into four pieces, taking one 25 milligrams piece per day at first, then after a few days increasing to two per day, and later up to four of the 25 milligrams pieces per day, one before each snack or meal. Once the body adapts to this dose, you may increase to one or more 100 milligrams tablets per day, and so on. If at very high doses (1,000 milligrams per day or higher) you note changes in your vision, especially in the central region (the fovea and macula) that you use to read fine print, you may want to lower the daily niacin dose by 50 percent or more, to 1,000 milligrams per day or below, in divided doses. The vision problems may then disappear after a few weeks. This threshold effect has been reported by ophthalmologists who have studied the condition.[19] Of course, with any regimen of high-dose niacin, you should consult and work with your own physician.

Deaths from Vitamins?
What the Evidence *Really* Says[21]

Over a forty-year period, vitamin supplements have been alleged to have caused the deaths of a total of fifteen people in the United States. However, an independent analysis of U.S. poison control center annual report data indicates that there have, in fact, been **no** *deaths* from vitamins . . . none at all, in the nearly four decades that such reports have been available.[22]

First, the allegations: The American Association of Poison Control Centers (AAPCC) attributes annual deaths to vitamins as:

2020 (most recent report available at present time): zero (one, wrongly attributed to an unknown "miscellaneous" vitamin)[23]

2019: zero[24]	2008: zero	1995: zero
2018: zero[25]	2007: zero	1994: zero
2017: zero (one, wrongly attributed to vitamin D)[26]	2006: one	1993: one
	2005: zero	1992: zero
2016: zero[27]	2004: two	1991: two
2015: zero[28]	2003: two	1990: one
2014: zero[29]	2002: one	1989: zero
2013: zero[30]	2001: zero	1988: zero
2012: two alleged but not proven[31]	2000: zero	1987: one
	1999: zero	1986: zero
2011: zero[32]	1998: zero	1985: zero
2010: zero[33]	1997: zero	1984: zero
2009: zero	1996: zero	1983: zero

Even if these figures are taken as correct, and even if they include intentional and accidental misuse, even the number of *alleged* vitamin fatalities is strikingly low, averaging far less than one death per year for over two and a half decades. In 19 of those years, AAPCC reports that there was not one single death due to vitamins.[34] Still, one cannot help but be curious: Did eleven people really die from vitamins? And if so, how?

Vitamins Not *THE* Cause of Death

In determining cause of death, AAPCC uses a four-point scale called Relative Contribution to Fatality (RCF). A rating of 1 means "Undoubtedly Responsible"; 2 means "Probably Responsible"; 3 means "Contributory"; and 4 means "Probably Not Responsible." For example, in examining poison control data for the year 2006, listing one vitamin death, it was seen that the vitamin's Relative Contribution to Fatality (RCF) was a 4. Since a score of "4" means

"Probably Not Responsible," it quite negates the claim that a person died from a vitamin in 2006.

Vitamins Not A Cause of Death

In other years reporting one or more of the remaining alleged vitamin fatalities, studying the AAPCC reports reveals an absence of any RCF rating for vitamins in any of those years. If there is no Relative Contribution to Fatality at all, then the substance did not contribute to death at all.

Furthermore, in each of those remaining years, there is no substantiation provided to demonstrate that any vitamin was a cause of death.

If there is insufficient information about the cause of death to make a clear-cut declaration of cause, then subsequent assertions that vitamins cause deaths are not evidence-based. Although vitamin supplements have often been blamed for causing fatalities, there is no evidence to back up this allegation.

Interestingly, AAPCC Annual Reports prior to 2012 are no longer available for downloading. But they used to be, and I am glad I did before they were apparently scrubbed from their website archive. I have attempted to obtain AAPCC's reply as to why they are now unavailable, and have received no reply.

Again we say: niacin is not liver toxic. That is a myth. This myth, which is pervasive in medicine, is based upon a series of observations, some of which were dead wrong. Between 1940 and 1950, when the toxicity of niacin and niacinamide were studied, the LD_{50} (lethal dose, 50 percent) of rats was determined. The LD_{50} is the amount of compound that will kill one half of the population of animals used to test toxicity. If 100 mice are given the drug and half die, that dose is the LD_{50}. For niacin, the LD_{50} is very high, about 4.5 grams per kilogram. This is equivalent to 225 grams (nearly half a pound) for a 110-pound female and 360 grams for a 176-pound male, approximately 100 times the normal recommendation. Whether anyone will ever find an LD_{50} for people is extremely unlikely. At necropsy, the animals in the early studies of B_3 toxicity showed elevated fatty acids in the liver.

In 1950, deficiency of methyl groups was a popular topic. It was accepted that this deficiency caused fatty livers. Niacin and niacinamide are methyl acceptors, so it made sense to consider that too much vitamin B_3 would cause fatty acid livers by producing a methyl deficiency syndrome. However, Professor R. Altschul, at the University of Saskatchewan, could not confirm these findings. In his animal studies he found that the vitamin had no effect on the fatty-acid levels in the liver.

The second observation, which is still routinely made, is that niacin will increase liver function tests in some patients. It is assumed, incorrectly, that elevated liver function tests always mean underlying liver pathology. Many other medicines cause the same elevations of liver function tests. Usually after a few days off niacin the test results become normal. Therefore, it is best to stop the niacin for five days and then do the tests to avoid confusing liver damage with increased liver function activity.

Dr. William Parsons Jr. first reported that medical professionals at Mayo Clinic examined the livers of a series of their patients being treated for high blood cholesterol, who were taking niacin. They found no evidence of pathology. Parsons points out that increases in the liver function tests do not indicate liver pathology unless they are very substantial. There are many compounds that elevate liver enzymes, including all the statins. In most patients with elevated liver function tests, the values become normal in a few days even if the niacin is not discontinued.

I advise doctors that they should stop the niacin for at least five days prior to doing a liver enzyme test. With real liver pathology, the results will not become normal in five days, but when they are elevated due to niacin, they will be normal within these five days. Liver enzymes are commonly elevated by many modern drugs. Gonzalez-Heydrich et al.[35] gave twelve children a combination of olanzapine and divalproic acid. Everyone had an elevated enzyme peak, and in five it remained elevated for many months. Two children had to be removed from the study because of severe pathology, pancreatitis in one child and steatohepatitis in the other.

Over forty years ago there were a few reports of liver damage and one or two deaths caused by niacin and/or niacinamide. But it is possible that the liver function test results may be raised due to methyl depletion. According to Dr. David Capuzzi, a specialist in diabetes, metabolism, and endocrinology in Philadelphia and one of the world's authorities on niacin and cholesterol, this can be prevented by giving patients 2,400 milligrams of lecithin divided twice daily. Betaine may also be effective for this purpose.

It is uncommon, but another possible side effect of high-dose niacin use is increased gastric acidity. This is probably because niacin stimulates the secretion of gastric juice.

DOES NIACIN "MASK" TESTS FOR ILLEGAL DRUGS?

The answer is no. In a personal communication with niacin researcher Todd Penberthy on this topic, he says, "'Masking' claims would appear to describe attempts to interfere with drug test assays. Niacin does not do this. The belief that any pill somehow masks a drug test indicates a lack of understanding of such tests."

However, Dr. Penberthy adds, "Niacin is without a doubt a powerful detoxifying agent. For example, when we are exposed to toxic environmental chemicals or cigarette smoke, there is a tremendous increase in the expression of certain P450 enzymes, particularly CYP1A1. This is especially true in response to PCBs. PCBs and some other inducers are known to cause so much CYP1A1 to be made that it can comprise 10 percent of a liver cell's total protein, and that is a lot. Ultimately, this leads to a situation where you have boatloads of substrate and enzyme, but not necessarily a needed cofactor. The rate of any enzyme-catalyzed reaction is proportional to the concentrations of everything involved in the reaction, i.e., the substrate, enzyme, and cofactor. One key cofactor is derived from niacin: NADPH (Nicotinamide adenine dinucleotide phosphate). It is very important and used for many reactions; indeed, hundreds of proteins use NADPH. We need more niacin to make more NADPH."

A new review indicates that there have been quite a few niacin detoxification studies.[36] Detoxification is further discussed in chapter 11 of this book.

DARKENING OF SKIN

In rare instances, high-dose niacin can cause increased brown pigmentation of certain areas of the skin, usually the flexor surfaces (the skin in the underside of a joint). This is *not* acanthosis nigricans, even though it has been erroneously labeled as such. This is never a problem for patients if they are told the truth about what is occurring, but it is a problem for some doctors who are not familiar with it. This niacin-related reaction is a harmless pigmentation change, unlike acanthosis nigricans, which is a very serious, almost cancer-like condition. Dr. William Parsons Jr. correctly called it a skin change which *resembles* acanthosis nigricans. It does, but only in color, not in pathology. The browning effect of niacin in a very few subjects is entirely different. It is transient, usually lasting only a few months, and when it is clear the skin is perfectly normal. Like an old tan, it washes off if the skin is rubbed when moist. It never recurs even with continued use of niacin. It is likely due to the deposition of melanin-containing indoles from tyrosine and adrenalin. It occurs most commonly in schizophrenic patients and is part of the healing process.

WHAT ABOUT NEGATIVE NEWS MEDIA COMMENTS ABOUT VITAMINS?

Nutritional information that does make news generally stays far from the headlines, unless, of course, it is critical of vitamins. The most widely publicized vitamin therapy trials tend to be low-dose, worthless, negative, or a mix of all three. Mass media attention to a given nutritional research study appears to be inversely proportional to its curative value. As a result, the public and not a few physicians remain unaware of the power of simple and safe natural methods, due to contradictory, inadequate, or just plain biased media reporting. When the press touts the "dangers" of vitamin "megadoses" while simultaneously overlooking Ritalin's carcinogenic potential, it strains at a gnat and swallows a camel. While drug side effects fill the *Physicians' Desk Reference* to bursting, I think we could truly say that the chief side effect of vitamins is failure to take enough of them. Perhaps the very concept of "megadose" needs to be rethought, and re-presented to the public. The quantity of a nutritional supplement that cures an illness indicates the patient's degree of deficiency. It is therefore not a megadose of the vitamin, but rather a megadeficiency of the nutrient that we are dealing with. By way of analogy, a dry sponge holds more milk.

WHAT ABOUT NEGATIVE MEDICAL JOURNAL VITAMIN STUDIES?

Neither rhetoric nor mere estimates are involved here—there is clear evidence that the major medical journals are heavily influenced by their advertisers. A 2008 study showed that journals with the most pharmaceutical ads have the most negative reports about vitamins. The authors wrote that "In major medical journals, more pharmaceutical advertising is associated with publishing fewer articles about dietary supplements" and that journals with more pharmaceutical advertising had more articles with "negative conclusions about dietary supplement safety."[37] The following journals were specifically named as having the most pharmaceutical ads and the most negative articles about vitamins:

Journal of the American Medical Association

New England Journal of Medicine

British Medical Journal

Canadian Medical Association Journal

Annals of Internal Medicine

Archives of Internal Medicine

Archives of Pediatric and Adolescent Medicine

Pediatrics and Pediatric Research

American Family Physician

The results were statistically significant:

[Medical] journals with the most pharmads published no clinical trials or cohort studies about supplements. The percentage of major articles concluding that supplements were unsafe was 4 percent in journals with fewest and 67 percent among those with the most pharmads. . . . The impact of advertising on publications [is real, and] the ultimate impact of this bias on professional guidelines, health care, and health policy is a matter of great public concern.[38]

The flip side of this problem is that medical research and the very data it generates is biased by pharmaceutical advertising cash. The *Washington Post* reported that "Drug studies skewed toward study sponsors. Industry-funded research often favors patent-holders, study finds."[39]

In the *American Journal of Psychiatry* study the *Post* was referring to, the authors said, "In 90.0 percent of the studies, the reported overall outcome was in favor of the sponsor's drug. . . . On the basis of these contrasting findings in head-to-head trials, it appears that whichever company sponsors the trial produces the better antipsychotic drug."[40]

Even the former editor-in-chief of the *New England Journal of Medicine* agrees. Dr. Marcia Angell says,

> [One of the] common ways to bias trials is to present only part of the data—the part that makes the product look good—and ignore the rest. . . . [Pharmaceutical] industry-sponsored research was nearly four times as likely to be favorable to the company's product as NIH [National Institutes of Health]-sponsored research. . . . The most dramatic form of bias is out-and-out suppression of negative results.[41]

This bias extends deeply into the medical schools themselves. Too many of tomorrow's doctors are bought and paid for with drug company money. Dr. Angell describes how Columbia University obtained manufacturing patents for Epogen and Cerezyme and received close to $300 million in royalties in just 17 years. National Institutes of Health (NIH) money—taxpayers' money—paid for this research. And, Dr. Angell adds, "The combined profits for the ten drug companies in the Fortune 500 were more than the profits for all the other 490 businesses put together."[42]

The *Washington Post* article quoted above said: "When the federal government recently compared a broader range of drugs in typical schizophrenia patients in a lengthy trial, the two medications that stood out were cheaper drugs not under patent."[39] Niacin works even better, and is cheaper, too. Niacin is a clinically proven therapy for serious mental illness, and yet the medical profession has refused to recommend it for over half a century.

Yet drugs are not the answer. A double-blind study of schizophrenics showed that three-quarters of patients stopped taking their pharmaceutical medication, either because the drug's side effects were unbearable, or the drug just plain did not work.[43]

The Orthomolecular Medicine News Service commented,

Perhaps drugs are not the answer because mental illness is not caused by drug deficiency. But much illness, especially mental illness, may indeed be caused by nutrient deficiency or nutrient dependency. Only nutrients can correct this problem. This not only makes sense, it has stood up to clinical trial again and again. Vitamins like niacin are cheap, safe and effective. Modern "wonder drugs" are none of those. But they do make money. Especially when the drug makers control the research, the advertising, and the doctors. No wonder which approach you've heard more about.

Principles of Orthomolecular Nutrition

- Most nonaccidental illnesses are due to malnutrition. This not only includes chronic diseases, but also viral and bacterial acute illnesses, which are greatly aggravated by inadequate nutrition. Conventional physicians are valuable for persons needing treatment of traumatic injury.

- Adding pharmaceutical drugs to a sick body to cure it is like adding poison to a polluted lake to clean it. Killing microorganisms or masking the cause of symptoms is no more than a temporary answer in either case.

- Restoring health must be done nutritionally, not pharmacologically. All of our cells are made exclusively from what we drink and eat. Not one cell is made from a drug.

- Nutrient therapy increases individual resistance to disease. Drug therapy generally lowers resistance to disease. Healthy plants, healthy animals, and healthy people do not get sick. Doctors do not like to admit this, because healthy people do not go to doctors.

- The quantity of a nutritional supplement required to cure an illness indicates the patient's degree of deficiency. It is therefore not a megadose of the vitamin, but rather a megadeficiency of the nutrient that is the problem. Uncorrected deficiency leads to vitamin dependency.

- The number-one side effect of vitamins is failure to take enough of them.
- With vitamin therapy, speed of recovery is proportional to the dosage given. Just as there is a certain, large amount of fuel needed to launch an aircraft or a spacecraft, there is a certain amount of nutrients needed to cure a sick body.
- The reason one nutrient can cure so many different illnesses is because a deficiency of one nutrient can cause many different illnesses.
- In high doses, a nutrient can act as a drug, but a drug can never act as a nutrient.
- Vitamin supplementation is not the problem—it is undernutrition that is the problem. Vitamins are the solution.
- Nutritional therapy is inexpensive, effective, and, most important, safe. (See chapter 6 for more about vitamin safety.)

MOST NIACIN SIDE EFFECTS ARE POSITIVE

If a patient takes niacin to normalize mental function, and as a result of the vitamin activity feels very much better in other areas such as more energy and faster healing, then this is a positive side effect. There are other positive side effects that often occur. For example, if the patient takes niacin to deal with his arthritis and at the same time his cholesterol levels decrease, this result would be a major positive side effect or, better still, side benefit. Niacin lowers C-reactive protein (CRP), one of the markers of inflammation. The statins also lower CRP but, in contrast to the statins, niacin is not toxic.

IS NIACIN TOO GOOD TO BE TRUE?

There is a recurrent problem with vitamins being perceived as "too useful." Frederick R. Klenner, MD, found vitamin C to be an effective and nearly all-purpose antitoxin, antibiotic, and antiviral. Is it possible to have one vita-min responsible for curing polio, pneumonia, measles, strep, snakebite, and Rocky Mountain spotted fever? Laypeople and professionals alike certainly struggle to wrap their minds around the possibility, especially considering the fact that Klenner also reported success with nearly four dozen other diseases. How did he do it? The explanation may be as simple as this: the reason that one nutrient can cure so many different illnesses is because a deficiency of one nutrient can cause many different illnesses.

> Each year in the United States, well over 100,000 patients in hos-pitals die from drugs that are properly prescribed and taken as directed. Many estimates are far higher. (Leape LL. Institute of Medicine medical error figures are not exaggerated. *JAMA*, 2000. Jul 5;284(1):95–7; Leape LL. Error in medicine. *JAMA*, 1994. Dec 21;272(23):1851–7; Lazarou J, Pomeranz BH, Corey PN. Incidence of adverse drug reactions in hospitalized patients: a meta-analysis of prospective studies. *JAMA*, 1998. Apr 15;279(15):1200–5.)
>
> Annual deaths from all hospital medical errors combined is over 225,000, making them the third largest cause of mortality in the U.S. It is interesting how this fact stays out of the news. (Starfield B. Is US health really the best in the world? *JAMA*. 2000 Jul 26;284(4):483–5. https://www.jhsph.edu/research/centers-and-institutes/johns -hopkins-primary-care-policy-center/Publications_PDFs/A154.pdf.)
>
> In sharp contrast, even the number of *alleged* vitamin deaths per year is less than one; we assert the true number to be zero.

This has led to something of a vitamin public relations problem. When pharmaceuticals are versatile, they are called "broad spectrum" and "wonder drugs." When vitamins are versatile, they are called "faddish" and "cures in search of a disease." Such a double standard needs to be exposed and opposed at every turn. Seemingly unrelated health problems may indeed be largely caused by a common nutritional deficiency. Treating accordingly was a good idea in the 1950s, when Dr. Hoffer was beginning his research. It is just as good today.

It is clear that vitamin B_3 is a very powerful yet benign substance that is involved in numerous reactions in the body, and which, in larger doses, is therapeutic and preventative for a large number of apparently unrelated diseases. It is highly likely that if any human community increases their population's intake of vitamin B_3 by even a few hundred milligrams per day (and to much higher levels in people already suffering from a number of pathological conditions), they will find a substantial decrease in mortality and an increase in longevity.

CHAPTER 7

Pandeficiency Disease

*Health is the fastest growing failing business
in western civilization.*
—Emanuel Cheraskin, MD

Doctors educated to dispense drugs using the "one drug, one disease" concept cannot understand any substance that is effective against more than one condition. It is looked upon as snake oil, not a real therapeutic compound, and one that is only a placebo. If modern medical schools gave their medical students more than an hour or two of nutrition instruction for every four years of education (instead of so much surgery they will seldom do, or pathology they will leave to pathologists, or a whole lot of other material they will never use), students would graduate with a modern understanding that there is nothing more important than food, and the proper intake of nutrients to maintain and restore health, and to fend off the invading organisms that look upon the human body as food. Medical schools also seldom emphasize other important subjects such as the history of medicine, the patient-doctor relationship, and how to be healers rather than merely laboratory-obsessed technicians, taught to remember but not very often to think and reason. If they understood pellagra clinically—once a major scourge around the Mediterranean and the Southeastern United States—they would have a perfect example of how one simple compound, vitamin B3, can cure a large number of conditions, disorders, or diseases that apparently are not related to each other.

THE CONCEPT OF PANDEFICIENCY DISEASE

All the conditions we have found to be responsive to the orthomolecular program can be considered subsets of *pandeficiency disease*, a deficiency of several vitamins. The recent report by Marini[1] refers to a large number of mild to moderate enzyme problems that can be corrected by proper doses of the vitamins. The vitamins we use for all pandeficiency diseases are the B-complex vitamins, vitamin B_3 in much larger doses, vitamin C, selenium, often zinc, sometimes vitamin E, and omega-3 essential fatty acids. This suggests that these are the main vitamins and minerals that should be investigated and followed up. There may be no advantage in analyzing the personal genome at this moment in history, as these vitamins and minerals are relatively cheap and easily available. Marini wrote: "I wouldn't be surprised if everybody is going to require a different optimum dose of vitamins depending on their makeup." No surprise was necessary. If he had been familiar with orthomolecular medicine, he would have anticipated this.

Pellagra is characterized by the four D's: dermatitis, diarrhea, dementia, and death. It is caused by a diet deficient in protein, essential fatty acids, and minerals and vitamins, especially B_3. It is cured by a good diet reinforced with the same vitamin.

Suppose a professor lectured to her medical students for one hour on skin lesions, one hour on gastrointestinal lesions, and one hour on psychoses ... but did not tell her students that these were all symptoms of one disease called pellagra, which is caused by one deficiency. During her fourth lecture she tells the students that one vitamin cures all of these illnesses, without teaching them the concept of deficiency diseases and pellagra in particular. The students would be mystified, would probably think she was nuts, and certainly would have major difficulty understanding how one drug could be so versatile. This was the situation before serological tests became the diagnostic criterion for syphilis. Old textbooks used forty or more pages of valuable space to describe its many symptoms and ways of treatment since there was no true treatment until penicillin came along. Now syphilis is rarely mentioned. It is diagnosed by a blood test and is treated by one drug. In times past, it was said that if you understood syphilis, you understood all of medicine. I think the same can be said about pellagra.

Diagnosis classifies disease for two main reasons: (1) to improve prognosis, and (2) to improve treatment. Prognosis is very important so patients and family can prepare for the future, especially if the future is very dim. Estimating when a person will die may be extremely important for all sorts of reasons. Before specific treatment was discovered, doctors were judged on their ability to prognose correctly. It would be very bad for the physician's reputation if his prognosis was wrong. Many years ago when I (AH) started to practice medicine, some of my patients, when giving me their history, would tell me that their doctor had told them they would die but the doctor died before they did. Good doctors were good prognosticators—and this depended upon accurate diagnosis.

Diagnosis became even more important when specific treatments were discovered. Diagnosis advised the clinician what treatment to use. It was assumed that patients with the same diagnosis would respond to a similar treatment already described by other doctors. I had pneumonia in my early teens. Our friendly family doctor (he was also surgeon, emergency doctor, obstetrician, and so on, as he was the only doctor in the community) told my mother I had pneumonia and ordered mustard plasters. It must have been very effective or else my pneumonia was very mild, as I was well in a couple of days. That was standard treatment for a disease that killed a large proportion of its victims. This type of diagnosis was a descriptive diagnosis. By listening to my chest, the doctor discovered something wrong and concluded that it was most likely pneumonia. No other diagnostic tests were available.

After it was discovered that many different lung lesions were possible, it became necessary to distinguish one lesion from another. Was it bacterial? If so, which bacteria, staph or strep? Today specific laboratory tests are used to determine this. Diagnosis is now etiologic—based on the cause of the condition. And until the causal diagnosis is made, the treatment cannot be very successful. This is the pathway diagnosis has traveled; from description of the site, the organ, and later to the cause when known. If the cause remains unknown, the diagnosis remains descriptive. Psychiatric diagnosis is almost entirely descriptive.

Medical schools teach medical students the use of medicines, not nutrients. From their nutrition lectures, if any, students will be told that only small amounts of niacin are ever needed by the human body, and that large doses do virtually nothing but result in "expensive urine." Yet it is widely known that a small amount of niacin prevents pellagra. It is less well-known that much larger doses of niacin cure the more dreadful symptoms of advanced pellagra: dermatitis, psychosis, dementia, diarrhea, and heart enlargement.

We willingly concede the successes of crisis medicine, while sticking to our guns that nutritional medicine is better for the prevention and treatment of chronic illness. Pharmaceutical medicine has a near-monopoly on health care service delivery. Such a monopoly probably results in more use of drugs than of nutrients.

THE ROLE OF SUGAR, DIET, AND CONSTIPATION

During World War II, Royal Navy Surgeon Captain T. L. Cleave was concerned about the ill health of many of the sailors. From his studies, he concluded that most of them suffered from one overall disease he called the "Saccharine Disease" in 1956.[2] The saccharine disease has no relation to the synthetic sweetener. Saccharine in this case refers to a detrimental craving for sweet tastes and consequent overuse of sugar. (And no, we do not recommend sugar substitutes. Artificial sugar substitutes have problems of their own, not the least of which is that they may stimulate people to want still more sweet foods.)

Cleave presented evidence that the various diseases of civilization are one disease, not a large number of discrete diseases.[3] I (AH) had a copy of his original publication, but it was worn out by constant use. This book turned my life around. I became a full-time nutritionist. Cleave's experience as a physician convinced him that overconsumption of sugar and processed carbohydrates was the root cause of diabetes, coronary disease, obesity, malabsorption, peptic ulcer, constipation, hemorrhoids, varicose veins, E. coli infections, appendicitis, cholicystitis, pyelitis, diverticulitis, renal calculus, many skin conditions, and dental caries.[4]

This nutritional disease affected all the organs and systems, which were then diagnosed and named according to the organ or malfunction of that organ. The cause is the modern diet, which is too rich in sugars and refined carbohydrates and too deficient in food containing its original fiber. It is also deficient in essential fatty acids, vitamins, and minerals, relating it to pandeficiency disease. This diet typically relies on refined cereals devoid of their bran and germ such as white bread, polished rice, and a heavy intake of sugar, averaging about 125 pounds per person each year. Cleave considered the role played by the deficiency of essential nutrient factors, and emphasized the problems with excessive intake of sugar and a deficiency of fiber. In other words, he emphasized the value of whole foods.

The massive evidence Cleave presented had little impact, except for a sudden interest in bran, as if it were a drug especially designed for people with constipation. Cleave did give bran to the sailors under his care, but he was much more concerned with the white flour they were eating. His message was clear: what was needed were the original whole grain cereals, as in whole wheat and rice. Just adding bran only provided a partial answer. In 1972 Professor John Yudkin published his book *Sweet and Dangerous*.[5] He presented the evidence that proved sugars were the culprit. His work was ignored.

Ever since reading Cleave's book many years ago, I have advised my patients to follow a sugar-free, refined carbohydrate-free diet. I think most of those who followed my advice have been grateful. There is nothing more pleasing than feeling good.

How could this one explanation account for such an amazing number of diseases? This is how: constipation is the main outcome of a diet deficient in fiber-rich foods, not in a simple deficiency of fiber. If it were a simple deficiency of fiber, one could eat fiber made from wood. This will certainly increase the fiber intake, but will do little for one's health. Chronic constipation leads to the other diseases of the intestine. In South Africa, it was said you had to be English to get appendicitis—the natives, who still ate high-fiber foods, did not. The remaining diseases come from high sugar intake. These are diabetes, coronary disease, and metabolic disease.

Everyone knows that the major problem with modern foods is that they are too high in fat. But is this really true? When I said "everyone," I was exaggerating; a few of us instead thought that too much sugar and not enough fiber-rich food were much more pathological. But the sugar industry has been more adept at deflecting blame from their source of revenue, and the meat and fat industries have been a bit lax in fighting and followed the same idea. Reviewing the recent evidence, Challem concluded that high-protein diets, still very controversial but more popular than they were when they were highlighted by Robert Atkins, helped people lose weight, improve their blood sugar levels, and normalize blood lipids.[6] Of three diets tested in Israel, the best results were obtained with the high-protein, high-fat diets. This included the levels of blood lipids. High cholesterol and high triglyceride levels do not come from high fat intake. They come from too much sugar. Again, stone-age diet advocates are vindicated.

The saccharine disease is also characterized by a deficiency in vitamins and minerals. The foods richest in these nutrients are not consumed. There is really no question about this, and it is well recognized by government as well as by the public. If governments concluded that diets were adequate they would not have mandated the addition of three vitamins and iron to white flour—and I would not have gotten my first job as a control chemist in a flour mill. Vitamin C, thiamine, riboflavin, niacinamide, vitamin D, iodine, and calcium are some of the nutrients that enrich our foods. But the most striking was the eradication of pellagra in the United States within two years after the addition of niacinamide to white flour was mandated in 1942. The Canadian government would not permit this. The American law was considered an adulteration by Canada, except that it had to ship the enriched flour overseas to the allied troops and the Canadian Commissioner of Indian Affairs insisted that it be given to Canadian natives who used it to make bannock (flat bread).

The enrichment of flour was one of the most beneficial public health measures ever, not only in preventing physical disease but in preventing mental disease. Before enriched flour became available, up to one-third of admissions to mental hospitals in the Southeastern United States were pellagrins, who could not be differentiated from schizophrenia by clinical examination alone. Pellagra—characterized by the four D's: dermatitis, diarrhea, dementia, and death—was gone. In the whole history of psychiatry, there has never been a public health measure as effective. The addition of a few pennies' worth of B_1 and B_3 to flour saved the United States and the rest of the world billions of dollars of disease-generated costs. The addition of folic acid to flour has done the same.

Yes, the fortification of processed food was one of the most beneficial public health measures in history. Still, only *some* of the necessary nutrients are replaced by fortification. For this reason, we think it's important to reduce your carbohydrate intake, especially that of simple carbohydrates. The solution is a diet of unprocessed whole foods. Such a diet automatically provides much more fiber, more vitamins and minerals, and far less sugar. Most nutritionists in the past and ever since have largely ignored the importance of this. It remains difficult for anyone to obtain an adequate intake of vitamins on a refined-carbohydrate dominated diet.

Roger Williams' demonstration that we are biochemically different has not been taken seriously by the medical and nutritional establishment even when they have been aware of it. This in spite of the fact we differ in our blood types, in our fingerprints, and more. The concept of individualization is so strong in our culture that nothing will stop people and make them stare more than three identical triplets walking down the street. I think that individualization is a key to the formation of the parent-infant relationship, and yet the worldwide nutritional standards do not take individuality into account. Indeed, standard-setters act as if we all have the same needs, except in a few clear-cut situations such as pregnancy.

Recent research from the University of California at Berkeley provides a clear scientific explanation for what Williams hypothesized. Marini and colleagues reported in the *Proceedings of the National Academy of Sciences* that there are many genetic differences that make people's enzymes less efficient, and that simple supplementation with vitamins can restore some of these deficient enzymes to normal.[7] This work follows that of Bruce Ames, who found that you can cure genetic disease in babies by giving them vitamins.[8] Each person has a unique genome. It follows that all the clinical nutrition research over the past half a century, where very small doses and a limited dose range were used, have been a waste of money and time. They have also poisoned the attitude toward vitamins, except among the general population, over half of whom are taking them. It appears as if the scientists were wrong, but not the public. One day the genome may be used to determine which vitamins should be used, and how much. The work by Marini et al. following the work of Ames is itself a major follow-up of Linus Pauling and his concept of orthomolecular medicine. We in this field who have been practicing this concept, based upon clinical observations going back sixty years, are now bolstered by this research, which establishes the genetic mechanism for individuality.

In our book *Orthomolecular Nutrition*,[9] we described some of the psychiatric symptoms associated with the saccharine disease, caused by excess sugar intake. These are anxiety and depression. The patients were referred to me

(AH) by their family doctors because of these symptoms. When I first read about the role of hypoglycemia in causing mental disease, I was very skeptical, but I was also curious. A young female was referred to me for depression. She told me that her main problem was that she was frigid. Psychoanalysis was riding high many years ago, and it occurred to me that she would be a perfect candidate for psychoanalysis or deep psychotherapy to explore why she was having this problem. However, since I felt it was unlikely that this was caused by hypoglycemia, she would be ideal to disprove its effect. I ordered the five-hour glucose tolerance test. The curve was typically hypoglycemic, to my surprise. She was equally surprised. Not expecting that it would help, I still advised her to avoid all sugar and increase her intake of protein. To my amazement, she was normal in one month. I was now more interested than skeptical. I began to routinely have patients with anxiety and depression take the test, and found that over 75 percent had the typical abnormal glucose tolerance curves. I no longer remained skeptical. Since then, I have placed every patient on a sugar-free and refined-carbohydrate-free diet without doing any more tests. The condition was present in every one of three hundred alcoholics tested by the five-hour glucose tolerance test. I did not realize it then, but sugar created disease by playing havoc with the metabolism of sugar, raising it up and down. Many patients are allergic to it. Other foods, like milk, to which patients are allergic will also give the typical glucose tolerance curves. Over the years I concluded that if every doctor who referred their patients to me were to test them and treat them with the special diet first, I would lose half of my psychiatric practice.

Indeed, whatever health problem you may have, sugar will make it worse. Health crusader Paul C. Bragg was right: "The best part of a donut is the hole." Americans' consumption of sucrose and high-fructose corn syrup grew from 127 pounds per person in 1986 to a teeth-chattering 153 pounds in 1996.[10] A sugar industry magazine advertisement from the 1970s actually said, "If sugar is fattening, why are kids so thin?" Perhaps the "fat" industries were too lax in competing with this message, and ultimately lost the information war. In the last two decades, people are, in fact, eating somewhat less fat and more sugar. And now, the envelope, please: kids today are much fatter. Childhood obesity is epidemic. We can easily accept that the sugar industry was wrong. It is much more difficult to accept that the medical and nutrition professions backed the wrong horse.

THE B VITAMINS

Decades ago, Cleave considered the fact that the "saccharine disease" diet was also deficient in the B vitamins. Nutritionists since have ignored this, even though massive surveys have shown that it is impossible to obtain enough vitamin B with this diet. Nor did it occur to me (AH) until I had many more years of experience using large doses of the B vitamins. We treated schizophrenic patients with large doses of niacin or niacinamide and ascorbic acid. This treatment was based on our hypothesis that schizophrenia was caused by the excess conversion of adrenalin to adrenochrome, a product of oxidation. We used niacin to decrease the formation of adrenalin and ascorbic acid to inhibit its oxidation. Other catecholamines could also be oxidized in the body due to superoxidative stress. Over the following years it became clear that many other diseases also responded to increased doses of some of the vitamins. Eventually my objective in treating patients changed. I no longer aimed at just curing their disease; I was now interested in much more. I planned on giving them a multinutrient program, that would not only help them get well but would keep them well until they died, as long as they remained on the program. Extra niacin remains one of the nutrients that is especially valuable.

Life extension also became an objective, as it had already been shown that niacin would decrease death and increase longevity. Finally, I concluded that I would no longer adhere to the "one drug, one disease" concept that permeates medicine and the drug industry. Instead, I would do what I could using nutrition and relevant nutrients to help patients regain their ability to deal with stress and with disease. People heal themselves if they are given the right tools with which to do so. I have been using the same therapeutic program for many years and have seen a large number of patients recover from different physical and mental disorders using it. In the same way that added sugar and refined carbohydrates will cause saccharine disease,[11] a multiple deficiency of vitamins will cause what I now call the pandeficiency disease. Pandeficiency disease is a general disorder that can affect any organ, system, or function, or any combination of them. About half of the population suffers from this chronic pervasive disease, caused by the overall deficiencies present in modern high-tech diets. If the psychiatric profession were to look carefully at the diagnostic system it now uses, it could eliminate hundreds of psychiatric disorders right along with their DSM numbers.[12] Almost all of the ADD (attention deficit disorder) diagnoses of children could be eliminated.

In a recent editorial,[13] Dr. Sidney MacDonald Baker discusses the term "biomedical." He points out that with every patient there are two essential questions: (1) Does the person have a special need, and (2) Does the patient need to avoid or get rid of something to be healthy. It is a "get and get rid of" approach. Getting the question right is more valuable than trying to decide what the diagnosis is. Dr. Baker describes three main biochemical problems: detoxification, oxidative stress, and inflammation. These three factors describe the major diseases of modern civilization. He concludes: "The term biomedical should convey a sense of rejection of the utter nonsense of at least one aspect of current mainstream medicine: the acceptance of the notion you can take a group of people who are sick in similar ways, give a descriptive name such as autism, colitis, depression, etc. to the group, and then say that the symptoms are caused by the name." The term pandeficiency should be considered a biomedical description.

The treatment of pandeficiency syndrome includes restoration of a nutritious diet, attention to the intestinal flora, and the following few nutrients: vitamin B3, both niacin and niacinamide, ascorbic acid, a strong B-complex preparation like 50 milligrams or 100 milligrams B-complex, selenium, zinc, calcium, magnesium, and omega-3 essential fatty acids. The doses depend on the symptomatology.

ACCESS TO INFORMATION, OR CENSORSHIP?

These conclusions are based upon my (AH) personal experience in treating many patients with many conditions. I've described case histories, beginning in 1960, in 30 books and in 600 publications in the establishment press and in the alternative press, mostly in the *Journal of Orthomolecular Medicine* (*J Orthomolecular Med*). Curiously enough, 50 years of *J Orthomolecular Med* have been blacked out by MEDLINE. Specifically, the taxpayer-supported U.S. National Library of Medicine refuses to index five decades of this peer-reviewed journal. Consequently, we consider MEDLINE to be the official censoring organization of the medical establishment. Our correspondence with NLM-MEDLINE confirmed that they actually do receive this journal by mail, but presumably keep it properly hidden in some dark closet and classified as top secret. But their censoring role is coming to an end, as Google and other search engines now provide easy access to *J Ortho-molecular Med* papers.

In our (AH and Harold Foster) book, *Feel Better, Live Longer with Vitamin B₃*, we summarized the epidemiological literature and reviewed clinicians' experience in treating these vitamin-deficient conditions. Our conclusion was that about half of the population, the sick half, would benefit by taking extra vitamin B3. About half of the population suffers from one or more chronic conditions. The fact that a nutrient, such as niacin, can act on more than one disease sometimes results in it not being taken seriously as therapy. It may be derided as "a cure in search of a disease" and dismissed out of hand.

Whether it is some kind of a conspiracy or not, it is clearly in the interests of pharmaceutical medicine to see that people continue to be advised that all the nutrition they need can be obtained from a regular, "balanced," unsupplemented diet. This official misinformation will likely continue until the public demands change.

The U.S. Recommended Dietary Allowance (RDA) for a given vitamin does not really apply to any specific person. Rather, it is a political judgment based on a theoretical average. And as RDAs demonstrate, the "average" is so low it resembles a mandated minimum wage that may never be exceeded. Should everyone work for minimum wage? Do we all really have pretty much the same nutritional needs? When is the last time you bought one-size-fits-all underwear that actually fit?

Niacin or Niacinamide?

by W. Todd Penberthy, PhD

It may be a great approach to do small doses of niacinamide throughout the day, but nothing is unequivocal at this point by a long shot. It's incredibly complicated NAMPT/visfatin is even secreted.

Dr. Joseph Mercola's comments are right that things like intermittent fasting, high-intensity strength training, and circadian training can increase the efficiency of the NAD salvage pathway (i.e., increase NAMPT activity), and this is huge for resilience in keeping cells alive after otherwise acute potentially deadly stress. This is really surprising when you think about it, but it is absolutely proven in many studies now that one can boost their NAD recycling levels without adding any precursors at all, by simply moving much more or fasting or high-intensity strength training. So, in response to an otherwise lethal NAD-depleting stress, cells from these individuals can survive and NAD precursors (vitamin B_3 isoforms/NMN/tryptophan boosting) have nothing to do with it. It has everything to do with the rapid recycling of niacinamide back to NAD. This occurs because the fasting/exercise/improved sleep causes increase in NAMPT/NAD salvage pathway efficiency.

However, I still prefer niacin (nicotinic acid; NA) and especially when starting from the condition of being a person that is about to have a heart attack.

NA activates a completely distinct and separate beneficial pathway (the flush pathway, starting with activation of GPR109a). None of the other precursors do this, and so none of the other precursors provide particularly impressive benefit to correcting the lipodystrophy (HDL, VLDL, triglycerides, LDL total cholesterol) associated with the number one cause of death, cardiovascular disease (CVD). However, niacin does, and it has been proven in many randomized controlled trials to save lives from death by CVD. None of the other precursors have. The flush pathway stimulates mitochondrial biogenesis and has effects on the immune system all mediated by the massive prostaglandins produced in the flush response.

Few have done the apples-to-apples experiment comparing the NAD precursors, but I actually did, using my zebrafish. One must compare NA, NAM, NAMR, tryptophan, NAD, and even perhaps quinolinic acid, and ±glutamine would be good too, as it is required for the final step. I did this in zebrafish and measured NAD levels and survival after an otherwise lethal stress, submerged in water that was preconditioned to have no oxygen. I also had compared resveratrol, and most shocking of all was that resveratrol was the best and it increased NAD levels. This was a huge discovery, and it is not well known at all, but it makes perfect sense because resveratrol is a well-established activator of Sirtuin activity, while Sirtuins are well known to use NAD as a substrate. The logic had been since 2004 that Sirtuins are directly activated by RSV (Respiratory Syncytial Virus), but this was later shown to be an artifact . . . Turns out it is increasing NAMPT, which increases NAD, which increases Sirtuins activity is what it looks like. And niacin was also better than the others in the few experiments that I did.

Niacin also has the interesting aspect that it does not feedback inhibit the NrPT enzyme (the first reaction on the way to NAD), but niacinamide does do this (to NAMPT). So, in theory, high-dose niacin can lead to more NAD after certain dose for which niacinamide cannot.

Also, the inherent niacin flush may have effects on influencing the absorption of co-supplements taken with niacin, i.e., the vasodilation, increasing the absorption of whatever is taken with it, including perhaps NAD precursors/niacin itself at the limits of the capillary beds, which may be exactly where supplementation is needed the most.

It's such an important perennial question: Which precursor is best and which indications are likely to be most responsive?

NAD+ versus Niacinamide versus NMN

A letter from Dr. Joseph Mercola, March 2022

I have done a very deep dive on NAD+, which is a vital life molecule and seems to be the reason why people die of niacin deficiency (pellagra). They simply don't have enough substrate to regenerate NAD+. So, it seems to me that while niacin deficiency affects many systems, the most crucial one is fueling NAD+.

This is important because if your goal is to increase NAD+, it is beyond clear that niacinamide is actually far superior to niacin.

NAD+ immediate breakdown product is niacinamide, and the enzyme NAMPT is the rate limiting enzyme in the salvage pathway. Many take NMN as a precursor, but it seems really foolish, and I believe primarily generated by manufacturers of NMN. It is far better to supply niacinamide in small doses, no more than 50 milligrams a few times a day, and higher amounts are actually counterproductive and will inhibit the Sirtuin longevity proteins. This is one instance where megadosing is not recommended.

Eighteen dollars will purchase a seven-year supply of niacinamide if you purchase the powder. Seven years. So, less than 21 cents a month. It is basically free. NMN in therapeutic doses is **hundreds** of dollars a month.

The other key is to activate NAD+, which can be done with:

- Time-restricted eating immediately followed by
- Exercising really HARD, especially resistance training compounded with
- Circadian optimization by going to bed at sunset and getting up at sunrise and avoiding blue light after sunset.

My guess is that if the general public knew this and applied the three principles above with niacinamide, they could radically improve their health for less than one cent a day!

CHAPTER 8

Reversing Arthritis with Niacinamide: The Pioneering Work of William Kaufman, MD, PhD

I noted that niacinamide (alone or combined with other vitamins) in a thousand patient-years of use has caused no adverse side effects.
—WILLIAM KAUFMAN, MD, PHD

Almost half the Canadian population older than seventy-five years has arthritis, and it is the third most common cause of disability in the country, costing some $4.8 billion each year. In 2010, direct and indirect arthritis costs to Canadians amounted to $33 billion. In the United States, over $300 billion. (see https://canadafreepress.com/article/new-report-indicates-arthritis -is-a-33-billion-burden-on-canadians and https://www.cdc.gov/arthritis /data_statistics/cost.htm)." Dr. William Kaufman was the second orthomolecular physician inducted into the Orthomolecular Hall of Fame in 2004. He proved that large doses of niacinamide healed arthritis and many of the changes of aging. He used at least 2,000 milligrams per day, divided into four or even eight smaller doses daily. One would think that this important discovery would be taken very seriously. It was not, even though it has been confirmed by one controlled study and by physicians who have seen what has happened to their patients. This chapter summarizes the discoveries and writings of Dr. Kaufman regarding vitamin B_3 (niacinamide) and its beneficial effect on arthritis.

ARTHRITIS AND NIACINAMIDE

The world was still deep in the Great Depression when William Kaufman, MD, PhD, had already begun treating osteoarthritis with two to four grams of niacinamide daily. Now, over eighty years later, his pioneering work in orthomolecular medicine is receiving the recognition it so well deserves.

In a 1978 radio interview with Carlton Fredericks, Dr. Kaufman described one patient's experience:

> I had one patient who was so severely arthritic that I could not bend his elbows enough to measure his blood pressure. He was one of my first patients. I gave him niacinamide for a week in divided doses, and then he could bend his arm. I took him off it and gave him a look-alike medicine (placebo). In a week he was back where he was before: his joints were stiff again.
>
> I arrived at my (megavitamin B_3 dosage) schedule by actually seeing the response of patients with varying degrees of arthritis. One cannot give a single large dose and get any really favorable results in arthritis. . . . It is necessary to divide the doses, so that the blood levels of niacinamide would be fairly uniform throughout the waking day.

Kaufman's findings were both plain and elegant. The greater the stiffness, the more frequent the doses. Severely crippled arthritic patients needed up to a total of 4,000 milligrams per day, divided into ten doses per day. After one to three months of this treatment, patients could get out of their chair or bed. "If continued, they would be able to comb their hair and be able to walk upstairs, so they would no longer be prisoners of the house. By the end of about three years of treatment, they would be fully ambulatory, and this was even in the older age groups."

Dr. Kaufman's book, *The Common Form of Joint Dysfunction: Its Incidence and Treatment*, includes highly specific niacinamide dosage information applicable to both osteoarthritis and rheumatoid arthritis, along with the doctor's meticulous case notes for hundreds of patients, and some remarkably prescient observations on the antidepressant-antipsychotic properties of niacinamide. Kaufman, whom his widow has described as a conservative physician, nevertheless was the first to prescribe as much as 5,000 milligrams niacinamide daily, in many divided doses, to improve range of joint motion.

Dr. Kaufman's book states:

> Theoretically, optimal nutrition must be continuously available to bodily tissues to ensure the best possible structure and function of tissues. While we do not know what constitutes optimal nutrition, it has been demonstrated empirically that even persons eating a good or excellent diet according to present-day standards exhibit measurable impairment in ranges of joint movement which tends to be more severe with increasing age. It has also been demonstrated that when such persons supplement their good or excellent diets with adequate amounts of niacinamide, there is, in time, measurable improvement in ranges of joint movement, regardless of the patients' ages. In general, the extent of recovery from joint dysfunction of any given degree of severity depends largely on the duration of adequate niacinamide therapy.
>
> Whenever a patient taking the amounts of niacinamide prescribed by the physician, and eating a good or excellent diet, fails to make satisfactory improvement in his Joint Range Index, in the absence of excessive mechanical joint injury the niacinamide schedule must be revised upward to that level which permits satisfactory improvement. Failure of the patient to take niacinamide as directed will result in failure to improve at a satisfactory rate.[1]

Dr. William Kaufman's Notes on Niacinamide Therapy for Arthritis[1]

(Used with the kind permission of Charlotte Kaufman)

The (more frequent) 250 milligrams dose of niacinamide is 40 to 50 percent more effective in the treatment of arthritis than the (less frequent) 500 milligrams dose. As an illustration, see my Tom Spies Memorial Lecture: "Niacinamide, a Most Neglected Vitamin."

This illustrative case history begins on page 17 column 2 and continues on page 18 column 2.

Do not use hard gelatin capsules containing 250 milligrams niacinamide because they do not deliver niacinamide as efficiently as 250 milligrams niacinamide in thin gelatin capsules in the treatment of joint dysfunction (arthritis).

In my 1955 paper in the *Journal of the American Geriatrics Society*, I noted that niacinamide (alone or combined with other vitamins) in a thousand patient-years of use has caused no adverse side effects.[2]

Some brands of niacinamide on the market today contain excipients that act as preservatives, probably meant to prolong shelf life. Some patients have adverse reactions to these preparations, but most do not experience any ill effects.

Niacinamide has ungated entrance to the central nervous system. It has a strong affinity for the central nervous system's benzodiazepine receptors and causes a pleasant calmative effect. In addition, it improves central nervous system function in the kinds of central nervous symptom impairments noted in my 1943 book, starting on page 3.

Please keep in mind niacinamide is a systemic therapeutic agent. It measurably improves joint mobility and muscle strength, and decreases fatigability. It increases maximal muscle working capacity and reduces or completely eliminates arthritic joint pain. Niacinamide heals broken strands of DNA and improves many kinds of CNS functioning.

Some joints are so injured by the arthritic process that no amount of niacinamide therapy will cause improvement in joint mobility, but it takes three months of niacinamide therapy before you can conclude this, since some joints are slow to heal.

CHAPTER OVERVIEW OF *THE COMMON FORM OF JOINT DYSFUNCTION*[3]

Dr. Kaufman, whom his widow has described as "a conservative physician," was nevertheless the first to prescribe very large amounts of niacinamide daily, in many divided doses, to improve range of joint motion.[4]

Chapter 1: Dr. Kaufman presents his niacinamide treatment protocol, beginning with his rationale and measurement methods. He also used ascorbic acid, thiamine, and riboflavin, all in large doses. There is a fascinating passage about "decreased running" (Attention Deficit Hyperactivity Disorder—ADHD). The chapter closes with case histories and an insightful, practical discussion of patient management.

Chapter 2: Dr. Kaufman discusses "Four Complicating Syndromes Frequently Coexisting with Joint Dysfunction," specifically physical and psychological stresses, allergy, posture, obesity, and other factors that may interact or interfere with niacinamide-megavitamin therapy for arthritis.

Chapter 3: "Coordination of Treatment" is a brief presentation of Dr. Kaufman's practical recommendations for case management.

Chapter 4: The 42-page "Analysis of Clinical Data" contains Dr. Kaufman's meticulous patient records supporting megavitamin therapy with niacinamide. This statistical analysis contains fifty-three charts, tables, and graphs, which are not reproduced online.

Chapter 5: "Some Inferences Concerning Joint Dysfunction." Dr. Kaufman, writing in 1949, shows remarkable foresight of orthomolecular medicine half a century into the future. In this chapter he describes how the lack of a single nutrient can cause diverse diseases, the need for a new way of looking at arthritis, and reviews his treatment and what level of success to expect.

Given Dr. Kaufman's work, the authors of "The effect of niacinamide in osteoarthritis: a pilot study"[5], published in 1996, could have omitted the words "pilot study" from their title. Dr. William Kaufman had, forty-seven years earlier, already published his meticulous case notes for hundreds of patients, along with specific niacinamide dosage information applicable to both osteoarthritis and rheumatoid arthritis. In addition, the doctor added some remarkably prescient observations on the antidepressant-antipsychotic properties of B_3.

References to more of Dr. Kaufman's other writings can be found in the For Further Reading section at the end of this book.[6]

Method of Treatment of Joint Dysfunction

by William Kaufman, MD, PhD

After completion of a physical examination, the patient was apprised of the normal and abnormal findings revealed by the clinical study. Where problems other than joint dysfunction existed, these were discussed, and appropriate therapeutic recommendations were made. The subject of joint dysfunction was then presented. The meaning of the numerical value of the patient's Joint Range Index was explained to him in terms of the Clinical Classification of Joint Function,[7] and the dynamic nature of joint dysfunction was described. The patient was told that joint dysfunction was reversible in time when appropriate therapy was taken.

All patients with joint dysfunction who elected to accept treatment were given niacinamide in suitable doses, either alone or in combination with other vitamins. When indicated the appropriate vitamins were prescribed in addition to niacinamide. The water-soluble vitamins used were never prescribed in aqueous solution, but as tablets or as dry powders in capsule form. When vitamin A was used, it was usually given in conjunction with vitamin D. Vitamin D was always given in conjunction with vitamin A; when vitamin D was administered in this study, the daily dosage rarely exceeded 6,000 U.S.P. units per 24 hours.

Participation in the therapeutic program was entirely voluntary on the part of the patient. Some patients at the outset declined to accept treatment for their joint dysfunction. When a patient accepted therapy for his joint dysfunction, with each succeeding visit after the initial one, improvement or lack of improvement in his joint dysfunction was frankly discussed with him. No patient was chided if they were unwilling or unable to carry out the program of therapy as it was originally scheduled. Thus, because there was no "loss of face," most patients cooperated well and gave an accurate account of their deviations, if any, from the suggested therapeutic program. Some patients at the end of the first or second month of treatment, or at a later time, felt so much improved physically that they discontinued therapy for their joint dysfunction, mistakenly believing, in spite of advice to the contrary, that they were "cured," and required no further therapy or medical supervision. Some of these persons, who experienced a recurrence of their original pattern of symptoms upon premature cessation of therapy, returned subsequently for re-evaluation of their therapeutic needs. Other patients, who felt that they had not benefited from therapy for their joint dysfunction, did not continue with treatment, though objectively they responded satisfactorily to adequate therapy, as shown by increasing values of the Joint Range Index on serial re-measurements.

Therapy was always individualized. In the therapeutic program introduced for the treatment of joint dysfunction, each patient served as their own test object in the bio-assay of the dosage of niacinamide necessary to reverse their joint dysfunction. Therapy with niacinamide (used alone or in combination with other vitamins) was not deemed successful unless there was continuous, objective improvement, as judged by continuously increasing values of the Joint Range Index on consecutive reexaminations. (When a patient subsists on a low-protein diet, amounts of niacinamide that would ordinarily be adequate for the treatment of his joint dysfunction prove to be inadequate for satisfactory improvement. In this case, the dosage of niacinamide is continued at the same level, but the protein level of the diet is increased to adequate levels, with subsequent satisfactory improvement in the joint dysfunction.)

The clinical classification of joint function in terms of the numerical values of the Joint Range Index is listed below:

Clinical Classification of Joint Function

Degree of Joint Dysfunction	Joint Range Index
No joint dysfunction	96 to 100
Slight joint dysfunction	86 to 95
Moderate joint dysfunction	71 to 85
Severe joint dysfunction	56 to 70
Extremely severe joint dysfunction	55 or less

For each clinical grade of joint dysfunction, the initial dosage schedule of niacinamide suggested in the table effects improvement in joint dysfunction as to be clinically satisfactory. (However, since April 1947, it has been found that dosage schedules 50 to 100 percent greater than those recommended in the table [particularly in the more severe and extremely severe grades of joint dysfunction] are therapeutically superior, as judged by the patient's clinical response.)

While the initial dosage may be increased as necessary during treatment, it is not decreased, even though the Joint Range Index increases in response to adequate therapy.

The vitamins were administered orally, usually in equal doses at equal intervals during the day, and, in severe and extremely severe joint dysfunction, during the night when the patient would spontaneously awaken from sleep. In slight grades of joint dysfunction, the daily continuous ingestion of 100 milligrams of niacinamide after meals and at bedtime sufficed for treatment (400 milligrams per 24 hours). Usually adequate in moderate joint dysfunction was the continuous ingestion of 150 milligrams niacinamide administered every three hours, for six daily doses (900 milligrams per 24 hours). In extremely severe and severe grades of joint dysfunction, 100 to 150 milligrams niacinamide were prescribed every hour (1,500 to 2,250 milligrams per 24 hours), every hour and a half (1,110 to 1,650 milligrams per 24 hours), or every two hours (800 to 1,200 milligrams per 24 hours), depending on the severity of the joint dysfunction, the more frequent schedule being used in more severe cases.

It has been found in the treatment of joint dysfunction that the manner in which the daily dosage of niacinamide is divided has an important bearing on the therapeutic results achieved; e.g., 300 milligrams niacinamide given three times daily (900 milligrams per 24 hours) is inferior in its therapeutic action to 150 milligrams niacinamide administered every three hours, for six daily doses (900 milligrams per 24 hours). Therefore, to define the type of therapy used, the data was recorded as: (a) the number of milligrams or units administered per dose, and (b) the total number of milligrams or units administered per 24 hours.

No untoward effects or clinical signs of toxicity were noted when niacinamide (alone or in combination with other vitamins) was administered according to the dosage schedules appearing in the table, to individuals for short or long periods of observation. Before 1943, mild hypoglycemia had been noted clinically in a few persons when niacinamide exceeded certain dosage levels, but this phenomenon has not been observed since that time.

"Adequate" and "Optimal" Dosage Levels of Niacinamide in the Treatment of Joint Dysfunction

"Adequate" dosage of niacinamide is defined as that clinically safe dosage of niacinamide which, when ingested in divided doses throughout the day, by a person with joint dysfunction whose ordinary diet is not inadequate in protein or calories, and whose joints are not subjected to excessive mechanical joint injury, will effect in time what is considered to be a satisfactory pattern of increasing values of the Joint Range Index.[8]

"Optimal" dosage of niacinamide is defined as that clinically safe dosage of niacinamide which, when ingested in divided doses during the day by a person with joint dysfunction, would permit the most rapid recovery in joint function, as demonstrated by the largest possible increments in the values of the Joint Range Index in the shortest possible period of time. At present, the optimal dosage of niacinamide for the treatment of joint dysfunction has not been determined clinically, although it is hoped to approximate such a dosage level eventually. Since **adequate dosages of niacinamide have given clinically satisfactory results without producing any untoward symptoms or signs of acute or chronic toxicity**, no attempt has been made in this study to determine the optimal level of niacinamide therapy in the treatment of the various clinical grades of joint dysfunction.

However, as the higher dosage levels of niacinamide have been cautiously explored, it has been found in severe and extremely severe joint dysfunction that divided doses of niacinamide totaling 4 or 5 grams (4,000 to 5,000 milligrams) per 24 hours are therapeutically superior to the lower dosage schedules which previously had been considered adequate. Even these higher dosage levels of niacinamide may not be optimal for the treatment of joint dysfunction.

The optimal dosage of niacinamide for the treatment of joint dysfunction, as well as the limit of human tolerance for niacinamide, can be established only in those medical centers equipped to provide careful clinical supervision, and to conduct such chemical, metabolic, and clinical laboratory studies as would reveal the earliest signs of toxicity, should these occur with the administration of progressively higher dosage levels of niacinamide.

Description of Joint Dysfunction and Its Treatment for the Patient

Since the cooperation of the patient is a prerequisite for the successful therapy of joint dysfunction, it was found desirable and necessary before treatment of joint dysfunction was instituted to discuss with the patient his various clinical problems (including the dynamic nature of joint dysfunction, and its response to niacinamide treatment, and the dynamic nature of certain complicating syndromes, and their appropriate treatment), and the therapeutic goals. During the course of therapy, it may become necessary to review and amplify this discussion for the benefit of the patient as various clinical problems arise.

Joint dysfunction is the articular aspect of a generalized, usually slowly progressive metabolic disorder which is corrected in time by adequate niacinamide therapy. Since the retrograde changes in tissue structure and function which characterize this disorder occur insidiously over a period of years, many of its symptoms and signs are incorrectly attributed by laypeople and physicians alike to the so-called "normal" aging process. But these retrograde changes in morphology and function of bodily tissues are usually reversible in time when adequate levels of niacinamide are supplied continuously to bodily tissues. The patient who takes continuously adequate amounts of niacinamide experiences, in addition to improvement in joint function, an improvement in his general health.

Theoretically, optimal nutrition must be continuously available to bodily tissues to ensure the best possible structure and function of tissues. While we do not know what constitutes optimal nutrition, it has been demonstrated empirically that **even persons eating a good or excellent diet according to present-day standards exhibit measurable impairment in ranges of joint movement which tends to be more severe with increasing age.**[9] It has also been demonstrated that **when such persons supplement their good or excellent diets with adequate amounts of niacinamide, there is, in time, measurable improvement in ranges of joint movement, regardless of the patients' ages.** In general, the extent of recovery from joint dysfunction of any given degree of severity depends largely on the duration of adequate niacinamide therapy.[10]

With the ingestion of adequate amounts of niacinamide continuously for a sufficient period of time, a patient whose ordinary diet is not inadequate in protein or calories, whose joints are not subjected to excessive mechanical trauma, will recover from joint dysfunction at the satisfactory rate of 6.0 to 12.0 Joint Range Index units, or better, in the first month of therapy, and 0.5 to 1.0 Joint Range Index unit, or better, for each month of therapy thereafter, until a Joint Range Index of 96 to 100 is reached. (Rarely, when a patient has one or more ankylosed joints, they may have no appreciable active or passive movement of these ankylosed joints, even after two years of adequate niacinamide therapy, although their other joints recover the full ranges of movement in response to such therapy. In such cases, the Joint Range Index cannot reach 96 to 100; e.g., when one wrist is ankylosed and has not shown increased movement in response to niacinamide therapy, the maximum Joint Range Index attainable is 90.9; and when both wrists are ankylosed, the maximal Joint Range Index attainable is 81.8.)

In general, the more severe and more chronic the patient's joint dysfunction, the slower is the rate of recovery in response to adequate niacinamide therapy, and the slower his subjective appreciation of improvement. The rate of recovery for each patient must be established empirically from serial determinations of the Joint Range Index. In order to ensure a continuously satisfactory rate of recovery from joint dysfunction, the physician must re-examine the patient at intervals during the course of niacinamide therapy. **Whenever a patient taking the amounts of niacinamide prescribed by the physician, and eating a good or excellent diet, fails to make satisfactory improvement in his Joint Range Index, in the absence of excessive mechanical joint injury the niacinamide schedule must be revised upward to that level which permits satisfactory improvement. Failure of the patient to take niacinamide as directed will result in failure to improve at a satisfactory rate.**

When a patient has joint dysfunction associated with obvious arthritic deformities, they are told that the physician cannot predict whether or not their articular deformities will resolve with adequate niacinamide therapy. However, in response to adequate niacinamide therapy for a sufficient period of time, other patients have shown partial or complete resolution of their arthritic joint deformities. Some patients with arthritic deformities show resolution of some of their joint deformities, but not of others. Only careful observation of the patient's deformities on serial re-examinations will indicate whether or not the patient's deformities are resolving in response to adequate niacinamide therapy. In most instances, the rate of resolution of the deformities will be slow, if it occurs at all.

It cannot be predicted whether or not a given joint that appears to be completely ankylosed clinically will recover any degree of movement. It has been observed many times that joints appearing to be clinically ankylosed prior to therapy tend to have partial or complete recovery of movement in response to adequate niacinamide therapy, although some ankylosed joints have not shown any degree of movement as a result of therapy during an observation period of several years. In response to adequate niacinamide therapy over a sufficient period of time, some patients have partial or complete recovery of movement in some of their ankylosed joints, but not in others. Only careful observation of the ranges of joint movement on serial re-examinations will demonstrate whether or not a given ankylosed joint can recover any degree of movement in response to adequate niacinamide therapy.

In general, in the absence of complicating factors, the higher the patient's Joint Range Index rises in response to adequate niacinamide therapy, the fewer articular symptoms he will have; and the better he will feel. However, even though the Joint Range Index increases satisfactorily in response to adequate niacinamide therapy, the patient may not feel well because of complicating syndromes which are not on the basis of aniacinamidosis. Careful clinical study is necessary in order to establish the etiology of whatever complicating syndromes may be present and, with appropriate therapy, the patient is likely to become free from articular symptoms and to feel well. However, at any time symptoms of bodily discomfort may recur, which must be studied and given appropriate treatment as promptly as possible, if the patient is to feel well again. While the patient may obtain temporary relief from articular and other symptoms through the use of analgesics, narcotics, sedatives, antihistamines, and local anesthetics, only adequate treatment of joint dysfunction and the complicating syndromes is likely to give more lasting benefits.

In order to assess the effects of niacinamide therapy on joint dysfunction and on the patient's general status, the patient is usually re-studied one month after continuous niacinamide therapy has been instituted. If good progress in recovery from joint dysfunction is noted at that time, the patient is reexamined in two months, and thereafter every three to six months. For the most part, this schedule of re-examination is found to be satisfactory for the supervision of the therapeutic program of patients presenting the chronic problems of joint dysfunction, although when the individual's problems are of unusual complexity, or when intercurrent problems arise, the time interval between visits is shortened.

When a patient with joint dysfunction fails to make the anticipated progress in response to niacinamide therapy, he is asked if he has taken the medication as prescribed; if not, he is urged to do so. When a patient has taken multiple vitamin capsules as prescribed and has not made satisfactory improvement in his Joint Range Index in response to such therapy, the pharmacist is asked how the vitamin powders were compounded. The clinical effectiveness of niacinamide seems to be lessened when niacinamide is mixed with ascorbic acid by vigorous trituration, since this favors inter-molecular reactions between niacinamide and ascorbic acid in the dry powder state. The occurrence of such inter-molecular reactions between niacinamide and ascorbic acid is hindered by the preliminary admixture of each dry powder separately with a small amount of calcium stearate (0.2 percent) before the final admixture by sieving.

It is always emphasized that the patient must take their medication continuously, as prescribed, until such time as the supervising physician may decide, on the basis of objective clinical evidence, that it is necessary to increase the level of niacinamide therapy in order to produce continuously satisfactory improvement in the Joint Range Index.

However, certain factors other than the ingestion of inadequate amounts of niacinamide may tend to depress the Joint Range Index. These include (a) transient or persistent mechanical joint injury resulting from unusual or physical exertion[11] or from psychogenically sustained hypertonia of somatic muscle,[12] (b) rapid and excessive gain in weight to obesity levels, (c) excessive ingestion of alcohol, and (d) inadequate dietary protein. When any of these factors is operative, it is of limited value to increase the amounts of niacinamide taken by the patient in an effort to effect satisfactory improvement in the Joint Range Index. Instead, treatment should be directed toward lessening the degree of mechanical joint injury, reducing the patient's weight to the normal range, interdicting alcohol, and increasing the protein intake to adequate levels, respectively.

When indicated, the physician describes for the patient four complicating syndromes frequently coexisting with joint dysfunction, and their treatment.[13] Most of the articular and non-articular symptoms of a patient with joint dysfunction which are not corrected by niacinamide therapy usually originate as part of these four complicating syndromes. When the patient understands the etiologic basis of his symptoms, they will not have anxiety concerning the meaning of symptoms which would otherwise seem mysterious and alarming. The patient with joint dysfunction who has one or more of these complicating syndromes is told they will not feel well unless joint dysfunction and these coexisting syndromes are correctly identified and successfully treated, and that in order to accomplish this, their active participation in the clinical investigation and therapeutic program is required.

Typical Improvement in Mobility of a Single Joint in Response to Levels of Niacinamide Therapy Used Prior to April 1947

In serial determinations of the mobility of single joints in response to levels of niacinamide therapy used prior to April 1947, it was found that niacinamide-induced recovery of full joint mobility was an orderly process. (Since April 1947, **when higher-dosage schedules of niacinamide were introduced,**[14] **there has been a marked reduction in the incidence of articular pain and discomfort upon maximal passive movement of the moveable joints during various stages of recovery from joint dysfunction.**)

A Case History

There is described below typical improvement in joint mobility, in sequential stages occurring during niacinamide-induced recovery of full mobility of the metacarpophalangeal (knuckle) joint. On the initial examination before niacinamide therapy was instituted, the metacarpophalangeal joint of the forefinger of the right hand could be extended passively to 30 percent of the full range of extension for this joint. No pain or discomfort was experienced by the patient during this maneuver. The examiner noted the presence of palpatory resistance from the initiation of the movement of passive extension of this metacarpophalangeal joint, and this resistance progressively increased as the joint was extended from the range of 0 to 30 percent of the maximal extension; the palpatory resistance at the end of the movement was graded as firm. When at the 30 percent level of passive extension, a small increase of force in the direction of extension caused no further extension of this joint, 30 percent of the full range of extension was taken as the upper limit of maximum passive extension of this metacarpophalangeal joint.

At the end of one month of continuous, adequate niacinamide therapy, maximal passive extension of this metacarpophalangeal joint increased to 60 percent of the full range of extension. No pain or discomfort was experienced by the patient when the metacarpophalangeal joint was extended from 0 to 40 percent of the full range of extension. The patient experienced localized joint pain, often severe, as the joint was passively extended from 40 to 60 percent of the full range of extension. The examiner's palpatory sensation indicated that movement of the joint in passive extension was free from 0 to 40 percent, and that there was soft, yielding resistance which progressively increased as the finger was extended at the metacarpophalangeal joint from 40 to 60 percent of the full range of movement. When a further small increase of the extending force did not increase the degree of extension, 60 percent of the full range of extension was taken as the upper limit of passive extension of this metacarpophalangeal joint. The palpatory resistance at the end of the movement of extension was rubbery.

After months of continuous, adequate therapy with niacinamide, maximal passive extension of the metacarpophalangeal joint reached 100 percent, or the full range of movement. Passive extension of the metacarpophalangeal joint from 0 to 85 percent was without pain or discomfort; passive extension from 85 to 100 percent was painful. The examiner's palpatory sensation indicated that the movement of this joint was free from 0 to 85 percent, and that there was soft resistance, which increased progressively with increasing extension of the metacarpophalangeal joint from the level of 85 to 100 percent. A small, additional force, in the direction of extension, when the 100 percent level was reached, did not cause further extension of this joint. The palpatory resistance at the end of the full range of movement (100 percent) was rubbery.

With a longer period of continuous, adequate niacinamide therapy, it was possible to achieve full, free, and painless extension of this metacarpophalangeal joint to the level of 100 percent. Slight additional palpatory force in the direction of extension with the joint fully extended did not increase the amount of movement beyond the full range of extension, the 100 percent level. The examiner's palpatory sensation indicated that the movement of extension was free from 0 to 100 percent of full extension, that the resistance met at the end of this movement was firm, and that the patient experienced no pain from this maneuver.

In November 1999, Dan Lukaczer, N.D., reported in *Nutrition Science*, "A few years ago, Wayne Jonas et al. (1996) from the National Institutes of Health (NIH) Office of Alternative Medicine in Bethesda, MD, conducted a 12-week, double-blind, placebo-controlled study of 72 patients to assess the validity of Kaufman's earlier observations that niacin was of great benefit to the elderly, reducing arthritis. Jonas reported that niacinamide at 3 grams per day reduced overall disease severity by 29 percent, inflammation by 22 percent and use of anti-inflammatory medication by 13 percent."[15] Patients in the placebo group either had no improvement or worsened.

Many of my (AH) patients with arthritis recovered or became much better when prescribed niacin.[16] The most dramatic case came into my office in a wheelchair, pushed by her very tired and sick-looking husband. She was sitting with her legs crossed over as she could not extend them. She had been sick for the previous twenty years and had received every known treatment for arthritis, including hormones and gold injections. Nothing had helped. Her hands were totally useless, and she was crippled. Her husband had to carry her around the house, even to the bathroom. He provided her with the equivalent care of four nurses, around the clock. No wonder he was totally exhausted and sick. I "knew" she could not be helped, since such very chronic deteriorated arthritis cases generally did not do well. She said to me, "I know that you cannot help my arthritis, but the pain in my back is terrible. All I want is some relief from it." I started her on a vitamin program, the main constituent of which was niacin, but I did not really expect to see much improvement. She returned a month later in her wheelchair, again being pushed by her husband. This time, however, she was sitting in her chair with her feet dangling straight down. Her husband looked relaxed and had lost his dreadful sick look. When I began to talk and ask her questions, she interrupted and said, "The pain is gone!" She was so much better that I began to think that maybe, with skillful surgery, some function might be restored to her hands. Six months later she telephoned. I asked her in surprise, "How did you get to the phone?" She replied that she was now able to get around on her own in her chair, and added that she was not calling for herself but for her husband, who had a cold. She wanted some advice about how to help him. This woman died several years later, having achieved her goal of a pain-free existence.

From Hoffer and Foster:

Arthritis recently has been at the centre of a vortex of controversy. In October 2004, Vioxx (rofecoxib), one of the main drugs used to treat it, was voluntarily withdrawn by its manufacturers, Merck and Co. It had been admitted that some 70,000 deaths, largely from cardiovascular episodes, had been associated with this drug's use. Such toxic side effects had been known by the industry for several years. In February 2005, a panel of the U.S. Food and Drug Administration voted to allow the possible return of Vioxx, provided it carried a striking black-box warning on its label about its cardiovascular risks. Patients who take it will be obliged to sign consent forms. 15 million prescriptions of Vioxx were filled in Canada before its withdrawal and it is not yet clear whether Health Canada will support its return to use. Interestingly, the *New York Times* reported that 10 of the 32 members of the U.S. Food and Drug Administration panel voting to allow the return of Vioxx were paid consultants for the drug's makers.[17] This panel also supported the continued use of other cox-2 drugs such as Celebrex and Bextra for arthritis despite their known cardiovascular risks, so long as they also carry a black-box warning. Given the evidence that arthritis can often be successfully treated with niacin or other nutrients, these decisions raise many interesting ethical issues.[18]

Here is a comparison between vitamin B$_3$ and Vioxx as it applies to arthritis:

TABLE SHOWING COMPARISON BETWEEN B$_3$ AND VIOXX FOR TREATMENT OF ARTHRITIS		
	VITAMIN B$_3$	VIOXX
What is it?	Vitamin	Drug
Cures?	Yes	No
Relieves pain?	Yes	Yes
Negative side effects?	Minor, not toxic	Major
Positive side effects?	Many	None
Toxic?	No	Yes
Causes deaths?	No	Many
Costly?	Cheap	Expensive
Patented?	No	Yes

Psaty and Kronmal examined pooled data from two studies that showed a significant increase in deaths from Vioxx:

[The study indicated] overall mortality of 34 deaths among 1,069 rofecoxib patients and 12 deaths among 1,078 placebo patients. These mortality analyses were neither provided to the FDA nor made public in a timely fashion. The data submitted by the sponsor to the FDA in a Safety Update Report in July 2001 used on-treatment analysis methods and reported 29 deaths (2.7 percent) among 1,067 rofecoxib patients and 17 deaths (1.6 percent) among 1,075 placebo patients. This on-treatment approach to reporting minimized the appearance of any mortality risk. In December 2001, when the FDA raised safety questions about the submitted safety data, the sponsor did not bring these issues to an institutional review board for review and revealed that there was no data and safety monitoring board for the protocol 078 study. The findings from this case study suggest that additional protections for human research participants, including new approaches for the conduct, oversight, and reporting of industry-sponsored trials, are necessary.[19]

Joseph S. Ross and his colleagues present a case-study review of industry documents that demonstrates that clinical trial manuscripts related to rofecoxib were authored by sponsor employees, but they often attributed first authorship to academically affiliated investigators who did not always disclose industry financial support. Review manuscripts were often prepared by unacknowledged authors and subsequently attributed authorship to academically affiliated investigators, who often did not disclose industry financial support.[20]

Based on these two reports, an article by DeAngelis and Fonanarosa concluded: "The profession of medicine, in every aspect—clinical, education, and research—has been inundated with profound influence from the pharmaceutical and medical device industries. This has occurred because physicians have allowed it to happen, and it is time to stop."[21] In another hard-hitting report, Taylor summarized these revelations of the drug industry's mode of operation as "Manipulated studies, conflicts of interest and threats to the public confidence in their medical system."[22] It is about time that the public is introduced to what really has traumatized it for so many years. The cost in deaths, disease, and failure to treat adequately has been enormous.

On Niacinamide as a Therapeutic Agent

A Memoir by William Kaufman, PhD, MD

(Dr. Kaufman died Aug. 24, 2001, at the age of 89. Dated the same year, this is Dr. Kaufman's final paper. It has never before been published.)

When I was in medical school in the 1930s, there were no automated blood chemistries of blood counts. There were no CAT, PET, MRI, or ultrasound scans. Electrocardiographic chest leads were just being invented. Coronary artery cauterization had not yet been attempted. There was no cardiac angiography. There were no coronary artery by-pass grafts. In cataract patients, there were no intra-ocular lens implants. There were no flexible gastroscopes and no colonoscopies. There were no antibiotics. Sulfanilamide had just been tried as an antibacterial agent, which proved to be mostly ineffective. There were no thiazide diuretics, no beta blockers, no calcium channel blockers. There were no renal dialysis centers. There was no cortisone. There were no tranquilizers, anti-psychotic agents or anti-depressants. There were no oral contraceptive agents.

The newest and most exciting development in the 1930s was the identification, structural analysis, synthesis, and ensuing commercial availability of such vitamins as ascorbic acid, thiamin, riboflavin, pyridoxine, pantothenic acid, nicotinic acid, nicotinic acid amide, vitamin K1, and alpha tocopherol.[23] In addition, there were those derived from natural sources such as vitamin A, vitamin D, and vitamin E complex which also were available commercially. As a result, the 1930s saw an explosive increase in research on animal and human nutritional deficiencies.[24] The frequency and scope of animal and clinical nutritional research resulted in large numbers of publications by the end of 1940. This can best be appreciated by scanning the bibliographies and references in some of the books dealing with the diagnosis and treatment of nutritional deficiency diseases in animals and humans that were published during the late 1930s and early 1940s.

I was a fortunate beneficiary of all this burgeoning activity in nutritional research. In my junior and senior years at the University

of Michigan Medical School in Ann Arbor (1936 to 1938), the cur-
riculum gave a new emphasis to nutrition. The Pathology Department gave intensive lectures on nutritional deficiency diseases
including their histopathology at various phases of their development and severity. The Departments of Physiological Chemistry,
Internal Medicine, Pediatrics, Neurology, and Psychiatry all gave
detailed lectures on nutritional deficiency diseases from the point of
view of their specialty. They also assigned readings of then current
articles dealing with the diagnosis and treatment of nutritional deficiencies. In addition, I was able to take an elective program dealing
with nutrition from the point of view of the dietitian.

Although I had intended to become a cardiologist, I was fas-
cinated by the power of nutritional therapy in ameliorating serious nutritional deficiencies. In addition to the assigned readings in
nutrition, I read as much as I could of non-assigned then-current
nutritional literature. I also began collecting and reading old books
on nutritional deficiency diseases. I became very interested in pellagra and the many attempts to find its cause and cure.

In 1937, Elvejhem and his associates found that nicotinic acid,
and in 1938, that nicotinic acid amide could cure canine black tongue,
an analogue of human pellagra. Thus, by the accident of earlier discovery of its possible anti-pellagra activity, nicotinic acid was used
in the therapy of pellagrous patients months before nicotinic acid
amide was. In 1938, I took 200 milligrams of encapsulated nicotinic
acid, a dose described as safe. In addition to the anticipated flushing, I experienced an extremely severe, acute, idiosyncratic adverse
reaction.[25] This is why when I finally started my private practice of
internal medicine, I always gave the patient an oral test dose of nicotinic acid in my office if I planned to use nicotinic acid for therapy,
a thing I rarely did. I would then observe for the next hour to be sure
that he or she did not experience a life-threatening reaction to it as I
had. If the patient had no early adverse reaction to it (excluding the
anticipated flush) only then would I prescribe nicotinic acid in his or
her therapy. In the latter part of 1938, I developed the courage to take
a 200 milligrams oral dose of nicotinic acid amide and experienced

no adverse side effects. However, I still took the precaution of giving each patient I wished to treat with niacinamide an oral test dose and for the next hour carefully observed the patient. This practice made it possible for me to record in detail some of the patient's earliest therapeutic responses to nicotinic acid amide.

In the course of my reading, I learned of an interesting ailment, "pellagra sine pellagra." The term pellagra comes from the Italian "pelle" and "agra," meaning "rough skin." People suffering from "pellagra sine pellagra" had the symptomatology of pellagra but not its skin rashes (Casal's necklace and the florid dermatitis on skin surfaces exposed to sunlight). This syndrome sometimes also was called "pre-pellagra," "incipient pellagra," "atypical pellagra," and "subclinical pellagra." But as you will soon see from my description of this syndrome, there was nothing "subclinical" about "pellagra sine pellagra."

In June 1938, I left the University of Michigan with a master's degree in Chemistry (1932), a PhD in Physiology (1937), and an MD (cum laude). I completed a rotating medical internship at Barnes Hospital in St. Louis (1938 to 1939); then an assistant residency and residency in private medicine at New York's Mount Sinai Hospital (1939 to 1940), and next held post-graduate fellowships for two years in the Physiology Department of Yale School of Medicine (1940 to 1942), joining a research group dedicated to researching the origins of the electrocardiogram. In addition, some mornings, I also taught students in Yale's medical outpatient department.

At the end of December 1940, I decided that in addition to continuing with my electrocardiographic research and medical outpatient teaching at Yale, I would begin my private practice of internal medicine in Bridgeport, Connecticut. I planned to see patients some afternoons, some evenings, and weekends. I would accept only those patients who wanted complete physical examinations. By the end of 1942, I practiced full time.

Without knowing what had been happening nutritionally to the American population in the 1930s, it may be difficult for you to understand how "pellagra sine pellagra" and other nutritional deficiencies I refer to in this memoir could have existed in such abundance even during the early 1940s. To give you an overview, I call your attention to the very important November 1943 report of The Committee on Diagnosis and Pathology of Nutritional Deficiencies of The Food and Nutrition Board of the National Research Council entitled "Inadequate Diets and Nutritional Deficiencies in the United States; Their Prevalence and Significance." The distinguished committee chaired by the late Dr. H.D. Kruse (who taught me nutritional biomicroscopy) concluded that in the previous decade malnutrition was widespread in the United States.

However, the extremely severe classic nutritional deficiencies such as beriberi, pellagra, scurvy, and xerophthalmia were relatively uncommon. The most frequent nutritional deficiencies were the milder, less acute, more moderate, more chronic forms. These abounded in the United States. Over the ten years preceding 1943, these nutritional deficiencies adversely affected persons of all ages in many locations and without exception led to the conclusion that a significant number of the diets were more than 50 percent deficient in the RDAs of several essential nutrients and most of the diets were less than 50 percent deficient.

"Accordingly, there is widespread prevalence of moderately deficient diets. All the data from numerous surveys with new methods among persons of all ages in many regions are entirely in accord that deficiency states are rife throughout the nation."

The severe economic depression of the 1930s played an important part in reducing the quality of the diet for many families. They could not afford to buy much meat, fresh fruit, or even fresh green or yellow vegetables. Bread was the "staff of life." The majority of people ate large amounts of white bread. Milling procedures used at the time robbed the white flour of much of its vitamin, trace mineral, and roughage content. Many families could barely afford to buy adequate amounts of milk for their children and thus had to forgo drinking milk themselves. It is clear how such inadequate diets could lead to various nutritional deficiency syndromes.[26]

But even the well-to-do families also had nutritional deficiency disorders arising from their poor habits of food selection. Many

preferred meat, potato, and apple pie suppers. These meals sometimes included green and yellow vegetables. There was always snack-
ing on fresh fruits when these were in season. The favorite fruit was
probably canned peaches in heavy syrup. Their breakfasts may have
started with a glass of orange juice and often included bacon, eggs,
and fried potatoes, followed by buttered white bread toast, some jam,
and coffee heavily sugared and loaded with heavy cream. The lunch
often was a hamburger—white bread sandwich and more coffee fixed
with a lot of sugar and heavy cream. Adults might sometimes have
a strong cheese with their apple pie, or have the pie à la mode, but
they rarely drank milk. Yet, they insisted that their young children
drink plenty of milk. Although these people were financially well off,
they too developed a variety of nutritional deficiencies, obesity, and
medical complications.

I had decided that before I began my private medical practice at
the end of December 1940, I would want to make a careful clinical
study of "pellagra sine pellagra," including the response of patients
to nicotinic acid amide therapy. To best accomplish this, I wanted to
dispense this vitamin and have look-alike placebos to use as controls. I also decided to rename "pellagra sine pellagra" "niacin amide
deficiency disease," and later "aniacinamidosis." Pellagra would then
become "aniacinamidosis" with skin rash. If there was a coexisting
thiamin deficiency, I would add "athiaminosis" to the diagnosis. If
there was a coexisting riboflavin deficiency I would also add "aribo-
flavinosis" to the diagnosis.

I sent out announcements in December 1940 that I was open-
ing my office for the practice of internal medicine in Bridgeport,
Connecticut, to community doctors. I was astonished to get so many
patient referrals from physicians who told me that I could keep the
referred patients as my own. Only some years later, a doctor friend
who was one of the referring physicians told me that he and a small
group of his doctor friends (who later also became my friends) saw
a way they could get rid of their most complaining, most difficult to
get along with, most obnoxious patients by sending them to me, and
they waited to enjoy hearing me complain that I found these referred

patients very difficult to manage medically. It was sort of a medical hazing ceremony and an initiation rite into the brotherhood of physicians. The majority of the referred patients had unrecognized aniacinamidosis. The comic outcome came into being because I could recognize, diagnose, and successfully treat aniacinamidosis, while at that time the referring physicians could not.

It was not easy to establish rapport with the patients during the initial part of their first visit. They frowned, scowled, looked and acted tired, anxious, and worried. They were circumlocutious, repetitive, and generally unfriendly. I treated these referred patients with kindness, respect, and adequate niacinamide, and they soon became easy to take care of medically. In a matter of days, they also had astonishing improvements in their health. They were basically good and decent people and not ogres. Because of their spectacular medical response to niacinamide therapy, some of their friends and neighbors sought appointments with me. Not long thereafter some of their relatives living in distant states (California, Georgia, Illinois, Indiana, Massachusetts, New Jersey, New York, Rhode Island, and even from Montreal) made appointments for medical consultations, and returned at intervals so that I could check on their progress.

My patients with aniacinamidosis had not felt well for many years. They were mainly middle-aged. There were one-third more women than men. There were many more elderly than children or teenagers in the group. Most adults were in the middle-income class. Most had at least a high school education. All had some occupation and daily responsibilities. Some were employees, some were owners of businesses that employed others. Some were self-employed, some were stay-at-home spouses, some were professionals, and some were schoolchildren and others college students.

The first visit generally took three hours, sometimes longer. Spending this amount of time was possible because the new patient was either the only patient I saw that day, or was the last patient I saw that day. This first visit was dedicated to getting acquainted with the patient, their health problems, medications they were taking, family problems, business or work problems, economic worries, and lastly what they expected from any medical treatment I might prescribe. Thus, this first visit included unhurried but detailed history taking, inventorying the patient's eating patterns, a brief psychologic survey, a careful physical and neurological examination, a careful examination of the skin, conjunctivae, lingual and buccal mucosa, lips, gums, the uterine cervix (in women) under magnification for possible signs of nutritional deficiencies, some laboratory tests, a discussion of the patient's health problems, and my recommendations for treatment and follow-up.

Early in the course of the first visit, most patients realized I was taking their complaints seriously, that I was not hurrying them to make their visit fit a limited time frame, and that when I questioned them, I was truly trying to understand their health problems, their dietary problems, their family and business problems, their lifestyle, and what they wanted to achieve healthwise from any medical treatment I might prescribe. Please remember that by December 1940, the United States had made considerable recovery from the depths of the great economic depression of the 1930s. This meant that most families were better off financially than they had been since the early 1930s, and that more people could afford to eat a nutritionally good diet, even if they did not do so. However, I did not make any recommendations that they change their diets. I wanted to observe what treatment with niacinamide alone (or sometimes combined with other vitamins) would do for them healthwise. Then, I made suggestions that some modifications of their usual pattern of eating might provide additional benefits.

Here is a description both of the symptomatology and of the coexisting clinical signs of aniacinamidosis based on my study of somewhat over 150 patients with this syndrome who consulted me between the end of December 1940 through March 1943 when bread was "enriched." Of course, no patient had all the symptoms or all the clinical signs. But most had enough symptoms to make it easy to conclude that their ailment fitted into the pattern of aniacinamidosis especially when correlated with the coexisting physical signs. The final test was that most of the symptoms disappeared with normal maintenance therapy and that simultaneously, most of the physical signs of aniacinamidosis were ameliorated to a significant degree and some vanished altogether. However, cessation of oral niacinamide maintenance therapy led to recurrences of the entire syndrome in a relatively short time.

Aniacinamidosis was independent of family income. No patient had the florid dermatitis of pellagra. No patient had dementia. Most had normal bowel movements. Some tended to be constipated. A minority had two or three loose stools a day.

***

Many patients had prolonged retention of suntan for five or more months after the last exposure to the sun. There was a tendency toward excessive, localized callusing in areas subjected to even mild recurrent pressure or rubbing. Many had calluses on the skin overlying their Achilles' tendons from the rubbing of the back of their shoes in this area. Nearly all had corns on several of their toes of each foot. Nearly all had calluses on the soles of their feet. Those who did manual labor also had marked occupational calluses on their hands. A secretary who sat a great deal of her working time in the office had callusing on her buttocks and skin overlying her sacrum, which she pressed against the back of the chair as she sat. The calluses were pigmented a dark shade of yellow and sometimes a deep brown. Middle-aged patients tended to have the wrinkled, reticular skin pattern of a much older person.

***

Many complained of excessive fatiguability. A goodly number of patients talked about muscular weakness. Some complained of muscle aching after relatively mild physical activity. Simple instruments made it easy to confirm that the patients had measurably increased fatiguability, impaired muscle strength and impaired maximal muscle working capacity. Many complained that when I pumped up the blood pressure cuff, it hurt them a great deal. This suggests that their muscles were tender to this kind of squeezing.

Physician's Notes on Taking the Case

A Closer Look into What Dr. William Kaufman Observed of New Patients That He Would Be Treating with Niacinamide Therapy

The patient says he feels tense. Is restless. Frequently changes sitting position in the consultation room facing me, as I ask questions.

Seems calm but as we talk, he or she often tell me that they are seething with resentment. They hate feeling so bad. They hate doctors who have not been able to help them and there is often a litany of other resentments against members of their family, friends, and people they work with. Can't relax. They often seem apathetic. They complain of mental sluggishness. Thoughts are slowed. Feel as if they are in a mental fog. Attention is easily distracted. Delays making decisions. Difficult to concentrate. The response to questions I ask often delayed although his hearing sense is normal. Not always sure he understands what he hears. May have to re-read an item in a newspaper or other reading material to get the meaning. Doesn't read as much as he did. Increased irritability. Frequently has unwarranted, prolonged anxieties which he can't get rid of. Some patients feel "nervous" and are tense and anxious all the time. Excessive worry and tension about small and often unimportant matters. Often feels that there is something drastically wrong with him and that's why he feels so bad. Can't shake his worries he may have cancer or is going to get a stroke or heart attack or die. Has recurrent feelings of other impending troubles. Has uncertainties about what his future will hold for him. He sometimes loses his former interest and pleasure in work, family, friends, hobbies. Adjusts poorly to unanticipated adverse life situations. Lacks initiative. Often uncooperative. Routine duties become particularly burdensome. Procrastinates. Often with a burst of enthusiasm, he starts projects which he never finishes. Frequently feels and acts opinionated, vindictive, quarrelsome, mean, unreasonable, and intolerant. Tends to act impulsively without considering the possible consequences of what he does. Emotional instability. Easily startled when I make a sudden movement to pick a pen off my desk. Flares "off the handle" when their feelings are hurt by trivial but reasonable criticism of some of his actions. Women and some men often feel like crying but hold back. Both men and women sometimes burst into tears and sob for no reason they can explain. Tearful or not, both sexes tend to become belligerent at the least challenge to their amour propre. Many tend to have a poor self-image. Tends to scowl or frown during our interview. Rarely smiles. Tends to be repetitive in his complaints.

Some patients occasionally become quite unhappy for short intervals (for less than an hour) without apparent cause. Some are mildly depressed much of the time. Doesn't enjoy their work as they formerly did. Often feels aggrieved and unappreciated by their employer or family. Some complain that they have not been themselves for years and that their personalities have changed for the worse. Many felt they were aging too fast. I observed that many had an excessive startle reaction in response to an unexpected noise such as the ringing of a telephone in my consultation room. A surprising number were afraid of being hurt when their blood pressure was taken or when a venipuncture was done. Many apologized after expressing their fear of being hurt by saying, "I guess I'm just a big baby."

Most had sleep problems. It was difficult to fall asleep. They turn, toss, twist at night They waken at intervals not because they need to urinate. They dream a lot but generally they have troubling dreams. Generally, doesn't feel rested when he wakens. After an intermittently wakeful night, in the morning when he has to go to work, he feels that if only he could sleep a little longer he would be rested. Barbiturates help put him to sleep but when he wakens in the morning, he feels groggy. In a short lime, sleeping pills are no longer very effective and again does not have restful sleep and wakes up tired and groggy.

Many have been told by one or more doctors they consulted that there was nothing wrong with them excepting they were neurotics. They were given a sedative, generally phenobarbital, advised to take a rest cure, or just to "snap out of it." Some were referred to distant famous name clinics for diagnosis and treatment The pattern of treatment generally was that the patient should rest as much as possible (never walk when they can sit, never sit when they can lie down). They were to take a barbiturate (to calm their nerves) and belladonna (to relax their stomach and intestines) three or four times a day. That was the total previous treatment.

Some patients complained of impairments in balance sense. This resulted in bumps into furniture or walls, severe enough to cause black and blue marks on the arms or legs. There were also many episodes of near falls on level ground. There were also falls. This was not associated with dizziness or vertigo.

Some also complained of awkwardness or clumsiness, dropping things they shouldn't have dropped. The explanation I received was that their fingers suddenly stopped holding the object that they dropped. I devised a simple test for detecting impairment of balance sense. With eyes open, the patient stood on one foot and elevated the other foot and positioned it so that its heel would be two inches in front of the knee of the contralateral leg. The patient would have to be able to remain in this position for at least thirty seconds. This maneuver then was repeated with the patient standing on his other limb. Then, this entire test was repeated with the patient's eyes closed. If a patient had impaired balance sense, I could ascertain if it was a one-sided or bilateral impairment of balance and if it was elicited both with eyes open and closed or only occurred with eyes closed. It was surprising how often the impaired balance sense was unilateral and only with eyes closed. In this case, the black and blue marks from bumping occurred only on the side that showed imbalance. Caution: In conducting this test of balance, one must have attendants beside the patient ready to prevent a fall from impaired balance sense.

When the sole of a patient's foot was stroked to elicit a plantar reflex, most patients experienced a persistent, disagreeable linear after-sensation on the sole lasting as long as ten minutes. However, simply passing my palm over the patient's sole with slight pressure would immediately "erase" these unpleasant sensations. I called this phenomenon "erasable paresthesias."

Many patients had spontaneous paresthesias mainly on the distal portions of the upper and lower limb and occasionally on the cheeks and around the mouth. These were in areas where there was significant decrease in light touch sensitivity but not of pain or temperature.

Many patients ate because they knew they needed to in order to sustain life. They did not have a good appetite. Food did not taste as good as it used to. Many ate small portions of food throughout the day, having six or seven small meals. They did this because regular-sized meals filled them up too much and made them feel uncomfortably distended. Some talked about their many digestive upsets. By this they meant that they did not feel well after eating, had water brash, belching, bloating, heart burn, indigestion, upper abdominal pain.

Many had loud intestinal rumbling and associated abdominal discomfort. Most patients had normal bowel movements. Some were constipated. A small number had loose stools.

Liver enlargement and tenderness was almost universal in both persons who never used alcohol and in those who drank social amounts. The liver edge was down one to two (rarely more) centimeters below the costal margin in the right mid-clavicular line and was soft and very painful to palpation.

The lingual membrane showed adverse changes in its morphology exhibiting some degree of atrophy of all of its papillae. This differed in degree of severity in different patients. In some patients there was additional increased redness at the tip and sides of the tongue. Sometimes the sides of the tongue had an indented pattern made by the sides of the patient's teeth and the tongue itself seemed swollen and larger than normal. Some of these patients told me that when they were tense and didn't want to say something that might hurt another person's feelings, they would almost automatically press their tongue forcefully against their front teeth while their mouth was shut. In some, the lingual muscles had undergone some degree of atrophy and in these patents the tongue seemed smaller than normal and there was the most advanced atrophy of the lingual papillae.

Virtually all patients had a specific type of non-dependent metabolic edema that affected non-articular cartilages including the aural, nasal, costal cartilages as well as the long bone's periosteum. All these swollen structures were very tender to digital pressure. (This edema also affected articular cartilages. Evidence for this will be given later.) But in addition, it also probably affected all tissues of the body to some degree. This metabolic edema was unique in that it would disappear upon the administration of a single oral 100 to 200 milligram dose of niacinamide starting within ten to fifteen minutes of administration.

This was accompanied by a duresis as copious as one would expect from a 40 milligrams oral dose of Lasix. Then, this metabolic edema would reaccumulate starting within an hour and a half of the time that the niacinamide tablet was ingested. Niacinamide has a half-life of about one hour and a half. If niacinamide was taken at intervals during every three hours during the day, this metabolic edema would not recur. The dosage pattern of niacinamide intake will be discussed in some detail later.

Some women complained of dyspareunia. Vaginal tissue was unusually red and tender to vaginal examination. No type of fungal, bacterial, or trichamonal infection could be demonstrated in most of these women. The syndrome disappeared with adequate oral niacinamide therapy.

Perhaps the chief complaint might be "I'm tired all the time," "I don't feel good," "I've got arthritis," "I think I'm losing my mind," "I'm very nervous and jittery," "I have stomach trouble," or women who might say "It hurts me to have sexual intercourse," meaning a tender and spastic vagina.

Careful, considerate questioning could elicit the symptoms and pattern of the patient's ill-health. The physical examination will contribute other data. The beneficial response of the patient to oral niacinamide therapy will contribute other data that will make it very likely that patient's illness was aniacinamidosis. Cessation of niacinamide therapy (or the administration of a placebo) will cause the niacinamide-induced improvements to disappear.

How It All Began for Dr. Kaufman

Dr. Kaufman became interested in the use of vitamin B_3, mostly niacinamide, for treating arthritis. In his own words, this is how his interest developed:

I began when I was still a student collecting some of the names which had been used to describe pellagra. These included formes fruste of pellagra, subclinical pellagra, pellagra sine pellagra, and atypical pellagra in addition to names used in European countries including mal de la rosa (used by Casal in 1730 in Spain when he described pellagra) and pella agra (a term used by Frapolli in Italy in 1771), plus 41 other names used in various provinces of various European countries to describe the nutritional deficiency disease we today call pellagra but should call aniacinamidosis. The reason for all the European names was because pellagra was endemic in large areas of Italy, Spain, and France and some of the Balkan countries.

I was carried away by reading about the superb results various investigators were having in the treatment of pellagra, a potentially fatal disease, using niacin. When I read an article by Spies and his associates in the *JAMA* 110: 461, 1938, I couldn't rest until I, myself, took 200 milligrams of nicotinic acid, a supposedly safe dose, to see what the flushing that this substance caused was like. Within 15 minutes, I flushed and itched alright, but I was also violently ill with uncontrollable alternate contraction of the large flexor and extensor groups of muscles in my arms and legs and periods of chest spasm creating apneic periods because I could not overcome the muscle spasm by willing to breathe.[25] This episode, lasting about half an hour, was terrifying. A few years ago, I tried the same dose of nicotinic acid, and had exactly the same violent reaction. However, this reaction never occurred with 250 milligrams of nicotinic acid amide taken every three hours for six doses a day. It was then that I first realized that niacin was not an innocuous material even though it was well tolerated by many. It made me feel that any patient given niacin should be given it in gradually increasing amounts if it is used at all. And, that there was no point in subjecting a patient to the flushing, itching, and other adverse reactions that nicotinic acid could cause when nicotinic acid amide would not cause such untoward effects and be just as therapeutic. As we now know from the pioneering work of Altschul, Hoffer, and Stephen, large divided doses of nicotinic acid will lower blood cholesterol in those with hypercholesterolemia whereas nicotinic acid amide will not do this. However, my major adverse reaction to nicotinic acid was not completely in vain. I noticed quite to my astonishment that the areas in which I flushed were exactly the major areas where the rash of pellagra occurred.

I had planned to become a cardiologist, and in my senior year in medical school, I worked in Dr. Frank N. Wilson Laboratory, with Franklin Johnston as my collaborator. Dr. Wilson suggested that I intern at Barnes Hospital, Washington University Medical School's teaching hospital, in St. Louis. I did so. Strangely, there was relatively little interest in the newer research using the vitamins. However, Robert Elman was researching the intravenous use of protein hydrolysates in surgical patients and was one of the pioneers who helped develop current total parenteral nutrition.

Because of recurrent infectious mononucleosis (I had two severe episodes of this in Ann Arbor), I switched from an 18-month straight medical internship to a 12-month rotating internship in medicine which included considerable work in the medical clinics and in radiology.

I rotated through the arthritis clinic and was horrified how little could be done for these sufferers. You could provide aspirin or other salycilates, hot paraffin dips, occasionally hyperthermia treatments in the "hot box," and more rarely helpful physiotherapy. Sometimes surgical ankylosis of painful joints helped relieve the pain but made the joint totally unmovable. I recommended losing weight, not injuring joints through daily activities, resting painful joints, applying heat and sometimes elevation to knee joints, and taking aspirin to a level that gave substantial relief without causing serious side effects.

In the x-ray department, I sat in at the reading of all the films that came through in a three-month period and I kept seeing all sorts of arthritic changes and developed some skill at interpreting such films.

One of the important learning experiences at Barnes Hospital was taking histories for Dr. David Preswick Barr of patients whom he wanted to use in his lectures to demonstrate certain clinical syndromes and diseases. When I took the routine history on ward patients, it was the conventional medical history that went into the

basic medical aspects of the patients' past and present health problems. But when I had a great deal of time to spend with the special
patients who were to be used in the teaching sessions, I was able to
ask questions, which gave me a very broad view of the patient in his
milieu at home, at work, at play and of his social status, his economic
problems, his interfamily problems, and the impact of his ill health
on his life and that of his family. It was astonishing how many health
problems would have escaped attention in the taking of a routine
medical history if more time was not spent with the patient and a
wider range of questions were not asked.

From Barnes Hospital, I went directly to an assistant residency
and residency in private medicine at New York's Mt. Sinai Hospital
and took care of the patients of many of the outstanding medical
leaders of our time including such physicians as Dr. George Baehr,
Dr. Burrill Crohn, Dr. Bela Schick, Dr. Arthur M. Masters, and leaders in neurology, and surgery, and surgical specialties. It was a very
good experience even though I was plagued by attacks of recurrent
infectious mononucleosis. When my residency was completed, July
1940, I started my Dazian Foundation Fellowship, and my concurrent
Emanuel Libman Fellowship, in the Physiology Department at the
Yale University School of Medicine. I worked in experimental canine
electrocardiography, with Drs. Louis Nahum and Hebbel Hoff, and
spent time teaching in the medical clinics. At the end of 1940, I was
licensed to practice medicine in Connecticut and started seeing private patients. What astonished me was that nearly all of the patients I
saw had the form of niacinamide nutritional deficiency disease that
I had learned of.

At that time, I did not have any idea why there was so much niacinamide deficiency around that was not classic end stage pellagra. It
was only in 1943, and finally in 1950, that I had a good idea why so
many people I saw as patients had nutritional deficiency diseases, primarily lacking niacinamide. And the results of treatment with niacinamide were absolutely astonishing because really sick people suddenly
developed a high degree of wellness and maintained this as long as
they continued taking niacinamide and relapsed when they stopped.

CHAPTER 9

Children's Learning and Behavioral Disorders

ADHD is not a disease; it is a nutritional deficiency.
—Lendon H. Smith, MD

An old "Shoe" cartoon strip shows an overweight, cigar-smoking old bird sitting at a diner counter. The waitress urges him to eat his carrots because it's been shown that they prevent cancer in rats. His response is, "Why would I want to prevent cancer in rats?" Then there is methylphenidate (Ritalin), which has been shown to promote cancer in mice. This drug is cheerfully given to millions of attention deficit hyperactivity disorder (ADHD) children every day. Yet as far back as 1995, the National Institutes of Health Toxicology Study stated, "There was some evidence of carcinogenic activity of methylphenidate (Ritalin) in male and female B6C3F1 mice based on the occurrence of hepatocellular neoplasms (liver cancer)."[1] This small but demonstrated carcinogenic potential of this commonly prescribed drug deserves more attention, and much more consideration of safer alternatives. Any bets on how many compliant parents have seen, let alone actually read, the full text of Ritalin's other side effects? Fortunately, there appears to be a vastly safer alternative: vitamins, particularly vitamin B_3.

TREATING ADHD WITH VITAMIN B_3 (NIACINAMIDE)

ADHD is not caused by a drug deficiency. But it may indeed be caused by profound nutrient deficiency, more accurately termed nutrient dependency.

Although all nutrients are important, the one that an ADHD child is most likely in greatest need of is vitamin B₃, niacinamide.

Over 60 years ago, niacinamide therapy pioneer William Kaufman, MD, PhD, wrote:

> Some patients have a response to niacinamide therapy which seems to be the clinical equivalent of "decreased running" observed in experimental animals. When these animals are deprived experimentally of certain essential nutriments, they display "excessive running," or hyperkinesis. When these deficient animals receive the essential nutriments in sufficient amounts for a sufficient period of time, there is exhibited a marked "decrease in running" ... [A person] in this group may wonder whether or not his vitamin medications contain a sedative. He recalls that before vitamin therapy was instituted, he had a great deal of energy and "drive," and considered himself to be a "very dynamic person." Analysis of his history indicates that prior to niacinamide therapy he suffered from a type of compulsive impatience, starting many projects which he left unfinished as a new interest distracted him, returning perhaps after a lapse of time to complete the original project. Without realizing it, he was often careless and inefficient in his work, but was "busy all the time."

This report appeared, almost as a side note, in Dr. Kaufman's 1949 book, *The Common Form of Joint Dysfunction*. So accurately does it describe the problems of ADHD children that it is difficult to believe that vitamin B₃ has been so thoroughly ignored for so long.

Dr. Kaufman continues:

> With vitamin therapy, such a patient becomes unaccustomedly calm, working more efficiently, finishing what he starts, and he loses the feeling that he is constantly driving himself. He has leisure time that he does not know how to use. When he feels tired, he is able to rest, and does not feel impelled to carry on in spite of fatigue... If such a patient can be persuaded to continue with niacinamide therapy, in time he comes to enjoy a sense of well-being, realizing in retrospect

that what he thought in the past was a super-abundance of energy and vitality was in reality an abnormal "wound-up" feeling, which was an expression of aniacinamidosis (niacin deficiency).[2]

Dr. Kaufman's observation that niacinamide is an effective remedy for hyperactivity and lack of mental focus is very important. With attention deficit hyperactivity disorder, orthodox medicine seems unwilling even to admit nutrient deficiency as a causal factor, let alone a curative one.

Dr. Kaufman advocated relatively modest quantities of niacinamide (250 milligrams) per dose but stressed the importance of the frequency (six or eight times a day) of those doses. Frequently divided doses are maximally effective. The precise amount of niacinamide that an ADHD child requires needs to be thoughtfully considered by parent and physician alike.[3] (To learn more about Dr. William Kaufman's clinical success with high-dose vitamin therapy, see Appendix 6: Vitamin Deficiency, Megadoses, and Some Supplemental History.)

Dr. Evan Shute began investigating the use of vitamin E for abruptic plancentae in 1936 and discovered it cured cardiovascular disease. Even before this, Max Gerson, MD, was treating migraine headaches with vegetable juices, and therein found an effective therapy for various forms of cancer. William Kaufman treated arthritis patients with niacinamide and noticed that it was also an effective remedy for hyperactivity and lack of mental focus. These and other natural health care milestones highlight just how dissimilar orthomolecular medicine and drug medicine truly are. While conventional medical authority would promptly admit malnutrition as one cause of cancer, and certainly as a cause of heart disease, there is a profound reluctance to allow that optimum nutrition could be curative of either. With ADHD, orthodox medicine seems unwilling even to admit nutrient deficiency as a causal factor, let alone a curative one.

Parents can change that. Just say "No" to drugs. Consider nutrition and niacin instead.

NUTRITION, NIACIN, AND CHILDREN

How many years does it take for a new way of treating behavior disorders in children to be generally accepted? The answer is forty, according to

Abram Hoffer. There are few physicians who have sufficient experience
to personally validate such a claim, but Dr. Hoffer could. He pioneered
megavitamin research and treatment back in the early 1950s, and, half a
century later, has still been largely ignored by the medical profession. In
fact, Hoffer had a seventeen-year jump on Pauling; vitamin B3 (niacin or
niacinamide) to treat behavioral disorders was first used by Hoffer and
his colleague, Dr. Humphry Osmond, in 1952. Niacin worked then, and
it works now.

I (AWS) knew of a ten-year-old boy who was having considerable
school and behavior problems. Interestingly enough, the child was already
on physician-prescribed niacin, with a total daily dose of less than 150 milligrams. Not a bad beginning, since the RDA for kids is under 20 milligrams
per day. But it wasn't enough to be effective, and the boy was slated for daily
medication. Dr. Hoffer suggested trying him on 500 milligrams niacinamide
three times daily (1,500 milligrams total). That's a lot, but niacinamide is a
comfortable, flush-free form of vitamin B3. So, they gave it a try.

What a difference!

People often ask, "If this treatment is so good, how come my doctor
doesn't know about it? How come it is not on the news?" The answer
may have more to do with medical politics than with medical science.
Consider Dr. Hoffer's views on attention deficit hyperactivity disorder:
"The DSM system [Multiaxial Diagnostic System, the standard of the
American Psychiatric Association] has little or no relevance to diagnosis.
It has no relevance to treatment, either, because no matter which terms
are used to classify these children, they are all recommended for treatment
with drug therapy" sometimes combined with other non-megavitamin
approaches. "If the entire diagnostic scheme were scrapped today, it would
make almost no difference to the way these children were treated, or to
the outcome of treatment. Nor would their patients feel any better or
worse."[4] Statements like these do not exactly endear one to the medical
community.

Criticisms and even lawsuits over the hazards of pediatric pharmaceuticals are on the rise, but neither court nor controversy can cure your
child. Badly beleaguered parents need to know what to do, and now. Saying
"No" to drugs also requires saying "Yes" to something else. That something
else is nutrition, properly employed. For those who say there is insufficient

scientific evidence to support megavitamin therapy for children's behavior disorders, we say they haven't been looking hard enough. Hoffer and his colleagues conducted the first double-blind controlled-nutrition trials in psychiatric history in 1952.

I (AH) have seen well over two thousand children under the age of fourteen since 1955.[5] The result of orthomolecular treatment in which vitamin B_3 is the main constituent has been very good, without the need to use any medication. In the early days I did on occasion use very small doses of antidepressants for children who were frequently wetting the bed. Later, I simply suggested that they eliminate the foods they were allergic to. Most of the children recovered. Recovery depended more on the cooperation of their parents, who were able to persuade even recalcitrant children that they should take their vitamins. More recently I have seen former child patients who brought their children in.

Here are a few examples to illustrate the results. One of the first was Mary (not her real name), who at age seven had been diagnosed as mentally retarded. This is too harsh a term for modern parents, and to please them, psychiatry adopted other equally erroneous names such as the ADHD series of diagnoses. Mary's mother was schizophrenic. Mary could not learn, she was developing behavioral problems, and she was being readied for classes for the retarded. I was asked to see her by a friend. At that time, I had little experience in treating children. I could not see anything wrong with her and had to accept her parent's observations. I started Mary on niacinamide, 1 gram after each of three meals. Two years later she was no better, and I saw her again. Not knowing what else to do, I suggested patience and that they should continue the supplementation. She recovered the third year. Mary completed university on the Dean's List, became a music teacher, married, raised her family, and has since retired. A small amount of a vitamin turned her life around.

In 1960, a physician phoned me, very worried about his twelve-year-old son, who was schizophrenic. His psychiatrist had advised him that he would never recover, and to lock him up and forget about him. Following my advice, he obtained niacin, but the psychiatrist refused to give it to him, stating that they had tried it, it had never worked, and it would fry his brain. All lies. So, his father began to visit him every day, and while they were walking about the grounds of the hospital, he fed his son jam sandwiches containing niacin. About twelve weeks later his son said, "Daddy, I want to go home." He later became a doctor, and one summer he worked in Professor Linus Pauling's laboratory. A small amount of a vitamin saved his life and family, and converted a tragic outcome into a happy one.

The next patient was a seven-year-old boy, who would race into his parent's bedroom at night. The boy told me that during the night, a huge vulture would fly through the closed door and that he ran into his parents' bedroom to save them from the vulture. I started him on a slow-release niacin, 1 gram taken after each of three meals. He recovered. He called me many decades later to touch base. He was a successful professional and still remembered that hallucination, as he now called it. He had forgotten why he ran into his parents' bedroom.

Another patient was a teenage boy, who came for treatment in 1973. He eventually became a professor at a major university. More recently, a man diagnosed as schizophrenic in 1976 at age sixteen came by to check whether he was still on the correct orthomolecular program. In the meantime, he had married, had two healthy children, and was working full time. He also tried to leave time for his art, which he enjoyed. I wonder how many orthodox psychiatrists can describe similar recoveries using only drugs?

The treatment of children has become even more toxic over the past five years. It has become fashionable to diagnose children, even babies, as bipolar.[6] Over one million children in the United States are being treated with adult atypical antipsychotic drugs. These drugs are poisoning huge numbers of unfortunate psychotic patients worldwide with the following side effects: diseases such as metabolic syndrome (diabetes, high blood cholesterol, high blood triglycerides), increased complications from cardiovascular pathology, neurological diseases such as tardive dyskinesia, deterioration of brain function, tranquilizer psychosis, permanent social incapacity, suicide, homicide, broken marriages and homes, homelessness, addictions to drugs and alcohol, increased prison population, more people on welfare, and more postsurgical delirious reactions of the aged on statins after surgery.

Why would anyone allow these toxic poisons to be inflicted on any population, child or adult?

NUTRITION AND CHILDREN WITH
SEVERE MENTAL CHALLENGES

There are literally hundreds of thousands of books and articles that illustrate the benefits of treating and preventing disease with high doses of nutrients. A few of the most spectacular of these publications describe the work of Dr. Ruth Flinn Harrell.[7] Initially, Dr. Harrell used nutrient-rich foods, and later, as they entered the marketplace, high doses of vitamins to treat children who had lost major parts of their brains to cancer and then to surgery. Beyond this, she treated Down syndrome and mentally challenged children in a similar manner. Her successes were spectacular. Most of these children, after nutritional treatment, returned to take their places in the local school system.[8] Improvements in IQ in some patients were in the 50 to 60 point range. One such child, who at the age of seven had never spoken a word and still wore diapers, learned to read and write at his appropriate elementary school levels, ride a bicycle and skateboard, and play team ball games. After forty days of high-dose nutrients, his IQ rose from the 25-to-30-point range to over 90. Dr. Harrell and her research team used nutritional dosages that were greatly in excess of those recommended for adults (see the table below for details). Her "super feeding" regimen for learning-disabled children included much larger doses of vitamins than other researchers are inclined to use: over 100 times the adult (not child) RDA for riboflavin; 37 times the RDA for niacin (given as niacinamide); 40 times the RDA for vitamin E; and 150 times the RDA for thiamine. Supplemental minerals and natural desiccated thyroid were also given. Harrell's team achieved results that were statistically significant, some with confidence levels so high that there was less than one chance in a thousand that the results were due to chance. Simply stated, Ruth Harrell found IQ to be proportional to nutrient dosage. This may simultaneously be the most elementary and also the most controversial mathematical equation in medicine.[9] Ruth Flinn Harrell's approach yielded smarter, happier children. Her results are sufficiently compelling justification for a therapeutic trial of orthomolecular supplementation for every learning-impaired child.[10]

DR. RUTH HARRELL'S NUTRIENT DOSES FOR LEARNING-DISABLED CHILDREN	
NUTRIENT	DOSE
Vitamin A palmitate	15,000 IU
Vitamin D (cholecalciferol)	300 IU
Thiamin	300 mg
Riboflavin	200 mg
Niacinamide	750 mg
Calcium pantothenate	490 mg
Pyridoxine hydrochloride	350 mg
Cobalamin	1,000 mcg
Folic acid	400 mcg
Vitamin C (ascorbic acid)	1,500 mg
Vitamin E (d-alpha-tocopheryl succinate)	600 IU
Magnesium (oxide)	300 mg
Calcium (carbonate)	400 mg
Zinc (oxide)	30 mg
Manganese (gluconate)	3 mg
Copper (gluconate)	1.75 mg
Iron (ferrous fumarate)	7.5 mg
Calcium phosphate	37.5 mg
Iodide (KI)	0.15 mg

FETAL ALCOHOL SYNDROME

Drinking alcohol while pregnant may result in a child having learning impairments and behavioral problems. This is known as fetal alcohol syndrome or FAS. Treatment is entirely psychosocial. Drugs commonly given to children to treat FAS, like Ritalin and Dexedrine, have been of no value. They are not even palliative. Two girls with FAS were given excellent psychosocial and nutritional care, but recovered only after supplements were added. This shows that the damage done by the alcohol is not permanent and can be corrected by giving these children the right doses of the B vitamins, especially B_3. It also suggests that had their mothers been taking more of the B vitamins, they would have given birth to babies free of FAS.

The B vitamin thiamine is also extremely valuable in correcting problems associated with alcohol poisoning, as seen in Wernicke-Korsakoff syndrome. There is, of course, a point of high-dose alcohol damage that can be irreversible. The best cure is prevention, and the best prevention is to stop drinking.

Hoffer and Foster wrote:

The sins of one's parents are often visited upon their children, and this applies particularly to fetal alcohol syndrome. These unfortunate, innocent children have not sinned. The metabolic derangement caused by the mother's use of alcohol during pregnancy surely is also present in the fetus and they are left with a major problem for which there appears to be no simple effective treatment. Hoffer treated several of these children with a multivitamin program with success. One of the main ones is vitamin B_3. The last two patients treated have shown convincingly that this is the right approach and of course will not do any harm. Here are their stories:

LR, born in May 1994 and seen September 2004, had been diagnosed with fetal alcohol syndrome. Her great-aunt took her for care. She had been neglected, later counseled, but continued to have major difficulty in focusing, frequently having to be asked the same question over and over again. She learned slowly and she suffered mood swings. She was hypervigilant and physically aggressive toward her younger sister. Dexedrine made her much worse and caused severe nightmares and visual illusions, and Ritalin, which was not as toxic as the Dexedrine, did not have any therapeutic effect.

Her aunt placed her on a dairy-free diet, which resulted in major improvement. Hoffer added niacin, 100 milligrams after each meal, ascorbic acid, 500 milligrams after each meal, the essential fatty acids, and a multivitamin complex. She did not like the niacin flush, so her B_3 was changed to inositol niacinate (no-flush niacin) 500 milligrams three times daily. When seen ten months later, she was almost normal. But because she had lost so much valuable learning experience, her aunt planned to have her go to a special school where she would be able to receive more attention from her teachers. She was cheerful, relaxed, and in Dr. Hoffer's opinion, was well on the way to complete recovery.[11]

By October 2008 she was a very good "A" student. Her personality was pleasant, helpful, and considerate. Her younger sister was born in March 2001. She was examined at the same time as her sister and appeared to be normal. It seemed likely that fetal alcohol syndrome might express itself later on. She was started on a similar program and when she was last seen she too showed major improvement and was normal.

Ieraci and Herrera found that injecting mouse pups with alcohol caused death of brain cells and behavioral changes. However, this damage was prevented when the pups were subsequently injected with nicotinamide. They recommended that "it is worth pursuing nicotinamide as a possible treatment for preventing FAS in situations where a pregnant woman is unable to stop drinking entirely."[12]

NUTRITION AND BEHAVIOR

Exceptionally high doses of nutrients can result in major positive changes in the behavior of children who have suffered significant brain trauma, in children with Down syndrome, and with other serious mental challenges. At lower dosages, it is apparent that such substances also can significantly improve antisocial behavior.

In May 2004, the Dutch Ministry of Justice provided the British Home Office with an evaluation of literature linking antisocial behavior and diet.[13] It argued that this novel approach was very cost effective, allowing both an improvement of services and an 18 percent cost savings.[14] Previous to this, in 2003, Gesch and colleagues from the University Laboratory of Physiology, University of Oxford, had reported on the results of a randomized, placebo-controlled trial.[15] Their study was designed to discover if adequate vitamin, mineral, and essential fatty acid intake reduced antisocial behavior in 231 young adult prisoners, inmates at HMYOI (Her Majesty's Young Offenders Institution) Aylesbury. For nine months, these "volunteers" were given either a placebo or capsules containing the generally accepted daily requirements of vitamins, minerals, and essential fatty acids. In addition, the subsequent number of proven offenses committed by each participant was recorded. When the trial code was broken, it was discovered that those prisoners who had received additional nutrients had committed an average of 26.3 percent fewer offenses than those in the inmate placebo group. The reduction of more serious offenses, involving violence, in the nutritionally enriched group was 37 percent. Both of these declines in antisocial behavior in the supplement group are statistically significant.

The realization that nutrition has a major impact on how humans behave is not new. As pointed out by Jack Challem[16] in the 1970s, Bill Walsh, a scientist at Argonne National Laboratory, was also working as a volunteer at Illinois' Stateville Prison. His experiences led him to compare mineral levels in the hair of twenty-four pairs of brothers. In each case, one brother was a well-behaved member of society, while the other was a "boy from hell." The results were amazing. The hair analyses showed that well-behaved males had normal mineral levels, but the imprisoned delinquents all showed one of two abnormal patterns. "Boys from hell" had either very high copper and very low zinc, sodium, and potassium levels in their hair; or they had very low zinc and copper, and very high sodium and potassium levels. In addition, the delinquents also had lead and cadmium levels that were three times greater than those of their well-behaved siblings.

Walsh subsequently found the same mineral abnormalities in a group of 192 adults, 50 percent of whom were incarcerated and the other 50 percent law-abiding. He also discovered that the two distinct, abnormal mineral and toxin levels in the hair of prisoners were linked to specific behavioral traits. Inmates with very high copper and very low zinc, sodium, and potassium levels in their hair had repeated uncontrollable temper losses. After their bursts of anger, such prisoners felt remorse for their actions. Prisoners with very low levels of copper and zinc combined with very high levels of sodium and potassium were always complaining, were mean, cruel, and defiant, and were never remorseful. Walsh eventually conducted hair mineral analysis on 28 mass murderers and serial killers. Each fell into one of the two abnormal mineral patterns. Although it is not entirely clear why some people have such unusual mineral levels in their hair and apparent associated antisocial behavior, Walsh believed that it reflected poor metallothionein function (metallothionein is a cysteine-based protein that transports metals such as copper, zinc, and cadmium in the body) that in infancy increased the probability of mercury, lead, and cadmium poisoning. Whether or not this interesting hypothesis is correct, it is clear that mineral and vitamin levels in the human body have a profound influence on human behavior, and this is still largely ignored.

CHAPTER 10

Mental Illness

For schizophrenics, the natural recovery rate is 50 percent.
With orthomolecular medicine, the recovery rate is 80 percent.
With drugs, it is 10 percent. If you use just drugs, you won't get well.
—ABRAM HOFFER, MD, PhD

The United States Patent Office delayed issuing a patent on the Wright brothers' airplane for three years because it broke accepted scientific principles.[1] This is actually true. And so is this: Vitamin B3, niacin, is scientifically proven to be effective against psychosis, and yet the medical profession has delayed endorsing it. Not for three years, but for nearly sixty.

In 1952, our late coauthor Abram Hoffer, MD, PhD, had just completed his psychiatry residency. What's more, he had proven, with the very first double-blind, placebo-controlled studies in the history of psychiatry, that vitamin B3 could cure schizophrenia. You would think that psychiatrists everywhere would have beaten a path to Saskatchewan to replicate the findings of this young Director of Psychiatric Research and his colleague, Humphry Osmond, MD.

You'd think so.

In modern psychiatry, niacin and schizophrenia are both terms that have been closeted away out of sight. And patients, tranquilized into submission or Prozac-ed into La-La Land, are often sitting idly at home or wandering the streets. In any case, it is highly doubtful that they will get much in the way of a daily vitamin intake. Those in institutions fare little better nutritionally. For everyone "knows" that vitamins do not cure "real" diseases.

For over half a century, Dr. Hoffer has dissented. His central point has been this: Illness, including mental illness, is not caused by drug deficiency. But much illness, especially mental illness, can be caused by a vitamin deficiency. This makes sense and has stood up to clinical trial again and again.

NUTRITION, NIACIN, AND MENTAL HEALTH

I (AWS) personally should have first become aware of a food-brain connection during the all-night, cookie-fired mah-jongg marathons that I indulged in all too regularly while attending Australian National University. Though arguably I was somewhat less than psychotic, my mind was nevertheless pretty whacked out on sugar, junk food, and adrenalin by 3:00 a.m. My mood was destroyed; my mind agitated; I was unable to sleep, sit still, or smile. Of course, I never entertained even the thought of a nutrition connection. For we've all been carefully taught that drugs cure illness, not diet.

And certainly not vitamin supplements!

But the truth will come out eventually. Three years later, I first saw niacin work on somebody else. He was a bona fide, properly diagnosed, utterly incurable, state-hospitalized schizophrenic patient. I did not see niacin work in the hospital, of course. The only vitamins given there are those your body can filter out of your tray of sweetened, overcooked, over-processed food. No, the patient was a fellow whose parents were desperate enough to try anything, even nutrition. Perhaps this was because their son was so unmanageably violent that he was kicked out of the asylum and sent to live with them. On a good day, his mom and dad somehow got him to take 3,000 milligrams of niacin and 10,000 milligrams of vitamin C. Formally a hyperactive insomniac, he responded by sleeping for eighteen hours the first night, and became surprisingly normal within days. It was an astounding improvement.

Sometime afterward, I tried niacin to see if it would help my own touch of sleeplessness. I found it worked nicely, and it only took a little to do so, perhaps 100 milligrams at most. Any more than that and I would experience a warm flush. But then I found that when I ate junk food or sugar in quantity, I could hold 500 milligrams or more without flushing a bit. And when I took all that niacin, instead of flipping out, I was calm. Dr. Hoffer[2] has explained why this is so:

1. Generally speaking, the more ill you are, the more niacin you can hold without flushing. In other words, if you need it, you physiologically soak up a lot of niacin. Where does it all go? Well, a good bit of it goes into making nicotinamide adenine dinucleotide, or NAD. NAD is just about the most important coenzyme in your body. It is made from niacin, as its name implies.

2. Niacin also works in your body as if it were an antihistamine. Many persons showing psychotic behavior suffer from cerebral allergies. They need more niacin in order to cope with eating inappropriate foods. They also need to stop eating those inappropriate foods, chief among them the ones they may crave the most: junk food and sugar.

3. There is a chemical found in quantity in the bodies of schizophrenic persons. It is an indole called adrenochrome. Adrenochrome (which is oxidized adrenalin) has an almost LSD-like effect on the body. That might well explain their behavior. Niacin serves to reduce the body's production of this toxic material.

I have taught nutritional biochemistry to high school, undergraduate, and chiropractic students. To most, it is not an especially gripping subject. But when even a basic working knowledge of niacin chemistry can profoundly change psychotic patients for the better, it becomes very interesting very quickly.

Dr. Hoffer treated thousands of such patients for over half a century. Medical fads come and go. But what we see today is what he saw all along: that even severely mentally ill people get well on vitamin B_3.

THE PHYSIOLOGICAL ROLE OF NIACIN

David Horrobin followed my (AH) observation that schizophrenic patients did not flush as much by developing a flush skin test, which has been amply corroborated. This increased researchers' interest in niacin receptors in the skin and elsewhere. Later the G protein-coupled niacin-responsive receptors HM74A and HM74 were identified. HM74A has a high affinity for niacin. Miller and Dulay[3] found that the protein for HM74A was decreased in schizophrenic brains compared with bipolar and normal controls. They suggest:

The possibility a deficiency in the high-affinity niacin receptor is a core feature of many individuals with schizophrenia provides a basis for research into more potent receptor agonists and therapies that might significantly increase expression of the fully functional protein.

This can be an explanation of the therapeutic value of niacin, which we discovered in 1952, and could account for the fact that so much is needed. Miller and Dulay wrote:

> In conclusion, one important implication of the data presented here is that the early clinical studies by Abram Hoffer reporting in a notable degree of success through treatment of unmedicated patients with niacin, but inconsistently, replicated in follow-up work by others, should now be reevaluated in the context of the limitations imposed by a deficient receptor. ... The possibility that a deficiency in the high affinity niacin receptors is a core feature of many individuals with schizophrenia provides a basis for research into more potent receptor agonists and therapists that might significantly increase expression of the fully-functional protein.

In 1973, I wrote in *Orthomolecular Psychiatry*, edited by Hawkins and Pauling: "It is possible and, if the views presented here are reasonably close to the truth, even highly probable, that the genetic errors which underlies the schizophrenias is an enzymatic block between tryptophan and NAD."[4] Later, Hoffer and Foster wrote:

> Niacin is not a true vitamin in the strictest sense of the term since it can be produced in the body from the amino acid tryptophan. Nevertheless, the synthesis of niacin from tryptophan is a very inefficient process and 60 milligrams of the amino acid are necessary to provide 1 milligram of niacin. This process also involves vitamins B_1, B_2, and B_6. If these are in short supply, the synthesis of vitamin B_3 will be even less efficient.

It must also be remembered that tryptophan itself is not usually very readily available in diet; especially in those eating high levels of maize.

It is clear, therefore, that humans have the ability to synthesize niacin, but this process is ineffective and is probably in evolutionary decline. Of course, vitamin B_3 is also available from many foods. If the diet contained enough of this vitamin to supply bodily requirements, there would be no need to convert tryptophan to niacin. This would liberate energy for other uses and free up tryptophan for the production of serotonin, a major neurotransmitter. It is argued that humanity has been depending more and more on vitamin B_3 derived from diet. However, recently, niacin has become less available from food. As a result, subclinical pellagra and other niacin deficiency disorders are becoming very widespread.

In a private communication to AH, Miller wrote:

A study of postmortem brain tissue was undertaken in this laboratory to quantify the protein for the high affinity niacin receptor. Although peripheral tissue bears more relationship to the blunted cutaneous flush response, it is obviously brain function that is most relevant to the schizophrenic condition. A comparison of postmortem brain samples derived from controls and schizophrenia patients revealed that the protein for the high affinity niacin receptor was significantly decreased in the schizophrenia group.

This raised the possibility of a genetic defect that would impair the amount of protein synthesized and thereby result in a compensatory upregulation of the mRNA transcript for the niacin receptor. Subsequent genetic association studies in a large cohort have confirmed that a polymorphism in the niacin receptor HM74 gene is associated with schizophrenia and bipolar disorder (Miller et al., submitted). Furthermore, the identified polymorphism affects gene expression in a manner consistent with the gene-expression difference seen between cases and controls.[5]

There is a great deal of evidence to support this argument. Some 50 percent of the population of the developed world seems to suffer from disorders or diseases that respond beneficially to niacin or niacinamide supplementation. This figure is probably an underestimate, as detailed in chapter 3. Indeed, the authors believe that the addition of 100 milligrams of niacinamide to the public diet would enormously reduce human suffering and have a major impact on the unnecessary escalation of health care costs. This additional niacinamide would probably nearly return the daily dietary intake to that of centuries ago, before the advent of food processing and widespread artificial fertilizer use. This suggested strategy is not new. During the Second World War, the United States government mandated the enrichment of flour with niacinamide. It is clear, however, that current dietary levels are still too low. Increasing the intake of niacinamide would not have any known risks, since it is not addictive or a narcotic, nor is it a euphoriant or an analgesic. In short, a small investment in niacinamide would provide huge economic and social benefits to society with no known associated risks. It must be recognized, however, that some people would require far more vitamin B_3 than others, either because of preexisting diseases and disorders, or as a result of their genetic inheritances.

> The question remains, "Why would a genetic aberration lowering niacin production in the body that could result in so many diseases or disorders become so widespread amongst the human population?" Perhaps the answer can be obtained by studying sickle-cell anemia. Roughly one out of every 400 Black Americans develops sickle-cell anemia. In those with this chronic hereditary disease, many of their red blood cells form rigid crescent or sickle shapes that cannot pass through capillaries. Affected children often die during adolescence of strokes, heart disease, and infections. Sickle-cell anemia also causes sufferers painful, unpredictable health crises. Those children that survive are underweight and slow to mature. How is it that a genetic, highly damaging disease can be so widespread amongst the Black population in the United States? What's in it for Darwin? Or more correctly asked, what is the evolutionary advantage that this mutation gives to Black people that makes its obvious disadvantages worthwhile? After all, as McElroy and Townsend point out, "It is only the phenotypic characteristics that give some advantage of degree of Darwinian fitness that are subject to selective action."[6]

So, what is going on? Vitamin B₃ (niacin or niacinamide) is involved in almost all the oxidation and reduction reactions in the body. Tryptophan is processed in the body into a number of very important substances. The overall pathway leading from tryptophan to NAD (nicotinamide adenine dinucleotide) and NADH (NAD plus hydrogen), the active antipellagra coenzymes, is not very efficient. It converts less than 2 percent of tryptophan into these enormously important substances. A major pathway for conversion is the kynurenine pathway. This enzyme is more active in schizophrenic brains, and this can account for the decrease in the formation of B₃ by diverting more of the tryptophan into this pathway instead of into B₃.[7]

A block between tryptophan and NAD might provide an evolutionary advantage, as long as dietary (exogenous) vitamin B₃ was high. It now appears that there are several possible genetic pathways. And among these we must include those needed to maintain NAD levels in the body, those that permit the production of excess amounts of adrenochrome, and those that prevent an optimum supply of the antioxidants. Modern views of the genes possibly involved are discussed by Foster and Hoffer in their reports. A deficiency of the NAD↔NADH system may be one of the most important causes. There are many triggers but most of them can be overcome with the use of adequate supplementation with vitamin B₃, which leads to an increased amount of NAD in the body.

Indoleamine 2,3-dioxygenase (IDO) is necessary for the degradation of tryptophan into B₃. We do not know if IDO activity is higher in schizophrenics. There is probably a higher-than-normal expression of the nicotinic acid G-protein coupled receptor.[8,9,10]

The discovery of nicotinic acid (niacin) receptors in the brain may help us understand why schizophrenic patients become so easily addicted to nicotine and find it so difficult to stop. This has been known about, and puzzling, for decades.[11] Nicotine, the poison, might be involved in the same biochemical reactions as niacin.[12]

There are probably several relationships between smoking (nicotine) and schizophrenia. I have advised clients who have schizophrenia not to stop smoking until they showed substantial progress on the orthomolecular program. If nicotine does attach to the nicotinic acid receptors, it may also act as a therapeutic imitator of niacin. If nicotine were not so toxic, it might be a very valuable treatment. But its toxicity overwhelms its benefits, and patients should discontinue its use as soon as it becomes possible. If they do not get well, they will not stop smoking. Luckily, schizophrenic patients do not get cancer of the lungs to the same extent as the rest of the population.[13] Nicotine may be considered a very toxic analogue of niacin. It is not surprising that taking niacin makes it easier for smokers to stop their habit.[14]

Psychiatric Disorders Need Niacin in Particular

To treat schizophrenia and schizoaffective disorder, the main emphasis should be on vitamin B$_3$. I have successfully treated over 5,000 patients this way.

Schizophrenia is not a multivitamin deficiency disease. It is pellagra, a vitamin B$_3$ dependency, and it will not be treated successfully, no matter how many dozens of vitamin pills are given, if these patients are not given the correct doses of this vitamin. You can give pellagrins every known nutrient, but if you do not give them B$_3$ they will still remain pellagrins.

I have always maintained that schizophrenia was a *B$_3$ dependency disease*, and not a multivitamin deficiency disease, and that large and sometimes very large doses are needed for treatment. I cannot believe that doctors could have failed so miserably to realize that while all the vitamins are helpful in restoring health, recovery will not occur if the schizophrenic patient (pellagrin) is not given the B$_3$ they require. A patient with pellagra can be given tons of vitamins, but they will not recover until the right amount of B$_3$ is added. And in most patients I have seen who failed to get well, most of the other vitamins they were taking were not needed, as they are available in food. In other words, they were forced to buy exorbitant amounts of pills they did not need. If your patients have scurvy, give them ascorbic acid, not niacin. If they are schizophrenic, give them vitamin B$_3$—but in the right doses.

Schizophrenia and pellagra differ in that pellagra needs small doses of vitamin B$_3$ in most cases, and schizophrenia needs large doses in most cases. As discussed in chapter 3, pellagra is a deficiency, and schizophrenia is a dependency.

Unfortunately, the vasodilatation (flush) caused by niacin when it is first taken has given niacin a bad name. Even today most doctors are more fearful of this vitamin, which kills no one, than they are of the major atypical antipsychotics, which kill many. The flush is a minor problem when niacin is used by doctors who know what they are doing. I had hoped that the results I have published—with hundreds of case histories, confirmed by every physician who used the same protocols—would have made other doctors comfortable with niacin by now. But unfortunately, this has not happened.

I foresee a major problem in getting physicians to accept this treatment if a large number of patients are only treated with multivitamins and do not get enough B₃. The establishment will believe they are correct in concluding that there is no connection between schizophrenia and the use of B₃, and this valuable treatment will be set back another forty years. If this happens, schizophrenic patients all over may lose a viable chance for healing. Instead, they will be given modern equivalents of mercury, alum, nitre, and, of course, ever more tranquilizers to correct the fanciful imbalances of "humors in the brain" (the neurotransmitters).

THE MAIN PSYCHOTIC DISORDERS

Of the $225 billion the United States spent in 2019 on psychiatric care, the lion's share went for drugs to treat psychotic disorders. This represents an increase of 52 percent since 2009 (accessed Sept 2022. https://openminds .com/intelligence-report/the-u-s-mental-health-market-225-1-billion-in-spending-in-2019-an-open-minds-market-intelligence-report/). Niacin can be useful to many of these patients. Niacin, given along with conventional drug therapy, reduces the amount of medication needed and reduces medication side effects. Niacin greatly reduces costs and increases treatment success.

The psychotic disorders are differentiated into primary groups, which can be identified by their characteristics.

THE SCHIZOPHRENIAS

Schizophrenic disorders are characterized by perceptual changes (hallucinations) and thought disorder (delusions). These are pellagra syndromes, including Huntington's disease, some Parkinsonism patients, schizoaffective patients, and LSD induced psychosis. I consider these conditions variants of pellagra. Schizoaffective patients have mood swings, and during their manic states will also have schizophrenic symptoms. These pellagra variants are responsive to vitamin B_3 when adequate doses are used. They will not respond to small doses or to other nutrients. They are B_3 *dependent* conditions, and should not be considered as deficiency diseases. Too many clinicians have ignored this and have tried to treat their patients with a multiplicity of nutrients but without using enough B_3. They therefore have not seen the therapeutic results that occur when the correct dose of this vitamin is used.

Patients with Parkinson's disease tend to develop psychosis, and this is more probable when they take L-dopa, which can be converted into dopachrome in the brain. Niacin protects them from the psychosis and coenzyme Q_{10} (CoQ_{10}) protects against neurological changes such as tremor.

Both niacin and niacinamide are antidotes to the LSD reaction.[15] If 100 milligrams of niacin is given intravenously to a person under the influence of LSD, most of the reaction will be gone in a few minutes. Many years back, when we were routinely using psychedelic treatment for alcoholics, we would terminate the experience with either IV niacin or oral niacin (500 milligrams three times daily) if it lasted too long or if it became too unpleasant for the patient.

Schizoaffective Disorder

Schizoaffective patients should be treated as if they were schizophrenic. Lewis and Pietrowski[16] found that half of a large series of manic-depressive (bipolar) patients, followed up during subsequent hospitalizations, were clearly schizophrenic by their final diagnosis. This important study has been overlooked or ignored by modern psychiatry, which tends to call anyone with a mood swing "bipolar" no matter how schizophrenic they are during their manic phase. I have seen the same change in diagnosis with repeated admissions.

I have written about the orthomolecular treatment of the schizophrenias over the past fifty years. A large literature of clinical studies is available in standard journals and in the *Journal of Orthomolecular Medicine*, beginning with our very first double-blind studies.

Letter from a Patient

I'm writing to thank you for changing my life. You may remember that I was in despair: I thought I'd have to quit my job, and most days were pretty miserable for me. Niacin changed everything. It enables me to enjoy my teaching once more, to be able to relate to the students and anyone else, to think and communicate clearly, and just to be a "normal" person. Like you said, it's not perfect, but the improvement has been incredibly great. I also take the other vitamins, and follow the other suggestions you made to me, but the niacin is at the heart of it all. If only I had called you years ago. But the niacin sure helped when things were at their worst. Thank you again.

Bipolar Disorder

Bipolar disorder is characterized by a series of mood swings, which swing from mania to depression, with normal periods in between. Most of the time, there are no perceptual symptoms or thought disorder. The cycle varies tremendously from once a month to once every few years. Modern drugs distort the typical cycle, and in many cases, convert depression into mania.

When normal or depressed, bipolar patients do not suffer the typical schizophrenic symptoms, but during manic episodes they may often hear voices and see visions, which clear as the mania clears. We therefore have at least two types of bipolar: those who never have any schizophrenic symptoms and those who do when they are manic. How, then, are we to differentiate the two types? Psychiatry got around this by giving those who suffer from schizophrenic episodes both diagnoses: they are called schizoaffective.

These types also respond differently to orthomolecular therapy. Non-schizophrenic bipolar patients need mood-stabilizing treatment, while the schizoaffective patients need this treatment plus treatment for the schizophrenic component of their disease. I find that schizoaffective patients are much easier to treat than bipolar or schizophrenic patients.

Diagnosis can be very difficult for these patients, and often it depends more on the orientation of the diagnostician than on the disease itself. The diagnosis, schizophrenia, is so dismal and carries such a poor prognosis that many physicians prefer not to consider it. If their patients have mood swings, minor or major, they will call them bipolar. A large proportion of the schizophrenic patients referred to me were originally diagnosed as bipolar, and their perceptual changes had either not been elicited or were ignored. In a major recent study, Weiser et al.[17] found that nearly 30 percent of a schizophrenic population had been diagnosed with affective disorder during adolescence compared with only 7 percent of the general population. This confirmed what I have been seeing for the past fifty years.

Niacin treatment is similar for all psychotic patients. Many years ago, I did not consider that vitamin B_3 would be useful in treating bipolar patients. I was still in my "establishment" stage, from which I have recovered. Over the years I have become more and more aware of the importance of niacin for bipolar patients. Several years ago, a middle-aged woman consulted with me. She had been diagnosed as schizoaffective, with two enforced admissions to the hospital. Each time she was force-treated with drugs, which she stopped taking when she was discharged. But after her last discharge she started to take niacin, an astonishing 30 grams in the morning and again in the evening. By the time I saw her six months later, she was normal. She told me she would rather take 120 pills of 500 milligrams niacin daily than any of the awful drugs she had been given in the hospital. Very, very few patients can take so much niacin without developing severe nausea and vomiting.

Delirium, Including Delirium Tremens

Dr. Humphry Osmond and I developed a treatment protocol for alcoholics in delirium tremens (DTs) or in a predeleriod state. On admission, they were given niacin (500 milligrams I.V. and 3,000 milligrams oral) and ascorbic acid (2,000 milligrams). On the first day, they received niacin (3,000 milligrams) after each of three meals, the same amount of vitamin C, and a sedative, if needed. This was to be continued until they were free of the delirium. The results were very dramatic. In most cases, delirium tremens and acute alcoholic intoxications respond well within twenty-four hours. For this purpose, it is as good as the tranquilizers that were commonly used at the time, but it has the added advantage that there is no sedation.

The patient remains more alert and, after a few hours, is cooperative. There are no toxic complications. Our studies in Saskatchewan corroborated Dr. Gould's observations in England. These doses were much larger than the usual recommended daily doses.

I have routinely given patients niacin to reverse delirium or to protect them from developing perceptual disturbances that predominate in deliria. These deliriod states, called DTs, are common in alcoholics and in other drug-induced toxic conditions. Niacin is also useful in protecting statin-induced delirium after surgery. Redelmeier et al.[18] found that patients are at greater risk for developing postoperative delirium if they were on statins. Mercantonio[19] concluded that the use of statins increased the incidence by 30 percent, even though the study his conclusion was based upon under-estimated the risk. However, being too cautious, they did not recommend stopping the statins. There is no need to use the statins at any time since niacin is much superior to any individual statin or combination of statins. It is the only compound that effectively increases high-density cholesterol levels in blood, which is the most important risk factor for vascular disease when it is too low. If patients were taking niacin instead of the statins, they would also be protected against postsurgical deliria.

POST-ELECTROCONVULSIVE CONFUSION

In 1952 a very unhappy man and very confused woman came to me for help. I could get no information from her, but her husband told me she had been very depressed and had been committed to a mental hospital where she had been given a series of electroconvulsive therapy (ECT) treatments. She was discharged home but had been totally confused for the next month. She displayed a typical organic confusional state, as if she were developing Alzheimer's disease. I had never seen a patient with this reaction to ECT and really did not know what to do, but I had read of niacin's use for confusional states in the 1940s and was certain it would do no harm. I started her on 1 gram taken three times daily after meals, and mailed her a supply from my office, as 500 milligram tablets were not available in stores. When I saw her again one month later, I saw an entirely different couple. He was cheerful and she had regained her previous normal personality. There was no evidence of confusion.

At the sixth meeting of the Saskatchewan Committee on Schizophrenia Research (June 11 to 12, 1953), I reported:

Often the underlying psychosis is banished by ECT and instead is replaced by a mental picture including memory loss, confusion, and aggressivity. EEG [electroencephalogram] records show some neuropsychological pathology; Lehmann first reported that these respond well to niacin. We have not run a series to further test this but plan to do so. Further, it may be successful in preventing the confusion following epileptic convulsions.

This was the beginning of my conviction that niacin must always be given with ECT, and this conviction has become stronger every year. Since then, I would never give any patients ECT without niacin. I consider that giving ECT without niacin should be looked upon as malpractice.

I have not needed to use ECT for many years, but there have been a few times when I recommended to patients that they should receive it from their psychiatrist. I think the art of giving ECT with minimum discomfort and minimum memory loss and maximum therapeutic effect is being lost. It causes much less harm than antipsychotic drugs.

CHAPTER 11

Cardiovascular Disease

Niacin is really it. Nothing else available is that effective.
—STEVEN E. NISSEN, M.D., PAST PRESIDENT OF THE AMERICAN
COLLEGE OF CARDIOLOGY, QUOTED IN THE NY TIMES, JAN 23, 2007

It is well established that niacin helps reduce harmful cholesterol levels in the bloodstream. Niacin is one of the best substances for elevating high-density lipoprotein cholesterol (the "good" cholesterol), and niacin provides other valuable cardiovascular benefits as well.

But you'd never know this from the headlines. A recent study has been frequently trumpeted to imply that niacin does not work, and that it is somehow detrimental. That, to put it scientifically, is a lot of baloney. Specifically, the researchers reported that the drug simvastatin worked better than simvastatin with Niaspan. Niaspan, an extended-release form of niacin, is alleged to have caused about a 1 percent increase in cardiovascular events. The drug somehow evaded suspicion, and blame was attached to the vitamin. That in itself is questionable. What's more, in this study there was no examination of Niaspan alone. There was also no consideration at all of immediate-release, plain old regular niacin. Regular niacin works just fine, and safely.[1]

NIACIN BEATS STATINS: SUPPLEMENTS AND DIET ARE SAFER, MORE EFFECTIVE

Statins for everyone? If media are to be believed, and if the drug industry has its way, the answer is "you bet." The American Academy of Pediatrics has stated that kids as young as eight years of age might take statin drugs. Specifically: *"As a group, statins have been shown to reduce LDL cholesterol in children and adolescents with marked LDL cholesterol elevation . . . when used from 8 weeks to 2 years for children aged 8 to 18 years."*[2]

Strangely enough, American Academy of Pediatrics projects appear to have received cash from Merck & Co., Pfizer, and Sanofi-Aventis, as well as from Procter & Gamble, Nestlé, and other large corporations.[3]

Statin drugs can produce serious side effects in adults. Such risk is of even more concern for the still-developing bodies of children. Statin side effects may include liver damage; elevated CPK (creatine kinase) and/or muscle pain, aches, and muscle tenderness or weakness (myalgia); drowsiness; myositis (inflammation of the muscles); rare but potentially fatal kidney failure from rhabdomyolysis (severe inflammation of muscle and muscle breakdown); memory loss; mental confusion; personality changes or irritability; headaches; difficulty sleeping, anxiety; depression; chest pain; high blood sugar and type 2 diabetes; acid regurgitation; dry mouth; digestive problems including bloating, gas, diarrhea or constipation; nausea and/or vomiting, or abdominal cramping and pain; rash; leg pain; insomnia; eye irritation; tremors; dizziness; and more.

What a list. Well, this is America, and you have the right to remain sick. Evidently you also have the right to be continually bombarded with exhortations to take statins, and to give them to your children as well. Statins for second graders? Sure! Do you want fries with that? The news media, television commercials, medical schools, and especially the pharmaceutical industry all want you and your family to be good, uncritical, daily consumers of pharmaceutical medicine.

However, **you also have the right to refuse drugs, and you have available nutrition-based alternatives**. Here are researchers and physicians who say "No" to statins, and their reasons that they provided me (AWS) with:

Robert G. Smith, PhD, Research Associate Professor, University of Pennsylvania

"Although statins can lower cholesterol, they lower the risk for heart disease mainly through their anti-inflammatory and anti-clotting effects. However, statins have many side effects, some very serious, and for most people do not greatly reduce the risk of heart disease. Niacin is a much safer way to lower cholesterol. A much more effective treatment to prevent heart disease is vitamin C taken to bowel tolerance (3,000 to 10,000 milligrams per day in divided doses), vitamin E (400 to 1,600 international units per day), niacin (800 to 2,000 milligrams per day in divided doses), magnesium (chelate, citrate, malate, chloride, 300 to 600 milligrams per day, divided doses), along with an excellent diet that includes generous servings of leafy green vegetables and only moderate amounts of meat."

Thomas E. Levy, MD, JD, Cardiologist

"The lower your cholesterol goes, the greater your risk of cancer, as cholesterol is a protective agent against toxins. Efforts to lessen the chances of morbidity and mortality of one major disease (coronary artery disease) should not substantially increase the chances of morbidity and mortality from another disease (cancer)."

Ralph Campbell, MD

"You have likely heard about the conclusions from Cleveland Clinic gathering of heart specialists. Their objective was to zoom in on LDL levels as they relate directly to heart disease. No mention of LDL/HDL ratio or of triglyceride levels. Again, niacin got very little recognition. Statins have some side effects that are serious, including rhabdomyolisis and kidney failure. The panel was made up of many with financial ties to industry, but 'it is practically impossible to find a large group of outside experts who have no relationship to industry.' This was followed (yes, actually) by stating the new guidelines are based on solid evidence and that the public should *trust* them."

Carolyn Dean, MD, ND, author of The Magnesium Miracle

"The mineral magnesium is the natural way that the body has evolved to control cholesterol when it reaches a certain level, whereas statin drugs are used to destroy the whole process. If sufficient magnesium is present in the body, cholesterol will be limited to its necessary functions—the production of hormones and the maintenance of membranes—and will not be produced in excess."

Jorge Miranda, PharmD

"Statin drugs are one of my favorite examples of a sickening drug. A fixation on cholesterol fails to address the importance of correcting the excessive oxidation of LDL, and fails to recognize the importance of correcting many other contributing risk factors such as homocysteine, lipoprotein(a) (LPa), and C-reactive protein (CRP). It is important to recognize that the reason we form cholesterol is because it's needed to form membrane, the eye's lens, hormones, and many other molecules including CoQ10. Decreasing cholesterol decreases CoQ10, which means less energy for a multitude of functions. The result can be neurologic disease and even cancer."

William B. Grant, PhD, SUNARC

"Statin use reduces CoQ10 concentrations and leads to myopathy (muscle weakness), which can lead to heart failure. Those taking statins should be aware of this problem and consider taking CoQ10 supplements."

Damien Downing, MBBS, MSB

"Statins overall succeed in reducing the risk of coronary events by about 17 percent—but that is *relative* risk. Taking a statin each day actually lowers one's chance of an event by about 0.16 percent—that is the absolute risk. But these figures are not lives saved; recent meta-analysis found only a non-significant reduction in mortality of 7 per 10,000 patient-years, or 0.07 percent. The difference between statins' effects on relative risk and absolute risk is about two orders of magnitude. Just ask any man in the street whether a reduction of

0.16 percent in the risk of a coronary event is 'significant' to him, and whether it warrants him taking statins. Unpleasant muscular side effects occur in up to 10 percent of statin-takers, which may rise to 25 percent if the person exercises; this is unhelpful to anybody seeking to improve their cardiovascular health. But because the primary threshold for acceptance under 'evidence-based medicine' is statistical significance, we are to accept that the benefit of statins has been proven. Data on worldwide sales of statins currently run at approximately US $30 billion per year."

Perhaps this helps explain the massive media blitz favoring statins. But drugs are not the answer, unless you are a drug company.[4]

Laropiprant Is the Bad One; Niacin Is/Was/Will Always Be the Good One

by W. Todd Penberthy, PhD

Niacin has been used for over 60 years in tens of thousands of patients with tremendously favorable therapeutic benefit.[5] In the *New York Times* best-seller *The 8-Week Cholesterol Cure*, the author describes his journey from being a walking heart attack time bomb to becoming a healthy individual. He hails high-dose niacin as the one treatment that did more to correct his poor lipid profile than any other.[6] Many clinical studies have shown that high doses of niacin (3,000 to 5,000 milligrams of inexpensive immediate-release niacin, taken in divided doses, spread out over the course of a day) cause dramatic reductions in total mortality in patients that experienced previous strokes.[7] High-dose niacin has also been clinically proven to provide positive transformational relief to many schizophrenics in studies involving administration of immediate-release niacin in multi-thousand-milligram quantities to greater than 10,000 patients.[8] Most importantly, after 60 years of use the safety profile for niacin (especially immediate-release niacin) remains far safer than the safest drug.[9]

Bad Reporting

So why has the media suddenly presented the following niacin alarm-ist headlines in response to a study in the *New England Journal of Medicine*?

> *"Niacin drug causes serious side effects, study says."*
>
> —Boston Globe, 7/16/14

> *"Niacin safety, effectiveness questioned in new heart study."*
>
> —Healthday News, 7/17/14

> *"Doctors say cholesterol drug risky to take."*
>
> —Times Daily, 7/16/14

> *"Niacin risks may present health risks, claim scientists."*
>
> —Viral Global News, 7/17/14

> *"Studies reveal new niacin risks."*
>
> —Drug Discovery and Development, 7/17/14

> *"No love for niacin."*
>
> —Medpage Today, 7/17/14

> *"Niacin could be more harmful than helpful."*
>
> —Telemanagement, 7/18/14

The truth of the matter is that the study quoted used laropiprant (trade names: Cordaptive and Tredaptive). Laropiprant is a questionable drug, and the results say next to nothing about niacin. The study compared over 25,000 patients treated with either niacin along with laropiprant, or placebo. The patients in this study had previous history of myocardial infarction, cerebrovascular disease, peripheral arterial disease, or diabetes mellitus with evidence of symptomatic coronary disease. The side effects observed in those who took the laropiprant-niacin combination were serious and included an increase in total mortality as well as significant increases in the risk for developing diabetes.

For responsible reporters, this should have raised the question of which compound, the drug laropiprant or the vitamin niacin, is the culprit.

Such side effects have not been seen in over 10 major clinical trials of niacin involving tens of thousands of patients, nor in over 60 years of regular usage of niacin in clinics across the country. In this study, niacin was given in combination with laropiprant, a drug that prevents the niacin flush. By including a dose of laropiprant along with the niacin to eliminate the flush, the thought was that more patients could benefit from niacin without complaint. But in fact the niacin flush is healthy. A reduced flush response to niacin is a diagnostic for increased incidence of schizophrenia, and this assay is now widely available.[10]

Problems with Laropiprant

So, what about the other half of the combo, the drug laropiprant?

Laropiprant has never been approved by the FDA for use in the United States, and when taken alone, has been shown to increase gastrointestinal bleeding. Laropiprant also interferes with a basic prostaglandin receptor pathway that is important for good health.

In 2013, Merck announced it would withdraw laropiprant worldwide due to complaints from continental Europe. Therefore, the clinical trials in this most recent study could only be performed in the UK, Scandinavia, and China. So why did so many media outlets and even some MDs conclude that niacin was the problem? Simple: none of the headlines mentioned laropiprant, which is quite clearly the real culprit that caused the side effects reported. The simplest way to put it is to say that sensational stories promulgated by the media are quite often completely wrong. This suggests a hidden agenda.

Confusing and fantastical headlines can increase readership for hysteria-based business models. Which headline is likely to garner the greatest attention: "Laropiprant is a Dangerous Medication that has Not Been Approved by the FDA" or "Niacin Causes Serious Side Effects"? The correct headline would be, "Niacin doesn't cause serious side effects; drugs do."

Why the B Vitamins Are So Important

The B vitamins were discovered due to terrible nutritional epidemics: pellagra (niacin/vitamin B_3 deficiency) and beriberi (thiamine/vitamin B_1 deficiency). We are very sensitive to a deficiency of niacin. Over 100,000 people died in the American South in the first two decades of the 20th century due to a lack of niacin in their diet. It was perhaps the worst nutritional epidemic ever observed in modern times, and was a ghastly testimony to how vulnerable humans are to niacin deficiency. The pellagra and beriberi epidemics took off shortly after the introduction of processed foods such as white rice and white flour. Poor diets, mental and physical stresses, and certain disease conditions have all been proven to actively deplete nicotinamide adenine dinucleotide (NAD) levels, causing patients to respond favorably to greater than average niacin dosing.

How is it possible that niacin can be useful for so many different conditions? It seems too good to be true. The reason is that niacin is necessary for more biochemical reactions than any other vitamin-derived molecule: over 450 different gene-encoded enzymatic reactions.[11] That is more reactions than any other vitamin-derived co-factor! Niacin is involved in just about every major biochemical pathway. Some individuals, who have a genetically encoded amino acid polymorphism within the NAD binding domain of an enzyme protein, will have a lower binding affinity for NAD that can only be treated by administering higher amounts of niacin to make the amount of NAD required for normal health. Genetic differences such as these are why many individuals require higher amounts of niacin in order for their enzymes to function correctly.[12]

It is a deadly shame that the media so often ignores this information. Fortunately, many physicians will see through the recent headlines that give misinformation about niacin, having already personally witnessed how effective high-dose niacin therapy is for preventing cardiovascular disease.

Nutrients Are the Solution, Not the Problem

So what is the solution? At the end of the day, the data on patients with problem cholesterol/LDL levels still support 3,000 to 5,000 milligrams of immediate-release niacin as the best clinically-proven approach to maintaining a healthy lipid profile. Niacin in 250- to 1,000-milligram doses can be purchased inexpensively from many sources. Extended-release niacin is the form of niacin that is most frequently sold by prescription, but it has more side effects than immediate-release (plain old) niacin. . . and it costs much more.

Tangential to niacin but pointed to cardiovascular disease, conventional medicine is finally beginning to respect chelation therapy as an approach owing to the recent unparalleled positive clinical results for cardiovascular disease patients with diabetes—up to 50 percent prevention of recurrent heart attacks and 43 percent reduction in death rate from all causes.[13] Sometimes chelation therapy can be expensive. However, an inexpensive approach that is yet to be conventionally appreciated includes high-dose IP6 therapy. Other supplements desirable for therapeutic treatment of individuals with cardiovascular disease include: vitamin C, magnesium, coenzyme Q, fat-soluble vitamins (A, D, E, and K2), and grass-fed organic butter. Your ideal intake varies with your individuality.

Nutrients such as niacin you need. Media misinformation you don't.

NIACIN IS THE SAFEST AND MOST EFFECTIVE WAY TO CONTROL CHOLESTEROL (BUT YOU'D NEVER KNOW IT FROM THE MEDIA)

The health benefits of niacin are again being challenged. Why? The simple answer is to follow the money. Cholesterol-controlling drugs are cash cows for the trillion-dollar-per-year pharmaceutical industry. Niacin is cheap, does not require a prescription, and safe. Drugs are much more dangerous and considerably less effective. Niacin is not being attacked because it doesn't work. Niacin is being attacked because it *does* work.

WHAT YOU ARE HEARING

"HPS2-THRIVE: No Benefit, Signal of Harm for Niacin Therapy"
—Forbes[14]

"ACC: HPS2-THRIVE May Signal the End for Niacin"
—Medpage

"Niacin Causes Serious Unexpected Side-effects,
but no Worthwhile Benefits, for Patients who are at
Increased Risk of Heart Attacks and Strokes"
—Sacramento Bee

"Niacin Therapy Unhelpful, Occasionally Harmful"
—Naharnet

"Niacin doesn't help heart, may cause harm, study says"
—USA Today

Sadly, these headlines ignore the full story, and are incorrect because they place the blame on niacin while ignoring the adverse effects of laropiprant and statins. Although statins are widely used, they have serious side effects in some people, and will not help most who take them.[15]

"Niacin is really it. Nothing else available is that effective."
—Steven E. Nissen, MD, Chairman of the Department
of Cardiovascular Medicine at the Cleveland Clinic
and past president of the American College of
Cardiology, quoted in the *New York Times*, Jan 23, 2007

THE REAL STORY

A recent widely publicized interventional study on the benefit of tredaptive, a compound drug containing an extended-release form of niacin and a drug called laropiprant, has been interpreted in the media as showing that niacin may have dangerous side effects. The study was designed to determine the advantage of tredaptive to participants who were already taking a dose of statins to reduce symptoms of high cholesterol and heart disease.[16] However, the study was focused on the benefit of a specific combination of drugs, and therefore cannot determine the efficacy of niacin. This essential vitamin is already known to be very safe and effective for lowering cholesterol. Rather, the study confounds the well-known benefits of niacin with the unknown dangers of incompletely tested drugs.

THE HPS2-THRIVE STUDY

The study on tredaptive was performed on two groups totaling 25,673 participants, in which one group took a dose of statin along with extended-release niacin plus laropiprant, and the other group took the same dose of statin along with a placebo.[16] The groups were followed for about four years, and the medical outcomes were tabulated. The group that received the niacin and laropiprant had a slightly increased amount of myopathy (muscle weakness), especially in a subgroup that tended to have increased rates of myopathy compared to the general population. This group did not show any advantage from niacin. In addition, those receiving niacin had a higher rate of stopping their medication, mainly because of its well-known effect of causing skin flushes.

The study of tredaptive was stopped prematurely, and it has been removed from the market. But this should not be taken as an argument against using niacin. Rather, it should be a notice for caution about the use of *extended-release* niacin in combination with these two other drugs that are known to have side effects. This is consistent with previous knowledge that prescription extended or slow-release forms of niacin are less safe than plain standard niacin. Further, there may also be a special problem in the combination with the statin and laropiprant drugs utilized in the study. This emphasizes that knowledge about laropiprant and its effects in combination with other drugs such as statins is insufficient. Although tredaptive is now unavailable for ordinary patients, and was never approved for sale in the USA, doctors continue to advise the use of niacin for its beneficial effects.

> *"Niacin is the best substance currently available for the control of cholesterol. It decreases the incidence of coronary disease and strokes and raises life expectancy."*
> —WILLIAM B. PARSONS JR., MD, MAYO CLINIC RESEARCHER[17]

WHICH IS THE CULPRIT: THE DRUG OR THE VITAMIN?

Which component of the tredaptive drug trial should be blamed for causing problems? Apparently, the headlines have implicated niacin by default. After all, it can cause flushes! Well, niacin, an essential nutrient, has been used very safely at very high doses (1,000 to 2,000 milligrams or higher) for over 60 years. It has been shown to reduce mortalities due to cardiovascular disease, even 10 years after patients stop taking it.[18–20] The effect of niacin in preventing dyslipidemia (to correct an unfavorable blood lipid profile) is known to occur through PGD1 (prostaglandin) pathways. In contrast, laropiprant is a relatively new drug that blocks PDG1 pathways. It was included in the compound drug tredaptive to prevent the niacin flush side effect that sometimes occurs in some patients. However, it was not included for any clinically beneficial effect on cardiovascular disease, and it may have even blocked the desired effects of niacin. The prostaglandin pathways inside cells are complex, and they are a current topic of intense research. In some studies, laropiprant showed a side effect on platelet DP1 receptors, which suggests that it may have adverse side effects on other receptors than on blood vessels within the skin, for example, in lung tissue and in the brain.[21,22]

The safety of laropiprant, when taken along with statins, has not been carefully studied. Pharmaceutical companies that design and manufacture these drugs, and the patients that use them, need to be very cautious about side effects, for they can be serious and unpredictable. Compared to laropiprant, niacin has been widely studied and shown safe in thousands of studies. Its use and effects are described in more than 7,000 publications in PubMed since 1943 (and in more than 35,000 as its alternate name "nicotinic acid"). For comparison, laropiprant is described in fewer than 100 studies within the last seven years. Thus, overall, the study provides no evidence of harm by niacin, and in testing a new combination of drugs has apparently discovered they can cause an adverse reaction in some people. Therefore, in combination with statins and extended-release niacin, laropiprant may be the culprit.

FORMS AND BENEFITS OF NIACIN

Niacin comes in several forms, including niacinamide and standard "fast-release" niacin. They both help to increase cellular NAD, an essential metabolic molecule for all life, but significantly, only niacin can raise HDL (good cholesterol) more than any statin while simultaneously lowering VLDL (very low-density lipoprotein), triglycerides (a risk factor for atherosclerosis), and total cholesterol. These outcomes are commonly desirable in most high-risk cardiovascular disease patients. However, niacin has also been shown to elevate NAD more than niacinamide in many cell types, making niacin superior to niacinamide for helping to prevent disease.

THE NIACIN FLUSH

A problem for some people is that niacin can cause the well-known side effect, the "niacin flush." This temporary (30 to 60 minutes) sometimes itchy redness of the skin occurs in some people after taking large therapeutic doses. Yet on the whole, the niacin flush is associated with beneficial health effects. Niacin specifically activates the high affinity G-protein coupled receptors, GPR109a and b, which then leads to release of a variety of prostaglandins that results in the flush response. This effect of niacin that causes vasodilation and the flush is widely understood to correct dyslipidemia. Although some people describe the niacin flush as a side effect, it means that the body is correcting its lipid metabolic lipid pathways, which may be important in preventing atherosclerosis.[23] Other forms of niacin, such as slow- or extended-release niacin, will not cause a flush but may also be less effective in prevention or treatment of atherosclerosis. Further, in some people slow release or non-flush niacin can result in an alarming increase in liver enzymes. Although in most accounts the niacin flush is associated with beneficial effects, it is perceived as uncomfortable by some people. For those who want to use niacin but avoid a flush, it is straightforward to find the largest dose that provides a minimal flush response. Niacin hardly ever causes a serious adverse response, but rather the response is temporary, and at worse mildly uncomfortable.

In order to slowly acclimate the body to niacin and minimize the flush, the following steps can be taken:

Anyone interested in this approach might go to a discount store and buy a bottle of 100 milligrams niacin tablets and a bottle of 1,000 milligrams vitamin C tablets.

One should expect to begin by taking 1,000 milligrams of vitamin C and 50 milligrams of niacin three times a day, preferably after each meal. Niacin tablets are scored, and a 100 milligrams tablet is easily broken along the score to produce two 50 milligrams half-tablets of niacin.

After three or four days, the niacin dosage is increased to 100 milligrams three times a day. One might continue increasing the niacin by 50 milligrams or 100 milligrams every three or four days until the dosage of 1,000 milligrams of niacin and 1,000 milligrams of vitamin C are taken three times a day.

It normally takes about three months on the higher dosage of niacin and vitamin C for cholesterol levels to stabilize at lower levels. How much does taking 3,000 milligrams of niacin and vitamin C cost? These two vitamins can be purchased for a total cost of about 50 cents a day.

HOW TO OBTAIN THE BENEFITS OF NIACIN

Niacin, like other B vitamins, is an essential nutrient required for cellular energy metabolism. It is available from a wide variety of foods, including whole grains, fresh fruits and vegetables, meat and fish, and beans and nuts. As an inexpensive and safe supplement, niacin is widely used for its effects on increasing HDL (good cholesterol) to lower cardiovascular risk, to prevent the pain and inflammation of arthritis, and to treat a variety of psychological disorders including anxiety and alcoholism. When used appropriately, niacin is very safe.

To obtain the benefits of supplemental niacin without the niacin flush, you can start by taking niacin at a low dose once a day and slowly increase the dose day by day. This allows the body to adapt to the increasing doses, which largely prevents a flush. An appropriate starting dose is 25 milligrams taken once per day with food. To obtain 25 milligrams doses, a good form to purchase is tablets of 100 milligrams of pure niacin. Break the 100-milligram tablets into four pieces and take one every day for several days. Then increase to two 25-milligram doses per day, taken in divided doses in the morning and evening with food. Gradually increase the dose over the next few weeks. Using this method, it is possible to achieve a dose of several hundred milligrams of niacin, taken as divided doses with meals, without noticeable flushing. If an occasional niacin flush occurs, reduce the dose by a small amount. You naturally should consult with your physician to discuss appropriate forms, cautions, doses, and benefits of niacin.

Niacin (Vitamin B$_3$) Lowers High Cholesterol Safely

There is a safe, inexpensive, nonprescription, convenient, and effective way to reduce high cholesterol levels and reduce heart disease risk: niacin. Niacin is a water-soluble B-complex vitamin, vitamin B$_3$. One of niacin's unique properties is its ability to help you naturally relax and to fall asleep more rapidly at night. It is well established that niacin helps reduce harmful cholesterol levels in the bloodstream. Niacin is one of the best substances for elevating high-density lipoprotein cholesterol (the "good" cholesterol) and so decreases the ratio of the total cholesterol over high-density cholesterol.

The finding that niacin lowered cholesterol was soon confirmed by Parsons, Achor, Berge, McKenzie, and Barker[24] and Parsons[25] at the Mayo Clinic, which launched niacin on its way as a hypocholesterolemic substance. Since then, it has been found to be a normalizing agent, meaning it elevates high-density lipoprotein cholesterol, decreases low-density and very low-density lipoprotein cholesterol and lowers triglycerides. Grundy, Mok, Zechs, and Berman[26] found it lowered cholesterol by 22 percent and triglycerides by 52 percent and wrote, "To our knowledge, no other single agent has such potential for lowering both cholesterol and triglycerides."

Elevated cholesterol levels are associated with increased risk of developing coronary disease. In addition to niacin, a typical diet generally recommended by orthomolecular physicians will tend to keep cholesterol levels down in most people. This diet can be described as a high-fiber, sugar-free diet which is rich in complex polysaccharides such as vegetables and whole grains.

With adequately high doses of niacin, it is possible to lower cholesterol levels even with no alteration in diet. E. Boyle, then working with the National Institutes of Health in Washington, D.C., quickly became interested in niacin. He began to follow a series of patients using 3 grams (3,000 milligrams) of niacin per day. He reported his conclusions in a document prepared for physicians involved in Alcoholics Anonymous by Bill W.[27] In this report, Boyle reported that he had kept 160 coronary patients on niacin for ten years. Only six died, against a statistical expectation that 62 would have died with conventional care. He stated, "From the strictly medical viewpoint I believe all patients taking niacin would survive longer and enjoy life much more." His prediction came true when the National Coronary Drug Study was recently evaluated by Canner. But Boyle's data spoke for itself. Continuous use of niacin will decrease mortality and prolong life.

Niacin Combined with Other Drugs Which Lower Cholesterol

Familial hypercholesterolemia is an inherited disease in which plasma cholesterol levels are very high. Illingworth, Phillipson, Rapp, and Connor[28] described a series of 13 patients treated with Colestipol 10 grams twice daily and later 15 grams twice daily. Their cholesterol levels ranged from 345 to 524 and triglycerides from 70 to 232. When this drug plus diet did not decease cholesterol levels below 270 milligrams per 100 milliliters they were given niacin, starting with 250 milligrams three times daily and increasing it every two to four weeks until a final dose of 3 to 8 grams per day was reached. To reduce the niacin "flush," patients took aspirin (120 to 180 milligrams) with each dose for four to six weeks. At these dosage levels of niacin, they found no abnormal liver function test results. This combination of drugs normalized blood cholesterol and lipid levels. They concluded, "In most patients with heterozygous familial hypercholesterolemia, combined drug therapy with a bile acid sequestrant and nicotinic acid (niacin) results in a normal or near normal lipid profile. Long-term use of such a regimen affords the potential for preventing, or even reversing, the premature development of atherosclerosis that occurs so frequently in this group of patients."

Fortunately, niacin does not decrease cholesterol to dangerously low levels. Cheraskin and Ringsdorf[29] reviewed some of the evidence which links very low cholesterol levels to an increased incidence of cancer and greater mortality in general.

Continuous use of niacin can be expected to reliably decrease mortality and prolong life.

Restoring health must be done nutritionally, not pharmacologically. All cells in all persons are made exclusively from what we drink and eat. Not one cell is made out of drugs.

FROM BLEEDING GUMS TO CORONARY DISEASE

In 1954, it was impossible to predict or even to think that my (AH) bleeding gums would one day, thirty-one years later, lead to additional useful life to people with coronary disease related to cholesterol and lipid metabolism. That year, malocclusion of my teeth had broken down the ability of my gum tissue to repair itself. My incorrect bite caused too much wear and tear on tooth sockets, and my gums began to bleed. No amount of vitamin C and no amount of dental repair helped. Eventually I reconciled myself to the idea I would soon have all my teeth extracted.

But at the time, I had been treating patients with niacin who were suffering from schizophrenia, senility, and a few other diseases, and I also began to take the vitamin myself—1 gram after each meal, for a total of 3 grams per day. I did so because I wanted to experience the flush that comes when one first takes niacin as well as its gradual waning with continued use so I could discuss these reactions more knowledgeably with my patients. There was also a legal issue. Most doctors' defense against malpractice suits is that they were doing what other physicians would do in similar circumstances. If I were sued (I have never been) because of unusual discomfort or adverse effects from niacin, I would not be able to use that "standard of practice" defense since only a handful of physicians had ever used such large quantities of niacin. I concluded that if the unlikely occurred and I was charged with malpractice, one of my defenses would be that I had tried it myself for at least three months without suffering serious consequences. I must admit I did not discuss this with a litigation lawyer, but it made sense to me. My reasons were therefore both practical and paranoid—but either way, initially I had no intention of treating myself for my bleeding gums.

Two weeks after I started taking niacin, my gums were normal. I was brushing my teeth one morning and suddenly awakened in surprise that there was no bleeding whatever! A few days later, my dentist confirmed that my gums were no longer swollen. I still have most of my teeth. Eventually I reasoned that the niacin had restored the ability of my gum tissue to repair itself faster than I could damage it by chewing with my crooked teeth.

A few months later I was approached by Rudolf Altschul, Chairman, Department of Anatomy, College of Medicine, University of Saskatchewan. I had been one of his students when he taught neurohistology. Professor Altschul had discovered how to produce arteriosclerosis in rabbits: he fed them a cake baked by his wife, Anna, that was rich in egg yolks. Rabbits fed cooked egg yolk promptly developed hypercholesterolemia and later arteriosclerotic lesions on their coronary vessels.[30] Altschul had also discovered that irradiating these hypercholesterolemic rabbits with ultraviolet light decreased their cholesterol levels. He wanted to extend this research by irradiating human subjects, but not one internist in Saskatoon would allow him access to their patients. (People who bake in the southern sunshine may wonder why this "dangerous" treatment received such a negative response.) Professor Altschul thus approached me. As Director of Psychiatric Research, Department of Health, Saskatchewan, I had access to several thousand patients in our two mental hospitals. I agreed to this research, provided that Dr. Humphry Osmond, Superintendent of the Saskatchewan Hospital at Weyburn, also agreed. The treatment was innocuous, would not cost us anything, and would help us create more of an investigative attitude among our clinical staff. But before we started, I requested that Professor Altschul meet with our clinical staff and present his ideas to them.

A few weeks later he came to Regina by train, and I drove him to Weyburn to meet Dr. Osmond and his staff. On the way down and back we discussed our work. He gave me an interesting review of how he saw the problem of arteriosclerosis, which he considered to be a disease of the intima, the inner lining of the blood vessels. He hypothesized that the intima had lost its ability to repair itself quickly enough. As soon as I heard this, I thought of my bleeding gums and of my own repair hypothesis. I then told him of my recent experience. I asked him if he would be willing to test niacin, which might have antiarteriosclerotic power, if it had the same effect on the intima as it had had on my bleeding gums. Professor Altschul was intrigued, and agreed to look at the idea, if he could get some niacin. I promptly sent him one pound of pure, crystalline niacin from a supply I had earlier received, courtesy of Merck and Company.

One evening about three months later, I received a call from Professor Altschul, who began to shout, "It works! It works!" Then he told me he had given niacin to his hyperlipidemic rabbits and within a few days, their cholesterol levels were back to normal. He had discovered the first hypo-cholesterolemic substance. Drug companies were spending millions to find such a compound.

But did it also work in humans? The next day I approached Dr. J. Stephen, Pathologist at the General Hospital, Regina. I was a biochemical consultant to him. I outlined what had been done and wanted his help in some human experiments. I assured him niacin was safe and we would only need to give a few grams to patients. He promptly agreed. He said he would order his technicians to draw blood for cholesterol assay from a large variety of patients, would then give them niacin, and would follow this with another cholesterol assay. I suggested we discuss this plan with the patients' physicians, but Dr. Stephen laughed and said they did not know what went on in the hospital, and that to contact each one would probably make the study impossible. A few weeks later the data poured in: niacin also lowered cholesterol levels in people. The greater the initial or baseline level, the greater the decrease.

We published our results. This report initiated the studies which eventually proved that niacin increases longevity.[31] It was not a double-blind study, but patients did not know what they were getting or why they were getting it. This type of impromptu research is now impossible with ethics committees, informed consent, and so on. Thirty years ago, only the integrity of physicians protected patients against experimental harm.

At the same time we were examining the effect of niacin on cholesterol levels, Russian scientists were also measuring the effect of vitamins on blood lipids. However, they used very little niacin and found no significant decreases.[32]

The finding that niacin lowered cholesterol was soon confirmed by Parsons and his colleagues in a number of studies at the Mayo Clinic, which launched niacin on its way as a hypocholesterolemic substance. Since then, it has been found to be a normalizing agent in that it elevates high-density lipoprotein cholesterol, decreases low-density and very low-density lipoprotein cholesterol, and lowers triglycerides. Grundy and his colleagues found that niacin lowered cholesterol by 22 percent and triglycerides by 52 percent and wrote, "To our knowledge, no other single agent has such potential for lowering both cholesterol and triglycerides."[33]

THE CORONARY STUDY

The only reason for being concerned about elevated cholesterol levels is that it is associated with increased risk of developing coronary disease. The association between cholesterol levels in the diet and coronary disease is not nearly as high, even though the overall diet is a main factor. The kind of diet generally recommended by orthomolecular physicians will tend to keep cholesterol levels down in most people. This diet can be described as a high-fiber, sugar-free diet, rich in complex polysaccharides such as vegetables and whole grains.

Once it became possible to lower cholesterol levels with no alteration in diet, it became possible to test the hypothesis that lowering cholesterol levels would decrease the risk of developing coronary disease. Perhaps Dr. E. Boyle's study (see "Niacin (Vitamin B₃) Lowers High Cholesterol Safely") was one of the reasons the Coronary Drug Project was started in 1966. Dr. Boyle was an advisor to this study, which was designed to assess the long-term efficacy and safety of five compounds in 8,341 men, ages thirty to sixty-four, who had suffered a myocardial infarction (heart attack) at least three months before entering the study.

The National Heart and Lung Institute supported this study. It was conducted at fifty-three clinical centers, in twenty-six American states. It was designed to measure the efficacy of several lipid-lowering drugs and determine whether lowering cholesterol levels would be beneficial for patients with previous myocardial infarctions. Niacin, two dosage strengths of estrogens, Clofibrate, dextrothyroxine, and a placebo were tested.

Eighteen months after the study began, the higher-dose estrogen group in the study was discontinued because of an excess of new nonfatal myocardial infarctions that occurred among patients using this drug compared to those on the placebo. The thyroxine group was stopped for the same reason for patients with frequent ectopic ventricular beats. After thirty-six months, dextrothyroxin was discontinued for the rest of the group, again because myocardial infarctions were increased compared to the placebo. After fifty-six months, the low-dose estrogen group study was stopped. There had been no significant benefit to compensate for the increased incidence of pulmonary embolism and thrombophlebitis and increased mortality from cancer. Eventually only the niacin, Clofibrate, and placebo groups were continued until the study was completed.

Canner's Follow-up Study

Dr. Paul L. Canner, Chief Statistician, Maryland Medical Research Institute, Baltimore, examined the data that came out of the Coronary Drug Project Research Group trial. About 8,000 men were still alive at the end of the treatment trial in 1975. Canner's study began in 1981, to determine if the two estrogen regimens and the dextrothyroxine regimen had caused any long-term effects. As described above, the high-dose estrogen had been discontinued because it increased nonfatal myocardial infarctions, low-dose estrogen increased cancer deaths, and dextrothyroxine increased total mortality compared to placebo, Clofibrate, and niacin. None of the subjects continued to take the drugs after 1975.

The 1985 follow-up study showed no significant differences in mortality between the treatment groups that had been discontinued and the placebo or Clofibrate groups. However, to the investigator's surprise, the niacin group fared much better. The cumulative percentage of deaths for all causes was 58.4 percent, 56.8 percent, 55.9 percent, 56.9 percent, and 50.6 percent respectively for low-dose estrogens, high-dose estrogens, Clofibrate, dextrothyroxine, and placebo.

The mortality in the niacin group was 11 percent lower than in the placebo group. The mortality benefit from niacin was present in each major category or cause of death: coronary, other cardiovascular, cancer, and others. Analysis of life table curves comparing niacin against placebo showed that niacin patients lived two years longer. With an average follow-up of fourteen years, there were seventy fewer deaths in the niacin group than would have been expected from the mortality rate in the placebo group. Patients with cholesterol levels higher than 240 milligrams per 100 deciliters benefited more than those with lower levels.

What is surprising is that the niacin benefit carried on for such a long period, even after no more was being taken. In fact, the benefit increased with the number of years followed up. It is highly probable the results would have been much better if patients had not stopped taking niacin in 1975. Thus, Boyle's patients who remained on niacin for ten years and received individual attention had a *90 percent decrease in mortality*. In the huge coronary study, this type of individual attention was not possible for the majority of patients. Many patients dropped out because of the niacin flush and may have been persuaded to remain in the study if they had been given more individual attention. This level of attention is very hard to do in a large-scale clinical study of this type. Dr. Boyle mentioned this as one of the defects in the Coronary Drug Study in his discussions with me. I would conclude that the proper use of niacin for similar patients should substantially decrease mortality along with increasing longevity, especially in patients with elevated cholesterol levels.

In 1985 the National Institutes of Health released a conference statement, "Lowering Blood Cholesterol to Prevent Heart Disease,"[34] based on the conclusions reached by a consensus development conference in 1984 on lowering blood cholesterol to prevent heart disease. It reports that heart disease kills 550,000 Americans each year, and 5.4 million are ill. Total costs of heart disease (at that time) were $60 billion per year. Main risk factors for heart disease include cigarette smoking, high blood pressure, and high blood cholesterol. The NIH recommended that the first step in treatment should be dietary, and their recommendations are met by the orthomolecular diet. When diet alone is not adequate, drugs should be used. Bile-acid sequestrants and niacin were favored while the main commercial drug, Clofibrate, was not recommended, "because it is not effective in most individuals with a high blood cholesterol level but normal triglyceride level. Moreover, an excess of overall mortality was reported in the World Health Organization trial of this drug."

Since niacin is effective only in megavitamin doses, 3,000 milligrams (1,000 milligrams three times per day), NIH was at last promoting megavitamin therapy. The National Institutes of Health asked that their conference statement be "posted, duplicated, and distributed to interested staff." Since every doctor has patients with high blood cholesterol levels, they should all be interested. One reason why they may not be is because NIH seems to have cooled its enthusiasm, such as it ever was, for high-dose vitamin therapy. If you go to the NIH website to read the pro-niacin conference statement, there is a prominent, red-letter editorial warning that:

> This statement is more than five years old and is provided solely for historical purposes. Due to the cumulative nature of medical research, new knowledge has inevitably accumulated in this subject area in the time since the statement was initially prepared. Thus, some of the material is likely to be out of date, and at worst simply wrong. For reliable, current information on this and other health topics, we recommend consulting the National Institutes of Health's MedlinePlus.[35]

We question the neutrality of such commentary. NIH's MedlinePlus and Medline/PubMed online indexes are selective filters and a long way from comprehensive.[36]

How Reliable Is Medline Plus?

Both Medline and MedlinePlus have a history of bias in favor of pharmaceutical medicine and against vitamin therapy. Medline/PubMed is used primarily by doctors and academics. MedlinePlus is aimed at the general public. Both are taxpayer funded. Medline censorship has been the subject of several articles:

Saul, A. W. "NLM censors nutritional research: Medline is biased, and taxpayers pay for it." *Orthomolecular Medicine News Service* (Jan 15, 2010).

Saul, A. W., S. Hickey. "Medline obsolescence." *Journal of Orthomolecular Medicine*, 22(4) (2007): 171–174. Editorial.

Saul, A. W. "Medline bias." *Townsend Letter for Doctors and Patients* 277/278 (Aug-Sep 2006): 122–123. Editorial.

Saul, A. W. "Medline bias: update." *Journal of Orthomolecular Medicine* 21(2) (2006): 67. Editorial.

Saul, A. W. "Medline bias. *Journal of Orthomolecular Medicine* 20(1) (2005): 10–16. Editorial

As to the objectivity of MedlinePlus, you can check for yourself at their website.[37] A MedlinePlus search[38] for "orthomolecular" brought up zero results. That is down by four from when the first edition of this book came out in 2011. Yes, it has gone from four to zero. *There were no MedlinePlus search responses whatsoever to any book, journal article, or website.* MedlinePlus is paid for by your tax dollars. Is information selectivity something you wish to fund?

THE EFFECT OF NIACIN WHEN COMBINED WITH OTHER DRUGS THAT LOWER CHOLESTEROL

Familial hypercholesterolemia is an inherited disease in which plasma cholesterol levels are very high. Illingworth and colleagues described a study of a series of thirteen patients treated with Colestipol, 10 grams twice daily and later 15 grams twice daily. Their cholesterol levels ranged from 345 to 524 with triglycerides from 70 to 232. When this drug plus diet treatment did not decrease cholesterol levels below 270, they were given niacin, starting with 250 milligrams three times daily, and increasing it every two to four weeks, until 3 to 8 grams per day was reached. To reduce the flush, patients took aspirin (120 to 180 milligrams) with each dose for four to six weeks. Researchers found no abnormal liver function test results with this dose of niacin. This combination of drugs normalized blood cholesterol and lipid levels. The authors concluded, "In most patients with heterozygous familial hypercholesterolemia, combined drug therapy with a bile acid sequestrant and nicotinic acid (niacin) results in a normal or near normal lipid profile. Long-term use of such a regimen affords the potential for preventing, or even reversing, the premature development of atherosclerosis that occurs so frequently in this group of patients."[39]

At about the same time Kane and his colleagues reported similar results on a larger series of fifty patients. They also studied the combined effect of Colestipol and Clofibrate. Abnormalities of liver function only occurred when the dose of niacin increased rapidly. Patients took 2.5 grams per day the first month, 5.0 grams per day the second month, and 7.5 grams per day the third month and thereafter. Blood sugar went up a little (from 115 to 120 milligrams) in a few patients and uric acid levels exceeded 8 milligrams in six patients. None developed gout. All other tests were normal. They concluded, "The remarkable ability of the combination of Colestipol and niacin to lower circulating levels of LDL . . . suggests that this combination is the most likely available regimen to alter the course of atherosclerosis."[40] The combination of Colestipol and Clofibrate was not as effective. For the first time it was seen that it is possible to extend the lifespan of patients with familial hypercholesterolemia.

Fortunately, niacin does not decrease cholesterol to dangerously low levels. Cheraskin and Ringsdorf[41] reviewed some of the evidence that links low cholesterol levels to an increased incidence of cancer and greater mortality in general. Ueshima, Lida, and Komachi[42] found a negative correlation between low cholesterol levels and cerebral vascular disorders. Mortality increased for levels under 160 milligrams. Further research found that the hypocholesterolemic action of niacin was related to the activity of the autonomic nervous system. Niacin also lowered cholesterol levels of schizophrenic patients, but to a different degree than in normal patients.[43–45]

WHY DOES NIACIN LOWER CHOLESTEROL?

It is important to note that although all forms of vitamin B_3 are anti-pellagra, and are almost equally effective in treating schizophrenia, arthritis, and a number of other diseases, only niacin (not niacinamide) lowers cholesterol. The no-flush niacin ester, inositol hexaniacinate, is also effective in lowering cholesterol and triglyceride levels.[46] Niacin also differs from niacinamide in that it causes a flush, while niacinamide has no vasodilation activity in 99 percent of the people who take it. For reasons unknown, about 1 in 100 persons who take niacinamide experience skin flush. They must be able to convert niacinamide to niacin in their bodies at a very rapid pace.

In 1983 I (AH) suggested that niacin lowers cholesterol because it releases histamine and glycosaminoglycans. Niacinamide does not do this. A histamine-glycosaminoglycan-histaminase system had also been found to be involved in lipid absorption and redistribution in an earlier study by Mahadoo, Jaques, and Wright in 1981.[47] Boyle had found that niacin increased basophil leukocyte count; these cells store heparin as well as histamine. He suggested that the improvement caused by niacin is much greater than can be explained by its effect on cholesterol, and that improvement may be due to release of histamine and also to a reduction in intravascular sludging of blood cells.

It is possible the beneficial effect of niacin is not due to the cholesterol effect, but is instead due to a more basic mechanism. Are elevated cholesterol levels and arteriosclerosis both the end result of a more basic metabolic disturbance that is still not identified? If it were entirely an effect arising from lowered cholesterol levels, why did Clofibrate not have the same beneficial effect? An enumeration of some other properties of niacin may one day lead to this basic metabolic fault. Niacin has a rapid anti-sludging effect. Sludged blood is present when the red blood cells clump together. The clumps are not able to traverse the capillaries as well as regular cells, as they must pass through in single file. This means that tissues will not receive their quota of red blood cells and will suffer anoxemia. Niacin changes the properties of the red cell surface membrane so that they do not stick to each other. Tissues are then able to get the blood they need. Niacin acts very quickly and increases healing, as it did with my gums. Perhaps it has a similar effect on the damaged intima of blood vessels. Niacin appears to directly help reduce inflammation.

In the past few years, adrenalin, via its aminochrome derivatives, has been implicated in coronary disease. If this becomes well established, it provides another explanation for niacin's beneficial effect on heart disease. In a series of reports Beamish and his coworkers showed that myocardial tissue takes up adrenalin, which is converted into adrenochrome, and it is the adrenochrome that causes fibrillation and heart muscle damage.

Under severe stress as in shock or after an injection of adrenalin, a large amount of adrenalin is found in the blood and is absorbed by heart tissue. Severe stress is thus a factor whether or not arteriosclerosis is present, but it is likely an arteriosclerotic heart cannot cope with stress as well as a healthy heart. Fibrillation would increase demand for oxygen, which could not be met by a heart whose coronary vessels are compromised.

Niacin protects tissues against the toxic effect of adrenochrome, in vivo. It reverses the EEG changes induced by intravenous adrenochrome given to epileptics,[48] and also reverses the psychological changes.[49] In synapses (gaps between nerve cells), nicotinamide adenine dinucleotide (NAD) is essential for maintaining noradrenalin and adrenalin in a reduced state. These catecholamines lose one electron to form oxidized amine. In the presence of NAD, this compound is reduced back to its original catecholamine. If there is a deficiency of NAD, the oxidized adrenalin (or noradrenalin) loses another electron to form adrenochrome (or noradrenochrome). This change is irreversible. The adrenochrome is a synaptic blocking agent, as is LSD. Thus niacin, which maintains NAD levels, decreases the formation of adrenochrome. It is likely this also takes place in the heart, and if it does, it would protect heart muscles from the toxic effect of adrenochrome and from fibrillation and tissue necrosis. None of the other substances known to lower cholesterol levels are known to have this protective effect. Niacin thus has an advantage in lowering cholesterol and decreasing frequency of fibrillation and tissue damage.

NIACIN AS A TREATMENT FOR ACUTE CORONARY DISEASE

A number of practitioners have used niacin clinically, as soon as possible after an acute event. These include C. E. Goldsborough, who used both niacin and niacinamide in this way between 1946 and 1960.[50] Patients with coronary thrombosis were given niacin, 50 milligrams by injection subcutaneously and 100 milligrams sublingually. As the niacin flush developed, the pain and shock of the coronary subsided. Another injection was given if the pain recurred when the flush faded, but if the pain was not severe another oral dose was used. The patient was given 100 milligrams three times daily after that. If the flush was excessive, niacinamide was used instead.

Goldsborough treated sixty patients during this period, twenty-four with acute infarction and the rest with angina. Of the twenty-four patients, six died. Four of the angina patients also had intermittent claudication, which was relieved by the treatment. Two had pulmonary embolism and also responded favorably.

Niacin should be used before and after every coronary bypass surgery. Inkeless and Eisenberg reviewed the evidence related to coronary artery bypass surgery and lipid levels in 1981.[51] There is still no consensus that this surgery increases survival. In most cases the quality of life is enhanced, and 75 percent get partial or complete relief of angina. I believe a major problem not resolved by cardiovascular surgery is how to halt the arteriosclerotic process. Inkeles and Eisenberg report that autogenous vein grafts implanted in the arterial circuit are more susceptible to arteriosclerosis than arteries. In an anatomic study of ninety-nine saphenous vein grafts from fifty-five patients who survived thirteen to twenty-six months, arteriosclerosis was found in 78 percent of hyperlipidemic patients (elevated blood lipid, especially cholesterol). Aortic coronary-bypass grafting accelerates the occlusive process in native blood vessels.

If patients were routinely placed on the proper diet and, if necessary, niacin long before they developed any coronary problems, most if not all coronary bypass operations could be avoided. If every patient requiring this operation were placed on the proper diet and niacin following surgery, the progress of arteriosclerosis would be markedly decreased. Then surgeons would be able to show a marked increase in useful longevity.

Niacin increases longevity and decreases mortality in patients who have suffered one myocardial infarction. *The Medical Tribune* properly expressed the reaction of early investigators by heading their April 24, 1985, report, "A Surprise Link to Longevity: It's Nicotinic Acid." More recently, niacin has been demonstrated to reduce injury to the brain after strokes.[52]

Elevated cholesterol levels are associated with increased risk of developing coronary disease. In addition to niacin, we also recommend a high-fiber, sugar-free diet, high in vegetables and whole grains. However, with adequately high doses of niacin, it is possible to lower cholesterol levels even with no alteration in diet. Continuous use of niacin will decrease mortality and prolong life. Incidentally, abnormally low cholesterol is not a niacin effect. Niacin does not decrease cholesterol to dangerously low levels.

In 2007, the *New York Times* reported that inexpensive vitamin B3, niacin, "can increase HDL as much as 35 percent when taken in high doses, usually about 2,000 milligrams per day. It also lowers LDL, . . . (and) triglycerides as much as 50 percent."[53] The *Times* quoted Steven E. Nissen, MD, president of the American College of Cardiology, as saying: "Niacin is really it. Nothing else available is that effective."

Niacin was first used to successfully lower serum cholesterol in 1955. Since then, placebo-controlled studies have confirmed that niacin prevents second heart attacks, and niacin also reduced strokes. One study showed that after fifteen years, men taking niacin had an 11 percent lower death rate. Although a warm "flush" is a common side effect of niacin, the vitamin is safer than any drug.

Recently, the non-statin drug Zetia (ezetimibe) was seen to be greatly inferior to niacin in controlled drug trials. Niacin stomped Zetia (a multibillion-dollar drug) so badly they had to stop the clinical trials for the benefit of the patients.[54]

So, for decades, it has been established that niacin not only is the best single substance we know for reversing all the pathological lipid findings in patients with cardiovascular problems, it is the only one. It decreases total cholesterol levels because it decreases the low-density cholesterol, it increases high-density cholesterol, lowers triglyceride levels, lowers lipoprotein(a), and lowers C reactive protein (CRP) levels. CRP is a measure of oxidative stress. None of all the other substances used widely, such as the statins, can even come close to niacin's ability to improve these numbers. In spite of billion-dollar efforts to develop a patentable product with the same beneficial properties as niacin, all efforts have ended in failure, including some deaths. Niacin decreased deaths by 11 percent compared to placebo, according to the Coronary Drug Study described earlier in this chapter. It increased life by two years in middle-aged men who had already suffered at least one coronary. That huge study was the direct outcome of our original finding that niacin lowered total cholesterol and the subsequent confirmation of that finding by studies at the Mayo Clinic.

Our national patent system, which places profit as the only important objective, not the health of its clients, is largely responsible for the fact that these studies have been largely ignored. Governments have allowed Big Pharma to get away with this. It is not surprising that I (AH) have seen many patients given statins, which are not effective and cause serious side effects, when they should have been on niacin. It does take medical skill to prescribe niacin properly. Parsons stated that "One must know niacin in order to use it." Too few physicians have developed this skill. They have not been encouraged by their medical training and have been misled by overwhelming drug advertising.

Statins versus Niacin

A reader writes:

> "Almost every day I read or see an article on statins and how good they are for you, and how more people should be taking them. I wonder. I was put on Zocor to lower cholesterol and after some time I experienced pain in shoulders. I was told to take warm showers. But I wanted to stop taking Zocor. So, I was put on Pravachol, and after a time, every joint (and I mean *every* joint) in my body was in agony. I was told I wasn't getting younger, and the doctor wanted to prescribe pain pills. I said "No." I refused to take Pravachol anymore. Lo and behold, in a matter of months, my joints stopped hurting. For the most part, I have returned to my old self. However, I did lose muscle tone to a great degree. When I was going through this, I know my doctor thought, 'This one is paranoid,' but I know what I felt. Can you please tell me more about statins?"

If Pravachol sounds like a street near the Kremlin and Zocor sounds like a *Star Trek* Klingon, read on. Dr. Hoffer says:

> "I would love to see a double-blind, controlled study comparing niacin against any one of the modern statins to be run at least ten years. It would win the battle hands down. And it can be combined with the statins if this is necessary.

Diet by itself is relatively ineffective, difficult to follow, and according to Parsons not very practical as it is so difficult to alter people's ways of eating. I agree.

"In his book, *Cholesterol Control Without Diet: The Niacin Solution*, Dr. Parsons reviews the role of the statins and the drug companies that got them approved and placed upon the market. I think this is an important section. And it is not a pretty picture. If your doctor tells you that you have a cholesterol problem, or if you suspect that you might have it, be sure and talk to him about niacin rather than take the statins, and refer him to this excellent book. It will answer all his questions and reassure him that niacin is the right one. You will be better for having done so."

It is odd that Big Pharma scientists are not able to understand Roger Williams' argument. To visualize the complexity of reactions in the cell, Williams compared the cell to an orchestra. Each essential nutrient is like one member of that orchestra. A superb symphonic performance is a function of the quality of the musicians, a good conductor, and everyone reading the same music. These criteria are what the public demands. However, suppose during the performance the solo violinist faints. The conductor believes the show must go on, and calls upon the lead drummer to replace the violinist. At this point we will no longer hear a symphony—it will be a cacophony. Recently, in real life, young Kuerti, a conductor, discovered that the pianist for that evening's performance was not able to appear. He called on his father, Anton Kuerti, who was at the concert. The symphony was superb. But there is only one Anton Kuerti. In the cells of the body each nutrient has been selected by evolution to be like an Anton Kuerti. If thiamine is removed from the cell only another Kuerti, thiamine, can replace it. It must be replaced, and until this is done, the cell will not perform. It will eventually die if the replacement doesn't arrive. Giving a patient a xenobiotic to replace what is missing is like replacing the violinist or pianist with the drummer. It would be like replacing Anton Kuerti with you or me. The orthomolecular law is that xenobiotics cannot replace missing orthomolecular substances. The drug companies are wasting our money, looking for something they will never find.

CHAPTER 12

Other Clinical Conditions That Respond to Niacin

*The person who says it cannot be done should
not interrupt the person doing it.*
—CHINESE PROVERB

It is hard to justify denying a patient a therapeutic trial with a vitamin. Open-minded, inquisitive physicians never have. The observations, insights, dedication (and often just plain courage) of nutritionally-minded doctors are worthy of our continued appreciation, today, a time when some say there is little value in "anecdotal" physician reports and case studies. Medical drug dogma is out of date. Inadequate nutrition, an old problem that has failed to go away, should be addressed first. Doing so will prevent much illness. For existing disease conditions, physicians should begin a therapeutic trial of specific nutrients such as niacin. It is up to each person to insist that their doctor does so. True, this is not always easy. To strengthen both your interest and your resolve, this chapter provides an overview of niacin's many specific clinical uses.

AGING

In April 2008, Miss Kaku Yamanaka died in Japan. She was 113 years old. The oldest person alive in the world at that time was Edith Parker, Indiana, age 114. In Canada, Miss Mary MacIsaac, age 112, died on March 10, 2006. She was Saskatchewan's oldest person, second-oldest in Canada, and nineteenth-oldest in the world. But Miss MacIsaac differed significantly from the others. She had been taking niacin for forty years before she died. She had cross-country skied until 110 and was photographed playing a piano duet with her great-grandson just before she died. She was weaker, but her mind was clear when she died after a brief illness. She credited the niacin with her advanced age, and perhaps she was correct, because research shows that niacin does have remarkable antiaging and life-extending properties.

In a large-scale double-blind controlled trial comparing niacin against other substances, including a popular cholesterol-lowering drug Atromid, estrogens, thyroid, and placebo, only niacin decreased the death rate. It decreased it by 11 percent, and increased longevity by two years. The cohort (group of individuals sharing a characteristic) tested were men who had at least one coronary and who were followed for fifteen years.[1]

This does not mean that everyone taking niacin will live as well and as long. But the evidence is persuasive. I (AH) truthfully tell my clients that if they will take niacin, one of the side benefits will be that they will feel better and live longer.

We have already referred to one of my female patients who lived to age 112. In December 2004, I received the following note from her son:

> There is one person older in Canada, but only our mother has all her wits about her and can walk. I kidded my sister that General Foods have asked her to recommend their products, and asked her what should be the fee. Seriously, she has always said that she followed the Hoffer program. There is a three-page spread on her in a Saskatchewan paper showing her skiing, rafting, horseback riding etc.

In this brief section on aging, I will review the highlights of this evidence. There is growing support for the idea that with proper nutrition and the use of vitamins, people will live longer. Ames, in two stimulating reports,[2,3] suggests that people can live longer by "tuning up their metabolism." By this he means that by adding nutrients to their diets, including niacin, in amounts larger than the RDAs (Recommended Dietary Allowances), many diseases will be better treated, the incidence of cancer will decrease, and aging will be slowed. According to Gutierrez,[4] Bruce Ames, discoverer of the Ames test for mutation and cancer-causing chemicals, concluded that a modern high-calorie, nutrient-deficient diet forces the body into a crisis mode. This is beneficial for short term but harmful for long term, and leads to disease, including cancer. According to recent health surveys, 93 percent of the population failed to meet even the inadequate RDA standards for nutrition. Linus Pauling, molecular biologist and Nobel Prize winner, stated that these insufficient health standards helped maintain the state of poor health we find in the general population.[5]

This is not surprising, since niacin protects the heart and vascular system and the brain by inhibiting the deposition of plaque in the arteries. It is the gold standard of compounds that lower total cholesterol levels in that it elevates high-density cholesterol levels, lowers triglycerides and lipoprotein(a) [Lp(a)], and has anti-inflammatory properties. This has been known for a very long time, although it is not widely appreciated or utilized by the medical profession. The Women's Health Study found that higher blood levels of HDL cholesterol in women is associated with better cognitive functioning.[6] This is another unexpected way by which niacin can help stave off dementia. Of all the cholesterol-lowering compounds, only niacin increases HDL significantly.

Modern studies have revealed additional antiaging properties of niacin that work by direct action on a cellular level. To summarize a few studies in this area: Christoph Westphal and his fellow researchers concluded from their review of the literature that, "Sirtuins are anti-aging proteins that have therapeutic potential for a range of diseases of aging, including metabolic disorders, neurodegenerative disorders, cancer, and cardiovascular disease."[7] Sirtuins are NAD-dependent protein decarboxylases related to life extension. Since NAD [nicotinamide adenine dinucleotide] is the active coenzyme made from niacin or niacinamide, this vitamin is important. Kaneko and colleagues confirmed that niacinamide protects against Wallerian degeneration in a 2006 study.[8] Wallerian degeneration follows local damage to the axon of nerve cells. This is a significant component of multiple sclerosis, discussed later in this chapter. Sasaki and his colleagues concluded, on the basis of their studies, that stimulating the NAD pathway may be useful in preventing or delaying axonal degeneration.[9] Yang and his colleagues summarized their work as follows: "A major cause of cell death caused by genotoxic stress is thought to be due to the depletion of NAD from the nucleus and the cytoplasm."[10] Since major causes of death are vascular damage and neuron destruction, it shouldn't be surprising that a substance inhibiting all these toxic events will have antiaging properties.

Indeed, evidence is accumulating that niacin helps recovery of the damaged brain. For example, after experimental strokes in animals, Yang and coworkers found that nicotinamide could rescue viable but injured nerve cells within the ischemic area. Early injection of nicotinamide reduced the number of necrotic and apoptotic neurons. Later injections were not as effective. In their report Yang and Adams concluded, "Early administration of nicotinamide may be of therapeutic interest in preventing the development of stroke, by rescuing the still viable but injured and partially preventing infarction." They also found that this vitamin decreased the progression of neurodegenerative disease. It prevented learning and memory impairment caused by cerebral oxidative stress. According to these studies nicotinamide works more quickly than niacin, but both are interconvertible and, in my opinion, niacin will have an advantage because it dilates the capillaries.

Patients with damage to the brain have responded to niacin treatment. It is likely that "chemo brain"—forgetfulness, confusion, or lack of focus experienced by patients undergoing chemotherapy—can be prevented by niacin in the same way that it protects against radiation- and chemotherapy-induced cancers sometime after the initial treatment. As many as one quarter of patients complain of "chemo brain." These changes are subtle but real, according to Dr. Daniel H. S. Silverman.[11,12] Dr. Silverman is the head of the neuronuclear imaging section at the University of California Medical Center, Los Angeles. He studied women who had received chemotherapy five to ten years previously. They compared the brain activity of these women to healthy controls. Chemo patients had reduced rates of metabolism in specific regions of the frontal cortex—an area involved in memory recall. The chemo had damaged the brain.

I (AH) have seen very few brain-damaged patients, but the following two cases suggest that niacin can be helpful to brain-damaged individuals. One case was a woman around sixty years old. She had prided herself on her good memory, which was helpful in her study of English literature. I saw her about a year after she had a stroke. She was then anxious, frustrated, and depressed because her memory was no longer reliable as it had been before her stroke. After six months on niacin, 3,000 milligrams per day, and ascorbic acid, 3,000 milligrams per day, her memory was so much better that she was able to deal with the residual loss without anxiety and depression. Her doctor had originally advised her that she would have to get used to her memory loss. The second case was a thirty-eight-year-old man. He had been struck on the head by a 1,000-pound object, two-and-a-half years before I saw him. He was in a coma for several days and in a hospital for several months. Before his accident, he had been an avid reader and in the ninetieth percentile level for intelligence. Six months later, he could read only at a third-grade level and was in the thirtieth percentile. The last time I saw him after his treatment, he was content with the improvement in his ability to read.

A report in *Annals of the New York Academy of Sciences* concluded that niacin-bound chromium (glucose tolerance factor contains niacin and chromium) combined with grape seed extract improved insulin sensitivity, decreased free radical formation, and reduced the symptoms of chronic age-related disorders, including Syndrome X (a combination of insulin resistance, elevated cholesterol or triglycerides, overweight, and/or high blood pressure).

ALLERGIES

Many very serious allergic reactions can be avoided by removing the foods causing the allergy and supplementing the patient with the orthomolecular program, which must include vitamin C and niacin.

Ms. D.H., born in 1960, was very concerned about pain in her wrists and elbows which had been present for over five years. She also suffered from other allergic and autoimmune symptoms. Her skin was constantly itching, she was overweight, had Raynaud's disease (see below) affecting her fingers, had a leg tremor at night, and had dermatographia, a condition in which lightly scratching your skin causes raised, red lines. She also reacted severely to insect bites. These symptoms were partially relieved by antihistamines, but their side effects (drowsiness, dry mouth and nose, headache, dizziness) were not tolerable.

Allergic reactions began when she was twenty. At the time, testing found her to be allergic to some foods, pets, and many other substances. In mid-2005 she developed hives, which later became so severe she had to be treated in an emergency room. An antihistamine helped, but she still suffered from itching on face, arms, and back. In 1996 she was diagnosed with Raynaud's. She continued to suffer from an amazing variety of symptoms. She was under the care of her allergist and several rheumatologists who could not help her when she was advised to consult me. She did so regularly and frequently for advice. Allergies to foods were discussed. She was started on vitamin C, 3,000 milligrams daily, and a small starting amount of niacin, 100 milligrams three times daily after meals. She continued adjusting her diet and followed the supplemental program. The hives and skin reactions ended, and subsequently her physician reported that she was well. A follow-up revealed she was still well one year after I first saw her.

For more in-depth discussion of allergies, we suggest you read *Orthomolecular Medicine for Everyone: Megavitamin Therapeutics for Families and Physicians*.[13]

ALCOHOLISM AND OTHER ADDICTIONS

Ever since I (AH) met Bill W., the cofounder of Alcoholics Anonymous (AA), I have had a personal interest in the treatment of alcoholism. Bill taught that there were three components to the treatment of alcoholism: spiritual, mental, and medical. AA provided a spiritual home for alcoholics that many could not find elsewhere, and helped them sustain abstinence. But for many AA alone was not enough; not everyone in AA achieved a comfortable sobriety. Bill recognized that the other two components were important. When he heard of our use of niacin for treating alcoholics, he became very enthusiastic about it because niacin gave patients immense relief from their chronic depression and other physical and mental complaints.

Niacin is the most important single treatment for alcoholism, and it is one of the most reliable treatments. And it is safe, much safer than any of the modern psychiatric drugs. Niacin does not work as well when alcoholics are still drinking, but in a few cases, it decreased their intake of alcohol until they became abstinent. This conclusion is based on the work my colleagues and I have done since 1953.

I know of many alcoholics who did not want to stop drinking, but did agree to take niacin. Over the years, they were able to reduce their intake gradually until they brought it under control. Some alcoholics can even become social drinkers, on a very small scale. I have not found many who could, but I think that if started on the program very early, many more could achieve normalcy. I suspect that treatment centers using these ideas will be made available one day and will be much more successful than the standard treatment today. Current treatment all too often still consists of dumping patients into hospitals and letting them dry out, with severe pain and suffering. When they are discharged, most go right back to the alcohol, the most dangerous and widely-used street drug available without a prescription.

The alcoholic's body needs the proper nutrients in adequate quantities to return to normal metabolic functioning. Bill W. was one of the first alcoholic addicts to benefit from niacin. After his last drink he suffered from decades of anxiety, fatigue, and some depression but was able to make his remarkable contribution, which helped millions of drug addicts. We met at a meeting in New York and became close friends. When I learned of his discomfort, I told him about niacin. He began to take 1 gram after each of three meals, and was normal in two weeks. This was so surprising that he joined me in promoting niacin for members of AA—but first he persuaded thirty of his friends in AA to try it. He found that ten were well in one month, another ten at the end of the second month, and the last ten had not responded by the end of the third month. This was remarkably close to the data I had accumulated. Bill W. then determined to share the good news with doctors in AA. This association appointed a committee of three of their members who studied it and agreed that it was very useful.

Against the opposition of International Headquarters of AA, Bill W. prepared and distributed two communications to physician members of AA. Thousands of copies were distributed. A third communication was distributed after his death. Had Bill W. not died, there is no doubt that the therapeutic use of niacin would be much further advanced than it is today. Andrew Saul and I wrote a book about the treatment of addictions, with heavy emphasis on my relationship to Bill W., *The Vitamin Cure for Alcoholism*.[14] Several clinics in the United States are treating addicts using orthomolecular methods with great success and up to 80 percent recovery rates.

The orthomolecular program works best in conjunction with the steps of Alcoholics Anonymous, which we support. As Bill W. realized, niacin helps addicts recover from the anxiety, fatigue, depression, and other discomforts that they usually suffer. This, in our opinion, is the basis for their use of alcohol or drugs. Addicts are not well to begin with. Many alcoholics suffer from increased gastrointestinal permeability.[15] This leads to a decrease in antioxidant status. A daily dose of 100 milligrams of niacin returns gastrointestinal permeability back to normal when associated with abstinence and a proper diet. In my opinion, a healthy individual will not become an addict. They will drink but in moderation, they may try drugs, but eventually decide they do not like the effect. They will therefore not become addicted to whatever removes that state of being well. For less healthy persons who do become addicted, they maintain the addiction in order to prevent the withdrawal effects. We do not need fancy or elaborate theories of personality or psychology to account for their addiction. They are all forms of self-treatment using drugs. Some are socially acceptable, and some are not. AA deals with some of the problems that have been generated by the addiction over years, and helps remove guilt and restore relationships. This is seen even in animals. Low-status monkeys placed in a cage physically close to high-status monkeys choose to take cocaine rather than food, if given a choice. High-status animals, under less stress because of their status, are more apt to choose food rather than cocaine.[16,17] Further evidence that alcoholics will conquer their addiction more easily when they become well is evidenced by alcoholics who refused to give up alcohol but agreed to take niacin. We (AH and AWS) have seen that they stop drinking.

Treating addicts is very easy in principle. Simply help them get well, but not by adding still more addicting drugs, even though they may be socially sanctioned and easier to control, like methadone to replace heroin. Niacin is the best substance we know that will do this. The late Dr. Roger Williams, a chemistry professor at the University of Texas and former president of the American Chemical Society, also wrote extensively on alcoholism. Dr. Williams recommended large doses of vitamins and an amino acid called L-glutamine.[18]

The orthomolecular program is the treatment of choice for alcoholism. The following protocol for alcoholism outlines many of the nutritional factors that have been shown to be very successful in treating this condition.

William Griffith Wilson (1895–1971)

"Bill Wilson is the greatest social architect of the 20th century."

—Aldous Huxley

The man who would co-found Alcoholics Anonymous was born to a hard-drinking household in rural Vermont. When he was ten, his parents split up and Bill was raised by his maternal grandparents. He served in the Army in World War I, and although he did not see combat, Bill had more than ample opportunities to drink. In the 1920s, Wilson achieved considerable success as an inside trader on Wall Street, but a combination of drunkenness and the stock market crash drained what was left of his fortune and his capability to enjoy life. Hard knocks, religious experience, and a growing sense that he could best help himself by helping other alcoholics led Bill to create one of the world's most famous introductions: "My name is Bill W., and I'm an alcoholic." Even as Alcoholics Anonymous slowly grew, many of Bill's financial and personal problems endured, most notably depression. Abram Hoffer writes: "I met Bill in New York in 1960. Humphry Osmond and I introduced him to the concept of megavitamin therapy. Bill was very curious about it and began to take niacin, 3,000 milligrams daily. Within a few weeks the fatigue and depression that had plagued him for years were gone. He gave it to thirty of his close friends in AA. Of the thirty, ten were free of anxiety, tension, and depression in one month. Another ten were well in two months. Bill then wrote "The Vitamin B_3 Therapy," and thousands of copies of this extraordinary pamphlet were distributed. As a result, Bill became unpopular with the members of the board of AA International. The medical members, who had been appointed by Bill, "knew" vitamin B_3 could not be as therapeutic as Bill had found it to be. I found it very useful in treating patients who were both alcoholic and schizophrenic."[19]

The Orthomolecular Program for Treatment of Alcoholism

- High doses of vitamin C (as much as 10,000 milligrams per day or more) to chemically neutralize the toxic breakdown of the products of alcohol metabolism. Vitamin C also increases the liver's ability to reverse the fatty buildup so common in alcoholics.
- Niacin. Dr. Hoffer's most common prescription was 3,000 milligrams per day, in divided doses.
- B$_{50}$-complex tablet (50 milligrams of each of the major B vitamins) several times daily, with meals.
- L-glutamine (2,000 or 3,000 milligrams). L-glutamine is an amino acid that decreases physiological cravings for alcohol. It is one of the two primary energy providers that burn glycogen to provide fuel to the brain and stimulates many neurofunctions. L-glutamine is naturally produced in the liver and kidneys. Alcohol harms the kidneys and liver; thus, supplementation is vital. L-glutamine concurrently reduces cravings for sugar and alcohol.
- Lecithin (2 or 3 tablespoons daily). Lecithin provides inositol and choline, related to the B-complex. It also helps mobilize fats out of the liver.
- Chromium (at least 200 up to 400 mcg chromium polynicotinate daily). Chromium improves carbohydrate metabolism and greatly helps control blood sugar levels. Many, if not most, alcoholics are hypoglycemic.
- A good high-potency multivitamin, multimineral supplement as well, containing magnesium (400 milligrams) and the antioxidants carotene and vitamin E as d-alpha tocopherol.

We further discuss alcoholism and other addictions in *The Vitamin Cure for Alcoholism*.

ALZHEIMER'S DISEASE

Increasingly, research evidence makes it more and more plausible that Alzheimer's disease will be treated much more successfully in the near future. However, the obsessive attempts to find that blockbuster drug that will be the magic pill need to stop. Foster, in his recent book *What Really Causes Alzheimer's Disease*,[20] describes its astonishing descent on our aging population.

This is already general knowledge, as few families have not seen it attack one of their members.

Alzheimer's disease has traditionally been considered untreatable, except by a few drugs, which at best may slow the degenerative process a little. However, there is growing evidence that it can be prevented by the proper use of nutrients.

Specifically, niacin has been demonstrated to have a marvelously protective effect against the development of Alzheimer's disease and cognitive decline. A study of nearly 4,000 people age sixty-five and older showed that those with the lowest niacin intake (an average of 12.6 milligrams per day) were 80 percent more likely to be diagnosed with Alzheimer's disease than those with the highest intake (22.4 milligrams per day). The rate of cognitive decline was only about half as much among those with the highest niacin intake when compared to those with the lower intake. Since 22.4 milligrams of niacin per day achieves such results, it is reasonable to expect that larger doses are likely to be still more effective.[21] Further support for niacin's support of cognitive function was found in research by Green and coworkers, which found that nicotinamide restored cognition in Alzheimer's disease transgenic mice.[22]

We are not suggesting that niacin alone is the answer to Alzheimer's disease. Compelling evidence indicates that early memory loss can be reversed by the ascorbates (vitamin C). Increased risk of Alzheimer's disease has also been linked to low dietary intake of vitamin E and of fish. The elderly should continue to eat well-balanced diets high in calcium, magnesium, selenium, the B vitamins, and essential fatty acids. Foster has argued at length that Alzheimer's disease is caused by an excess of monomeric aluminum in people who are calcium and magnesium deficient.[23]

Alzheimer's disease and other conditions, such as repeated little strokes, are aging factors. A recent report from Rush Institute for Healthy Aging and Center for Disease Control and Prevention, Atlanta, concluded:

> In this prospective study we observed a protective association of niacin against the development of Alzheimer's Disease and cognitive decline with normal levels of dietary intake, which could have substantial public health implications for disease prevention if confirmed in further research.[24]

This study indicates two things: that a very little niacin goes a long way, and that many of the elderly are not even getting a little.

High HDL protects against dementia, according to the fifteen-year Women's Health Study, in which 4,081 women age sixty-six and older were divided into five quintiles for HDL levels. The highest group had an HDL level of 73 milligrams per deciliter, and the lowest 36 milligrams per deciliter. The women in the highest quintile had five times less chance of having cognitive impairment. The only substance that significantly elevates HDL is niacin.

The main B vitamin is niacin, but other nutrients are involved in lowering risk for development of Alzheimer's disease. Other B vitamins, vitamin E, and vitamin C, when taken together, decrease the incidence of Alzheimer's. Dr. Peter Zandi of Johns Hopkins School of Public Health said that "Vitamin E and C may offer protection against Alzheimer's disease when taken together in the higher doses available from individual supplements."[25] These nutrients decreased risk by 78 percent. Essential minerals such as selenium and zinc are also important, as they counteract the accumulation of toxic metals such as aluminum and mercury. Essential fatty acids also play a major role. In short, optimal nutrition will be the most decisive factor in slowing down the ravages of aging.

Niacin may inhibit the development of Alzheimer's disease, but unfortunately, I (AH) have not found it helpful in treating the condition once it is established. However, about one-third of all patients diagnosed with Alzheimer's disease will, at autopsy, not show Alzheimer's typical pathological findings. In these cases, the clinical syndrome is the same, but the causes are different. I suspect that these patients were more apt to have had a series of small strokes. Niacin will be more helpful for patients such as these. Their cholesterol levels may be an important clue. Alzheimer's patients often have elevated cholesterol levels, suggesting that cerebrovascular senile patients will have Alzheimer's disease more often than patients without this condition.

There are no plausible clinical claims or reports that patients with Alzheimer's disease ever recover spontaneously. For this reason, double-blind studies would be a waste of time and money since it is illogical to use this method when a condition has no natural recovery rate. Instead, each clinical report of a recovery must be taken very seriously.

During October 2007, Mary, age seventy-three, complained that under stress her memory failed, which made her depressed. She tended to become confused in space, but she was still able to drive her car. Until her memory began to fail, she had been able to deal with stress with little difficulty. She was advised to improve her intake of vitamins including niacin (1 gram after each of three meals) and minerals and to eliminate dairy products. One month later she was very much better. After ten months she wrote to express her gratitude for her recovery and said:

> Since I started the healing process with vitamins, I have been able to survive in my home when my family had been trying to convince me to sell and move into an apartment. I've lived here thirty-two years and I love my garden and was able to walk four blocks to market. Twice each week I watch my flowers come up, and weed my garden. My family refers to Alzheimer's, yet I know I am more aware and confident than I have been for years. If I hadn't had my meeting with you, I'd be in hospital and my house sold. With deep gratitude.

The universal rule that all crows are black is no longer a universal rule if one sees a crow that is white. The clinical belief that there can be no recovery from Alzheimer's is equally false.

Orthomolecular treatment tries to optimize shelter. In this case it was important for this woman to remain in her home, which had been her shelter for thirty-two years. I suspect she was more grateful for that than for any other single factor. The program also removed a negative factor: the dairy foods to which she had been reacting for many years. And it allowed her to retain her dignity and demand to be treated with respect and decency by those around her. She did not respond to just one factor. Niacin was only one of the important factors, as a member of a therapeutic team of nutrients.

Identical twins are ideal for comparison-controlled trials. In animal studies it is recognized that one identical twin pair is equivalent to two groups containing forty nonrelated animals. Therefore, what happened to an identical-twin pair of women is very instructive. In this case, one twin developed galloping Alzheimer's and died within a few years. Her identical twin sister then started on a comprehensive megavitamin program. She lived another thirty years, mentally normal, and then died of a stroke.

If Alzheimer's patients have too little dopamine and therefore too little dopachrome, it would make sense to treat them by giving them safe amounts of L-dopa and yet protecting them against excessive dopachrome formation. This would include using L-dopa as if they were Parkinson's cases, combined with at least 3 grams of niacin daily as the two main nutrients, with adequate amounts of calcium and magnesium and the elimination of aluminum. Of course, the entire orthomolecular program would be even better.

Henry Turkel, MD (1903–1992)

I know Dr. Turkel, and I can testify to his sincerity and conviction. The results that he reports are striking. There is evidence that the patients would receive significant benefit.

—Linus Pauling, PhD

Used with permission of the Linus Pauling Institute, Oregon State University.[26]

It was thirty-five years ago that Dr. Henry Turkel testified before the United States Senate Select Committee on Nutrition and Human Needs. His presentation was entitled, "Medical Amelioration of Down's Syndrome Incorporating the Orthomolecular Approach." Dr. Turkel was the very voice of experience, having pioneered the nutritional treatment for Down's syndrome in the 1940s. Since then, he had successfully employed a combination of vitamins and other nutrients, plus some medication, with over 5,000 patients. In addition, Dr. Turkel wrote two key books: *Medical Treatment of Down Syndrome and Genetic Diseases* and *New Hope for the Mentally Retarded*.

Regarding the work of Dr. Turkel, Abram Hoffer has written:

I first became interested in Down syndrome when I heard about the work being done by Dr. Henry Turkel in Detroit many years ago. I published many of his papers in the *Journal of Orthomolecular Psychiatry* and its earlier versions. Dr. Turkel suffered the fate of almost all early pioneers. He had the nerve to make his claims when everyone "knew" that children with genetic defects could not possibly be treated successfully.

Linus Pauling specifically recognized Dr. Turkel's work in his book, *How to Live Longer and Feel Better:*

> The physician who has made the greatest effort to amelio-rate Down syndrome is Dr. Henry Turkel of Detroit, Mich-igan . . . I know Dr. Turkel, and I can testify to his sincerity and conviction. The results that he reports are striking. Many of the children show a reduction of developmental abnormalities, especially of the bones. Their appearance changes in the direction of normalcy. Their mental ability and behavior improve to such an extent that they are able to hold jobs and support themselves. Rapid growth (increase in height) occurs during the period when tablets are being taken, and the growth stops during the periods when they are not taken. My conclusion is that there is little danger that this treatment or treatment with supplementary nutri-ents would do harm, and there is evidence that the patients would receive significant benefit. . . . I think that all (people with Down syndrome)—especially the younger ones—should try nutritional supplementation to see to what extent it ben-efits them.[27]

Jack Challem writes:

> Vitamin therapy in Down syndrome began in 1940, when Henry Turkel, MD, of Detroit became interested in treat-ing the metabolic disorders of Down syndrome with a mix-ture of vitamins, minerals, fatty acids, digestive enzymes, lipotropic nutrients, glutamic acid, thyroid hormone, antihistamines, nasal decongestants, and a diuretic. By the 1950s he had devoted his practice almost entirely to Down

syndrome patients, of whom he kept exceptionally detailed records, including serial photographs of their progress. Conventional medicine ignored Dr. Turkel and he eventually retired and moved to Israel. Turkel clearly demonstrated that one of the 'worst' genetic defects—trisomy, leading to Down syndrome—could be modified through what is largely a nutritional program with moderately high-dose supplements. The program never corrected the basic genetic defects in Down syndrome, of course, but it did correct much of the collateral biochemical consequences, leading to improvements in cognition, physical health, and appearance. Turkel was probably the first to show that nutrition could improve genetic programming, and that genetic predeterminism was limited.

Alzheimer's, Schizophrenia, and Down Syndrome

From my experience treating over 5,000 schizophrenic patients since 1952, I cannot remember having seen any schizophrenic patients develop Alzheimer's disease. (Of course, it is possible that Alzheimer's disease may be found in the chronic populations in mental hospitals, with whom I have not had nearly as much experience.) Nor would I have expected it, as schizophrenia had been identified as a disease with no known metabolic dysfunction, and Alzheimer's disease was known to be caused by brain damage, an organic rather than a functional disorder. In 1952 one of the patients in our psychiatric ward had been diagnosed with Alzheimer's disease. After a few weeks of observation, he was sent to the closest mental hospital for permanent care, but a few weeks after he arrived his behavior became decidedly uncharacteristic of Alzheimer's disease. He became very aggressive and difficult, and he was re-diagnosed as schizophrenic. He was given niacin, which we had just obtained, and he recovered. He surely had not had Alzheimer's disease.

Schizophrenia is characterized by major changes in perception and in thinking, with little memory loss, disorientation, and confusion. Organic psychosis is characterized by severe loss of memory, by disorientation with respect to time, place, and identity, and by confusion. Alzheimer's may also be confused with depression in the elderly. In my first-year residency in psychiatry in 1951, one of my patients clearly suffered from senile psychosis. I did not know how he might be treated. Dr. KcKerracher suggested I give him electroconvulsive therapy (ECT). This made no sense to me, but I went along with this advice. The patient made a complete recovery after having been demented for two years. I was really astonished at his recovery. Given the difficulty in diagnosing Alzheimer's disease, the failure to see any of the elderly chronic schizophrenic patients in my practice develop Alzheimer's is striking.

Down syndrome is a congenital condition that is associated with Alzheimer's disease. Alzheimer's tends to come early in these patients. Down patients also tend to suffer from depression more often, but the coexistence with schizophrenia is low. Three studies showed the following relationship: in the first study, 6 out of 371 Down patients had schizophrenia, and in the next two studies, of 119 and 315 patients, none were schizophrenic. From a total of 805 patients with Down syndrome, only 6 were also suffering from schizophrenia. Diagnosing schizophrenia in Down patients may be very difficult and the precise relationship between the two conditions may not be known, but it is clear that Down syndrome and Alzheimer's disease resemble each other a lot more than either resembles schizophrenia.

Dr. H. Turkel began to treat Down children early in the 1950s with a multivitamin, multimineral mixture plus desiccated thyroid. The results he saw and published, including pictures of recovered young patients, were very impressive. Dr. Turkel believed that properly treated Down syndrome children would not suffer from early Alzheimer's. His work was not taken seriously and the Food and Drug Administration (FDA) made very strenuous attempts to suppress this treatment. Eventually he was able to use his preparation legally only in Michigan, as long as the product did not cross state lines. Dr. Turkel was embittered by this blatant attempt to keep these children sick. Sporadic half-hearted attempts were made to confirm his evidence with mixed results. Dr. B. Rimland concluded, after examining the literature, that Dr. Turkel's method was not fairly followed by other researchers who denied his conclusions. Dr. Turkel is in the Orthomolecular Hall of Fame.

Thiel concluded:

Whether or not specifically due to the presence of a third 21st chromosome, metabolic disturbances are involved with Down syndrome. The nutritional profiles of the Down syndrome population do, in certain significant ways, differ from those of the general public. Various signs and symptoms associated with Down syndrome have been reported to improve when certain nutritional protocols have been tried (and there is no accepted medical treatment currently in existence for Down syndrome). Orthomolecular medicine has safely been treating people with Down syndrome for over sixty years. Orthomolecular medicine is a logical therapy to consider when Down syndrome is present.[28]

MacLeod is in full agreement with this conclusion. In his excellent 2003 book, *Down Syndrome and Vitamin Therapy*,[29] he recorded the phenomenal improvement seen in Down children when they were treated with the correct nutrients. He has advanced since Turkel in that his laboratory has been using some of the latest clinical laboratory tests to determine which of the nutrients have to be emphasized. The stories of some of the young people and their pictures offer proof that the orthomolecular approach pioneered by Dr. Turkel so many years ago is valid. As in so many other areas the medical establishment has once again shown a remarkable tendency to back the wrong horse.

Recently the findings by Li and his colleagues raised this question: Do schizophrenic patients get Alzheimer's disease? These researchers suggested:

Our findings have important implications for understanding protein deposition diseases, support the hypothesis that a common molecular mechanism may underlie development of pathological features of Parkinson's disease and Alzheimer's disease and suggests that common strategies of intervention could benefit patients suffering from these diseases.[30]

The adrenochrome hypothesis suggests that if schizophrenic patients have too much adrenochrome or dopachrome (from dopamine) this would protect them from the excessive formation of amyloid.

Religa and his coworkers reported levels of amyloid ß-peptide in the postmortem brains of schizophrenic and normal patients with and without Alzheimer's disease. Seven of the brains in their study came from patients with dual diagnosis.

They concluded:

In contrast to elderly schizophrenia patients with Alzheimer's disease pathology, those without Alzheimer's disease had amyloid ß-peptide levels that were not significantly different from those of normal subjects; hence amyloid ß-peptide does not account for the cognitive deficits in this group. These results suggest that the causes of cognitive impairment in "pure" schizophrenia are different from those in Alzheimer's disease.[31]

In a 1998 study, Purohit and colleagues examined 100 consecutive autopsy brain specimens of patients aged 52 to 101 years (mean age 76.5 years), 47 patients with nonschizophrenic psychiatric disorders from the same psychiatric hospital, and 50 age-matched control subjects.

Although 72 percent of the patients with schizophrenia showed cognitive impairment, AD [Alzheimer's disease] was diagnosed in only 9 percent of the patients and other dementing diseases were diagnosed in only 4 percent of the patients. The degree of senile plaques or neurofibrillary tangles was not different in the group with schizophrenia compared with the age-matched controls or the group with nonschizophrenic psychiatric disorders.... This study provides evidence that elderly patients with schizophrenia are not inordinately prone to the development of AD or to increased senile plaques or neurofibrillary tangle formation in the brain. Other dementing neurodegenerative disorders are also uncommon. The cognitive impairment in elderly patients with schizophrenia must, therefore, be related to some alternative mechanisms.[32]

Niacin and Schizophrenia:
History and Opportunity

by Nick Fortino, PhD

Schizophrenia is usually treated with prescription antipsychotic drugs, many of which produce severe adverse effects;[33-38] are linked to an incentive for monetary profit benefiting pharmaceutical corporations;[39-45] lack sufficient evidence for safety and efficacy;[41,46] and have been grossly misused.[47-52] Orthomolecular (nutritional) medicine provides another approach to treating schizophrenia, which involves the optimal doses of vitamin B_3—also known as niacin, niacinamide, nicotinamide, or nicotinic acid—in conjunction with an individualized protocol of multiple vitamins. The orthomolecular approach involves treating "mental disease by the provision of the optimum molecular environment for the mind, especially the optimum concentrations of substances normally present in the human body."[53]

Evidence for the Niacin Treatment of Schizophrenia

Vitamin B_3 as a treatment for schizophrenia is typically overlooked, which is disconcerting considering that historical evidence suggests it effectively reduces symptoms of schizophrenia, and has the added advantage, in contrast to pharmaceuticals, of mild to no adverse effects.[54-67] After successful preliminary trials treating schizophrenia patients with niacin, pilot trials of larger samples commenced in 1952, as reported by Hoffer, Osmond, Callbeck, and Kahan in 1957. Dr. Abram Hoffer began an experiment involving 30 patients who had been diagnosed with acute schizophrenia. Participants were given a series of physiological and psychological tests to measure baseline status and were subsequently assigned randomly to treatment groups. Nine subjects received a placebo, 10 received nicotinic acid, and 11 received nicotinamide (the latter two are forms of vitamin B_3). All participants received treatment for 42 days, were in the same hospital, and received psychotherapy from the same group of clinicians.

The two experimental groups were administered three grams of vitamin B_3 per day. Each of the three treatment groups improved, but the two vitamin B_3 groups improved more than the placebo group as compared to baseline measures. At one year follow-up, 33 percent of patients in the placebo group remained well, and 88 percent of patients in the B_3 groups remained well. These results inspired many subsequent trials, and those that replicated the original method produced similarly positive results.

Antipsychotic Drugs

That schizophrenia may be caused or aggravated by a deficiency of essential nutrients appears to have eluded the majority of the health care providers serving the schizophrenic population, as evidenced by the fact that "antipsychotic medications represent the cornerstone of pharmacological treatment for patients with schizophrenia."[68] Waves of different antipsychotic drugs have been developed throughout the last 60 years, which have not decreased the prevalence of schizophrenia; in fact it has increased.[47,69]

Although dangerous when taken in high doses and for a long period of time, the value of antipsychotics appears to be that in the short term they can help to bring some control to schizophrenic symptoms, not by curing the condition but by inducing a neurological effect that is qualitatively different from the schizophrenic state. Dr. Hoffer acknowledged their value and in his private practice he would introduce antipsychotics and vitamins simultaneously because antipsychotics work rapidly and vitamins work more slowly, so a person could benefit from the short-term relief from symptoms that antipsychotics provide while the vitamins slowly, but surely, healed the deficiency causing the schizophrenic symptoms. This also allowed for a much easier process of tapering from the drugs.

"For schizophrenia, the recovery rate with drug therapy is under 15 percent. With nutritional therapy, the recovery rate is 80 percent."

—Abram Hoffer, MD, PhD

ANXIETY

In my (AH) very first book on niacin in 1962, I discussed what little was then known of vitamin B3 as a sedative in chapter 3. The old term "sedative," which applied to the barbiturates, has been replaced by the term "antianxiety." The first report of niacin's antianxiety properties appeared in 1949, when it was reported that it was synergistic with some drugs. Later I found that it indeed had anticonvulsive properties if combined with anticonvulsants, and it was possible to achieve better control with less sedation by adding niacin to the anticonvulsant program. I also found that niacin increased the sedative effect of phenobarbital, a very common barbiturate, when they were combined. Further studies showed that it was also therapeutic for a mix of anxiety and depression and agitation. I have seen this frequently over the past fifty years. Niacin also sedated animals when a sufficient amount was administered.

Prousky described the orthomolecular treatment of anxiety in 2006.[70] Vitamin B3 is a major factor in this program. Currently the press, and perhaps the public as well, have recognized that the xenobiotic antidepressants used to treat depression and anxiety are seldom better than placebo. In addition, they are very addictive and toxic because the withdrawal effects are so severe and prolonged. Physicians concerned about the use of these drugs should study Prousky's book. They will be reassured that orthomolecular treatment of anxiety and depression is much more effective without the use of these dangerous drugs. Over the past ten years I have not started anyone on these drugs—indeed, I have done just the opposite. Most of these patients came because they wanted to eliminate them from their program.

Supplements Accelerate Benzodiazepine Withdrawal

A Case Report and Biochemical Rationale

by W. Todd Penberthy, PhD, and Andrew W. Saul

A middle-aged male had success rapidly reducing fast-acting alprazolam (Xanax) dosage by taking very high doses of niacin, along with gamma aminobutyric acid (GABA) and vitamin C. The individual had been on 1 milligram per day Xanax for two years, a moderate dose but of long duration. As a result, he had been presenting increased anxiety, personality changes, and ringing in the ears (tinnitus), all side effects likely due to long-term alprazolam use. Typical withdrawal from this drug would involve substitution medication, about a 10 percent dose reduction per week, and take a matter of months.[71] A fast withdrawal is a 12.5 to 25 percent reduction per week.[72] On very high doses of niacin, vitamin C, and also GABA, this individual reported being able to cut the dose 60 percent down to 0.4 milligrams in one week. The dose was reduced by 90 percent (to 0.1 milligram per day) in less than a month. He reported residual anxiety, but that it was substantially less than when fully medicated. After a total of five weeks, the medication intake was zero, with minimal residual anxiety.

Dosage

Niacin doses were between 6,000 and 12,000 milligrams per day. The individual reported reduced anxiety when taking the highest levels of niacin. Bowel-tolerance levels of vitamin C were taken daily, along with 750 milligrams of GABA twice daily. The individual also drank a quart of beet/cabbage soup broth daily for the first week, took 400 milligrams magnesium citrate per day, and took sublingual methylcobalamin (high-absorption B_{12}), 5,000 micrograms twice a week. During the initial total withdrawal from alprazolam, intake of GABA was 750 milligrams three times daily. The patient experienced side effects of daily but manageable anxiety. He also reported occasional nausea, possibly attributable to the GABA and almost certainly attributable to the extremely high niacin intake. He experienced increased frequency of urination, especially at night. Evening niacin doses as inositol hexaniacinate (a semi-sustained release, no-flush niacin) reduced nighttime urination. The individual used regular flush niacin about three-quarters of the time; inositol hexaniacinate constituted the balance. Dosage was divided into eight to ten 1,000 milligrams doses in 24 hours. Niacinamide was specifically not used, as its nausea threshold is low (under 6,000 milligrams per day).

Niacin Mechanism of Action

Dr. Abram Hoffer had observed beneficial anticonvulsant activity by performing coadministration of niacinamide with anticonvulsants to treat epileptics in the early 1950s (personal communication). The dosage of the anticonvulsant could be reduced by 50 percent when 1,000 to 2,000 milligrams of niacin was administered with each meal. Hoffer noted that this was beneficial to patients because at the lower dose of anticonvulsant they were not nearly as drowsy.

In the late 1970s niacinamide was reported to be a ligand for the benzodiazepine receptor with physiological activities. Later studies suggested that the effect is not based on a direct specific interaction between niacinamide and benzodiazepine receptors.[73–75] However, ten years later a completely different benzodiazepine-binding receptor was identified in the peripheral nervous system.[76] This peripheral benzodiazepine receptor, known as translocator protein (TSPO), can modulate neurosteroids, which can alter neuronal excitability through interactions with GABA neurotransmitter ion channels. This can enhance GABA receptor function.[77]

But how can GABA taken orally help if it does not readily cross the blood brain barrier (BBB)? While GABA receptors are primarily known for their CNS locations and functions, there are also GABA receptors in the liver, immune cells, and lung cells that are accessible to bind GABA without crossing the BBB. The peripheral benzodiazepine receptor TSPO, as mentioned above, is one example. This can activate neurons in peripheral nerves that ultimately affect the CNS as well.

This case report described, however, showed a positive result when using niacin. The common theme here is nicotinamide adenine dinucleotide (NAD) since both niacin and niacinamide are converted to NAD by the body. This indicates that therapeutic benefit is most likely being mediated via the increase in NAD levels, not through activation of the high affinity niacin G-protein coupled receptor, GPR109a, which niacinamide does not bind. NAD is used in over 450 reactions by the body, which is more than any other vitamin-derived molecule. The following are just a small list of the pathways that are dependent on it: drug/xenobiotic metabolism, steroid metabolism, basic glycolysis/TCA adenosine triphosphate (ATP) generation, and many more.

These pathways are quite complicated, but one thing is for certain. We are susceptible to niacin deficiency as exemplified by the deadly pellagra epidemics in the first two decades of the twentieth century, which killed over 100,000 people in the southern United States. Due to this epidemic, President Roosevelt commissioned epidemiologists to begin working on this serious problem. Many people with skin disorders were placed in sanitariums because common subclinical pellagra symptoms are dermatitis and sensitivity to sunlight.

Niacin is thought to help maintain homeostasis of neurotransmitters that are commonly unbalanced in the brains of those with anxiety,[78] and it may also alter the metabolism of Xanax. As a primary participant in the hydroxylation reaction characteristic of phase I drug-metabolizing enzymes, NAD can speed up the metabolism of toxic waste products arising from the metabolism of the foreign alprazolam molecule.[78,79]

Specifically, Xanax is metabolized by the enzyme CYP3A4. Xanax induces CYP3A4 expression, meaning the body responds to Xanax administration by making more of the enzyme that degrades the Xanax molecule. The enzymatic reaction is dependent on the presence of the cofactor NAD, which is derived from niacin in the diet. The drug metabolizing enzyme reaction cannot proceed without the presence of all three: the substrate (Xanax), the enzyme (CYP3A4), and the cofactor in NAD (derived from niacin). Individuals taking Xanax are likely to have high levels of the drug and the enzyme. But the metabolic reaction utilizing this enzyme that degrades the drug is commonly limited by insufficient levels of the cofactor, NAD.

By administering high doses of niacin, the concentration of NAD is increased, which then accelerates the rate of the drug-metabolizing reaction, ultimately clearing the drug from the body faster. The niacin flush / vasodilation is likely to aid in delivery to otherwise hard to reach anatomical locations as well as increase physical flow of the drug metabolites.

GABA

GABA seems likely to be a safer replacement to withdraw from as compared to simple weaning off of alprazolam. Using GABA is an orthomolecular approach, involving manipulating a substance normally present in the body. Ingested GABA will be metabolized by the normal endogenous mechanisms, for which humans have evolved to control properly. GABA will likely be cleared better than alprazolam and not be afflicted with the non-specific effects associated with the foreign molecule that GABA is.

GABA is one of the main inhibitory neurotransmitters in the brain. Oral GABA does not cross the blood brain barrier (BBB), but yet GABA oral ingestion still exerts the calming effect that is attributed to GABA activity. Low GABA is detectable in Xanax withdrawal, while plenty of GABA enables one to feel calm and to sleep better. GABA has been successfully used to assist with Xanax withdrawal.[80]

Another molecule, picamilon, is a niacin molecule bonded to GABA as one single molecule that may be useful. Picamilon crosses the BBB and then is broken down to niacin and GABA. Picamilon can help restore GABA receptor levels.

Also, GABA is degraded into succinate, which in its own right can provide a significant source of energy as it directly enters the TCA cycle. Even though the exact reason is unknown, people taking GABA have noticed calming effects. The placebo effect may be responsible for part of the benefit. However, it is likely at high doses some GABA does get into the CNS.

Vitamin C

Because ascorbate in high doses is a strong antitoxin,[81] it is considered to be an important inclusion. Flu-like symptoms common in benzodiazepine withdrawal may be ameliorated with vitamin C. Ascorbate also provides support for the liver, ranging from 500 milligrams per day preventing fatty buildup and cirrhosis to 5,000 milligrams of vitamin C per day appearing to actually flush fats from the liver, to 50,000 milligrams per day eliminating jaundice in under a week.[82]

Magnesium

Magnesium depletion is common in nearly all examples of people ingesting drugs. Thus, magnesium supplements are helpful. Nightly Epsom salt baths and 400 milligrams of magnesium citrate, once in the morning and once in the afternoon, can facilitate a smooth transition away from alprazolam. Also realize that if you desire to measure your magnesium levels, be sure to do either the red blood cell test or the ionized magnesium test. However, do not test for serum magnesium levels. Serum magnesium concentrations are so tightly controlled that the results are invariably normal, so the test has been removed from the standard blood test suite.

Conclusion

Collectively this case history and biochemical rationale indicate that very high doses of niacin, GABA, and vitamin C together may greatly speed detox and reduce withdrawal symptoms from alprazolam. Additional therapeutic trials are warranted. It is emphasized that every person is different and that this experience may not be applicable to all. Alprazolam is a seriously addictive drug and withdrawal symptoms may be severe. Every individual should work closely with their health care provider.

CANCER

Niacin is effective in decreasing the death rate of patients with cancer by protecting cells and tissues from damage caused by toxic molecules or free radicals. One of the most exciting findings is that *niacin will help protect against cancer*. A 1987 conference at Texas College of Osteopathic Medicine in Fort Worth was already the eighth conference to discuss niacin and cancer. The first was held in Switzerland in 1984.

In the body, niacin is converted to nicotinamide adenine dinucleotide (NAD). NAD is a coenzyme necessary to many reactions. Another enzyme, poly (Adenosine adenine phosphate ribose) polymerase, uses NAD to catalyze the formation of ADP-ribose. The poly (ADP-ribose) polymerase is activated by strands of DNA that have been broken by smoke, herbicides, and other toxins. When the long chains of DNA are damaged, poly (ADP-ribose) helps repair it by unwinding the damaged protein. Poly (ADP-ribose) also increases the activity of DNA ligase. This enzyme cuts off the damaged strands of DNA and increases the ability of the cell to repair itself after exposure to carcinogens.

Jacobson and Jacobson[83,84] discussed the anti-cancer properties of niacin at the Texas conference. They believe niacin (more specifically, NAD) prevents processes that lead to cancer. They found that *one group of human cells given enough niacin and then exposed to carcinogens developed cancer at a rate only one-tenth of the rate in the same cells not given niacin.*

It is not surprising that niacin also decreased the death rate from cancer in the National Coronary Drug Study. I gave both niacin, 3 grams per day, and ascorbic acid, 3 grams per day, to the first cancer patient I treated in 1960. He was psychotic and had been admitted to our psychiatric ward, Royal University Hospital in Saskatoon, Saskatchewan. I did not realize that I would see him recover from both of his diseases, the psychosis and his inoperable lung cancer.[85]

Niacin and Cancer:

How Vitamin B₃ Protects and Even Helps Repair Your DNA

by W. Todd Penberthy, PhD, Andrew W. Saul, PhD, and Robert G. Smith, PhD

Although an individual's DNA sequences cannot be changed, the expression of genes can be modified by diet, including supplementation with high-dose niacin to boost NAD levels.

Cells that have had DNA damage are frequently transformed into cancer cells due to mutation. When our tumor suppressor genes are mutated, they can no longer function, and cells can grow without regulation and become cancerous. In a healthy situation, when a cell has DNA damage, poly-ADP ribose (PAR) is added to the DNA, and the cell will stop dividing. If the DNA can be repaired, the cell may continue dividing normally. If the damage is too much, then the cell will die by apoptosis. If the DNA damage is too extreme and acute, then the cell will die by the uncontrollable and messy process of necrosis, which will then adversely affect neighboring cells, likely causing greater collateral damage to them. When the PAR polymer is formed, NAD can become depleted, and cell death occurs because cells cannot live more than a minute or two without NAD.

Niacin, PAR, and Sirtuins

Poly-ADP ribose (PAR) is a polymer that is made starting from NAD, which is made from vitamin B_3 (niacin, niacinamide).[86] PAR is produced especially in response to any damage to DNA as with radiation oncology treatments, UV sunlight, many chemotherapeutics, and other DNA damaging environmental toxins. When the DNA damage is extreme, unless there is adequate vitamin B_3 (niacin or niacinamide), NAD can become so depleted that cells die by apoptosis (programmed cell death) or with more extreme damage by necrosis. PARP1 is the enzyme responsible for this enzymatic activity, and inhibitors of PARP1 will prevent this as well, thus keeping the cell alive, but at great cost.

The two primary niacin/niacinamide concentration-responsive pathways are defined by poly-ADP-ribose polymerase-1 and the sirtuins.

While PARP1 is more studied in the context of DNA damage repair, genome stability, and cancer research, the other major NAD epigenetics pathway involves the sirtuins, of which there are seven genes in humans. These genes are most known for their roles in lifespan across the animal kingdom, even in yeast. Generally, there has been a tremendous amount of research focused on identifying small molecule activators of sirtuins for many types of therapeutics as well as longevity focused supplements, where resveratrol, pterostilbenes, and polyphenols in general are the most well-known molecules.

Sirtuins work on DNA by removing a 2-carbon molecule (deacetylation), from the higher order structure of DNA wrapped around histone solenoid-like structures on chromosomes. This activity resembles that which is seen in caloric restriction, the only method shown to increase lifespan in all animal models. Sirtuins use NAD as their substrate for their activity and sirtuin activity is increased simply by keeping NAD levels up—which can be accomplished by adequate doses of niacin.

Here's where niacin/niacinamide comes in: Vitamin B_3 is the essential molecular precursor to nicotinamide adenine dinucleotide (NAD). All roads in longevity research consistently point to the importance of NAD in controlling lifespan, the most bioenergetically demanding processes (muscle and nerve), and susceptibility to all disease, including cancer.

NAD is made starting from niacin/niacinamide. The NAD precursors are niacin (or chemically, nicotinic acid), niacinamide (nicotinamide), nicotinamide riboside, or nicotinamide mononucleotide. These are all commercially available as supplements, with niacin or niacinamide as the cheapest, oldest, and most studied forms.

Niacin or niacinamide was the first form of vitamin B_3 to be discovered. These have been fortified in flour since the 1940s eradication of the pellagra epidemics that were endemic during the first decades of the 20th century United States.

NAD

Basic biology courses include instruction related to the central role that NAD plays in bioenergetics, where NAD is shorthand for nicotinamide (or niacinamide) adenine dinucleotide. Its reduced form, NADH, is used to create the voltage gradient for mitochondria that generate energy for cells, ultimately producing 3ATPs per NADH with conversion to NAD+.

However, molecular genetics research also reveals that NAD is required for the function of over 400 genes, which is far more than any other vitamin.[87,88] Moreover, NAD is involved in most of the 55 human cytochrome P450 drug-metabolizing enzymes. This family of phase-I detoxification enzymes is widely known for its role in drug metabolism, but also functions normally in detoxification of environmental chemicals as well as the metabolism of steroids, prostaglandins, and some other vitamins. Research on NAD is ongoing and complex. Here we focus on NAD-related cellular transformation leading to the development of clinical cancer.

Niacin, Cancer, DNA, and Chemotherapy

The involvement of niacin in preventing cancer and chemotherapeutic side effects is not commonly recognized, but decades of research has established that niacin deficiency is common in cancer patients and cancer patients require larger amounts of niacin to correct deficiency.[89]

Generally, studies indicate that NAD functions as a preservative protecting cellular DNA from mutation and also preventing mutated cancer cells from surviving. Niacin deficiency promotes cancer by decreasing genomic stability, increasing the chances both for mutation and survival of mutated cancer cells.

Studies indicate that niacin deficiency delays DNA repair, promotes accumulation of DNA strand breaks, chromosomal translocations, telomere erosion typical of aging, and promotes cancer. Rat model studies indicate that most of these aspects of genomic instability are all minimized by the recommended levels of niacin.[90] Niacin deficiency also increases levels of the tumor suppressor.[91] Studies in mice indicate that mild niacin deficiency can cause an increased incidence of ultraviolet-B induced skin cancer.[92]

Kirkland concluded after decades of niacin deficiency cancer research, "With exposure to stressors, like chemotherapy or excess sunlight, supraphysiological [large] doses of niacin may be beneficial."[89]

Studies have found that essentially all cancer patients are niacin deficient at first diagnosis, and almost half are still deficient after supplementation with RDA levels of niacin.[90] This strongly supports supplementation with a high-dose NAD precursor (e.g., niacinamide

500 milligrams three times per day). Adequate dosing is likely to be beneficial for the health of all cancer patients.

Niacin and Chemotherapies

Most cancer chemotherapies work by damaging the DNA of the rapidly dividing cells. Like most cancer chemotherapeutics, studies in rats have shown that niacin deficiency on its own causes anemia,[92] and it also increases the severity of mutagen-induced anemia and the development of cancer.

Chemotherapeutics targeting the NAD biosynthetic enzyme NAMT (NAMPTi) are currently in clinical trials.[93,94] All NAMPTi clinical trials to date have shown dose-limiting toxicity presentations resembling severe niacin deficiency, or pellagra. Pellagra killed over 100,000 people in the southern United States from 1900 to 1920, and prompted the discovery of niacin.[94] Moreover, no NAMPTi trial has demonstrated a reduction in tumor burden. Thus, the results of NAMPTi clinical trials do not support the idea of NAMPT targeting as a beneficial approach to treating cancer.

The amino acid glutamine plays an interesting role in cancer as there are glutamine-dependent tumors, and glutamine is required in the final step of biosynthesis to NAD starting from niacin or tryptophan, but not from niacinamide.

Thus, niacinamide or niacin supplementation is critically important for cancer patients. The beneficial effect of adequate niacin supplementation has been proven by studies showing that niacin supplementation can protect a cancer patient's bone marrow cells from the side effects of genotoxic chemotherapy drugs.

The role of NAD in the bioenergetics of cancer is huge. Cancer cells perform glycolysis at exceptionally high rates, demanding and taking glucose at the expense of healthy cells. There are distinct advantages and differences in the NAD precursor pathways as related to cancer. Niacinamide would appear to be most preferred with respect to bioenergetic perspective of cancer. A suggestion that takes this into conclusion is included below.

Conclusion

Supplementation with vitamin B_3 (niacin), the precursor to NAD, can lower the risk of cancer. NAD deficiencies are observed in nearly all cancer patients, likely due to the energy-draining component of suffering from hyper-proliferative cells. Chemotherapeutics commonly cause additional NAD deficiencies. There have been concerted efforts and considerations of targeting the NAD biosynthetic pathways as a novel patentable approach to the development of chemotherapeutics, but the results to date are in no way encouraging or exceptional, where dose-limiting toxicities resemble that of the deadly NAD deficiency disease pellagra. Many decades of research focused on using NAD precursors to favorably alter epigenetics via PARP1 and now sirtuin pathways indicate that supraphysiological doses of niacin will preserve the integrity of the genome, prevent mutation, and help prevent the rogue survival and proliferation of transformed cancer cells. In short, niacin prevents cancer and metastasis. NAD research is both complex and likely highly rewarding, and we still have much to learn regarding which NAD precursors are the best for addressing cancer. Nonetheless, studies strongly support high-dose NAD precursor supplementation. That means taking niacin, starting with low dosages (100 to 200 milligrams) to get accustomed to the flush, and working up to 500 milligrams three times a day (1,500 milligrams total). During treatment for cancer, however, niacinamide may be the preferred form since it is not dependent on glutamine for the synthesis of NAD and glutamine restriction is helpful in treatment of cancer. The authors recommend this measure as potentially highly beneficial to saving the health of all cancer patients.

- NAD deficiency is associated with greater risk for mutagenesis with cancer, and this is likely best avoided using daily niacin, e.g., starting with 100 to 200 milligrams three time per day to get to the know the flush, and then working up to 500 to 1,000 milligrams three times per day.

- For cancer patients, chemotherapy commonly causes NAD deficiency, which is best rescued with niacinamide, e.g., 500 milligrams three times per day.
- Dietary relevance, glutamine restriction with niacinamide; glucose restriction, and ketogenic diet is recommended.[95,96]

Cancer, the Mauve Factor, and Niacin

We (AH and colleagues) discovered a substance in the urine of psychiatric patients that we called the mauve factor, as it stained the paper chromatograms mauve.[97] For comparison we analyzed the urine of normal subjects and patients suffering very severe stress, such as terminal cancer. A psychotic delirious seventy-five-year-old man with terminal lung cancer was admitted to the psychiatric ward. He had been treated with cobalt bomb radiation, and the cancer clinic concluded that he could not live more than a month or two. He excreted huge quantities of the mauve factor. Most of the lung cancer patients I tested excreted this substance in large amounts.

By then I knew from our previous therapeutic trials that psychiatric patients who excreted the mauve factor responded very well to treatment with large doses of vitamin B3 (niacin or niacinamide). I suggested to his resident that he start him on niacin, 3 grams daily. The patient was started on niacin on a Friday, and by the following Monday he was mentally normal. I was interested in seeing what the long-term effect of the vitamin would be on his psychiatric state. I offered to give him both niacin and vitamin C for free if he would come to my office each month to obtain it.

A year later, I was surprised when I was told by the cancer clinic that they could no longer see any lesions in his lung. Every three months they had seen a reduction in the size of his cancer. He died twenty-eight months after I started him on the vitamin. No autopsy was performed. I thought the niacin might have been the most important agent in the reduction of his cancer, since it was and still is my favorite vitamin. I had added vitamin C only because I did so routinely for my schizophrenic patients. The exciting work of Cameron and Pauling, however, suggested that the vitamin C was the more important single factor, but since then I included niacin in my program for treating cancers.[98]

Niacin and Chemotherapy

Recent studies have increased my confidence that niacin is important for cancer treatment. In 2008 Bartleman, Jacobs, and Kirkland[99] found that niacin supplementation in rats helped protect them from the long-term deleterious effect of chemotherapy, especially the nonlymphocitic leukemia. Secondary or treatment-related cancer occurs in 5 to 15 percent of chemotherapy patients due to DNA damage. Jacobson[100] reported studies of DNA damage in cultured mouse and human cells low in niacin, suggesting that niacin may be protective against cancer. She used a biochemical method based on the observation that with deficient niacin, NAD readily decreases and NADP remains relatively constant. She used the following algorithm to determine a "niacin number," which would indicate a healthy versus low level of niacin in the body: (NAD/NAD + NADP) x 100 percent from whole. Healthy controls showed a mean niacin number of 62.8 +/- 3.0. Analyses of women in the Malmo Diet and Cancer Study showed a mean niacin number of 60.4 with a range of 44 to 75, with an unpredictably large number of individuals having low values.

Moalem[101] reported that methylation (addition of a CH3 group) of genes is related to cancer. Investigators found a very high correlation between breast cancer recurrence and the amount of methylation of a gene called PITX2. In breast cancer patients with low methylation rates, 90 percent were free of cancer for ten years, while in patients with high methylation rates only 65 percent remained cancer free for that length of time. (Smoking increases methylation as does chewing betel nut, since both are carcinogenic.) Niacin provides one of a few natural powerful methyl acceptors in the body. Jacobs and Kirkland's very important observations strongly suggest that every patient receiving chemotherapy should also be given niacin. Oncologists are not overly accustomed to seeing recoveries. If they want to improve the outcome of treatment, they should not continue to ignore this work.[102–105]

Schizophrenia, Niacin, and Cancer

Dr. Foster and I (AH) discussed a hypothesis regarding why schizophrenic patients do not get cancer as frequently as patients who are not schizophrenic.

We suggest that excess production of adrenochrome, a derivative of adrenalin, creates the psychosis, as it is a hallucinogen. At the same time, it also protects them against cancer, as it is an inhibitor of cell mitosis. Out of about five thousand patients I have seen since 1955, only twelve developed cancer. One developed cancer only recently, fifty years after being cured from her schizophrenia. The literature does not show such a clear differentiation. My patients were all on niacin and most were also on vitamin C, while none of the literature series were. This might explain this difference. In other words, these vitamins protected these patients from cancer. Of the two vitamins, niacin is probably the more relevant because the amount of vitamin C given was three grams daily or less. But when my patients were treated with large doses of vitamin C, all but one recovered.

Skin Cancer, Sunscreen, and Niacinamide

Now here's something you may not have been expecting: Professor Darmian and colleagues recently reported that niacinamide was a better sunscreen against ultraviolet-induced cancers than the common sunscreens.[106] It protects against both UVA and UVB, while common sunscreens do not protect against UVA. Niacinamide does so by maintaining the immune defenses of the skin against ultraviolet radiation. If this vitamin can protect against melanoma, it becomes even more probable that it will protect against other cancers. Of course, the entire orthomolecular program, including selenium and antioxidants such as vitamin E and C, will provide even more protection. The common sunscreens decrease exposure to ultraviolet and therefore reduce the production of vitamin D_3 in the skin. This increases the number of people who will suffer from lack of vitamin D, especially because we are exposed to so many warnings about the dangers of the sun and the need to lather ourselves with these preparations. Niacinamide does not prevent the body from making vitamin D.

Cancer of the Stomach

In September 2008, a woman consulted with me (AH) to get nutritional advice for her stomach cancer. She had been treated for colon cancer six years earlier with the usual three components of modern cancer therapy (chemotherapy, radiation, and surgery) and was apparently well for five years. Then cancer of her stomach was diagnosed. She had surgery but no further treatment was offered. As I listened to her story, I could not help but wonder whether she would have had this second cancer if she had been given niacin when she was originally treated for her colon cancer. It could not have hurt her and may have saved her from terminal cancer.

Late-Effect Cancer and Niacin

The Canadian Cancer Society reports that two-thirds of children who survive after cancer treatment have one or more late-effect cancers, and of these, one-third are grave or life-threatening, including damage to the heart, lungs, and stomach.[107] The risk of later cancers is mentioned, but not the secondary cancers induced by radiation or chemotherapy. These may average around 10 percent of the total. This article discusses what is being done to decrease these late-effect cancers, but the use of niacin in conjunction with the original treatment is not mentioned.

To understand why niacin can help to reduce cancer risk, it is necessary to understand some basic biochemistry. Niacin, niacinamide and nicotinamide adenine dinucleotide (NAD) are interconvertible, via a pyridine nucleotide cycle. NAD, the coenzyme, is hydrolyzed or split into niacinamide and adenosine dinucleotide phosphate (ADP-ribose). Niacinamide is converted into niacin, which in turn is once more built into NAD. The enzyme which splits ADP is known as poly (ADP-ribose) polymerase, or poly (ADP) synthetase, or poly (ADP-ribose) transferase.

Poly (ADP-ribose) polymerase is activated when strands of deoxyribonucleic acid (DNA) are broken. The enzyme transfers NAD to the ADP-ribose polymer, binding it onto a number of proteins. The poly (ADP-ribose) activated by DNA breaks helps repair such breaks by unwinding the nucleosomal structure of damaged chromatids. It also may increase the activity of DNA ligase. This enzyme cuts damaged ends off strands of DNA and increases the cell's capacity to repair itself. Damage caused by any carcinogenic factor such as radiation or chemicals is, as a result, neutralized or counteracted. Jacobson and Jacobson hypothesized that this is why niacin can protect against cancer. They illustrated this by treating two groups of human cells with carcinogens. The group given adequate niacin developed tumors at a rate of only 10 percent of that seen in the group that was deficient in niacin. Dr. M. Jacobson is quoted as saying, "We know that diet is a major risk factor, that diet has both beneficial and detrimental components. What we cannot assess at this point is the optimal amount of niacin in the diet. . . . The fact that we don't have pellagra does not mean we are getting enough niacin to confer resistance to cancer."[108] About 20 milligrams of niacin per day will prevent pellagra in people who are not chronic pellagrins. The latter may require twenty-five times as much niacin to remain free of pellagra.[109]

CATARACTS

Larger than dietary quantities of all of the B-complex vitamins, including niacin, appear to help prevent cataracts, as does vitamin A. Recent research involving 2,873 persons taking supplemental amounts of these nutrients showed a 30 to 60 percent reduction in nuclear or cortical cataracts.[110]

Antioxidants such as lutein and vitamins C and E are also important for cataract prevention. A review of the literature recommended that people take "considerably higher than the current recommended daily intakes"[111] of vitamin C and four times the RDA of vitamin E.

CHOLERA AND DIARRHEA

Niacin is protective in a strikingly large variety of diseases. Niacin also inhibits and reverses intestinal secretion caused by the cholera toxin and E. coli enterotoxin. A randomized controlled clinical trial showed that 2,000 milligrams of niacin per day, in divided doses, reduced fluid loss in cholera patients. It did so in less than half a day, and was described as "well-tolerated" by patients.[112] Niacin also reduces diarrhea associated with pancreatic tumors in humans. Niacinamide does not appear to have this fluid-loss reducing effect.[113]

DETOXIFICATION

L. Ron Hubbard, the controversial founder of Scientology, combined induced sweating by heat (for example, sauna) with niacin as a way of treating patients. Each technique by itself has been widely used with no danger and with many positive effects. It is clear that niacin is safe and effective.

Sweating lodges have been and are being used by native North Americans as part of a well-established ritual. It has been found to be very effective. Hubbard put these two treatments together by placing patients on niacin and then having them use heat to induce sweating. The method has been helpful, but the Hubbard detoxification program has been vilified and critically condemned simply because Hubbard was the original proponent. The main criticism is that his explanations for why it works are not scientific. I (AH) find this criticism rather simplistic, since the entire psychiatric profession has accepted psychoanalysis for many years although it has not been shown to work and has some very bizarre explanations to explain why it should work. Logically, the only important questions for any program of therapy are, "Does it work?" and, "Is it safe?" If it is eventually shown to be effective it will be easy to develop hypotheses, most of which will be wrong, to explain why. We have never been short of explanations like the stress hypothesis of peptic ulcers, which in the vast majority of cases turned out to be caused by an infection. The battle over Hubbard's detoxification treatment is a matter of one church called Medicine attacking another church called Scientology. You might wonder what happened to evidence-based medicine, until you realize that to be accepted as evidence the work has to come from a prestigious institution like Harvard, has to be done by well-established scientists, has to be published in standard journals (whose club of editorial committees keep out really new ideas), has to be accepted by the governing bodies of the traditional medical profession, and, of course, must be double-blind.

EPIDERMOLYSIS BULLOSA

In *Harrison's Principles of Internal Medicine*,[114] an inherited zinc deficiency disease is described. The symptoms and signs include severe chronic diarrhea, muscle wasting, alopecia (loss of hair), and rough, thick, ulcerated skin around the body orifices and on the extremities.

When I first saw CC, in December 1989, he appeared to be about ten years old, was very short and physically immature. Mentally he appeared to be normal. There were no perceptual changes or thought disorder, and his mood was surprisingly cheerful and upbeat. After CC was born, his skin, which had been under pressure from a forceps delivery, began to slough off.

A few days later lesions, which later blistered, developed on his face, mouth, chest, and limbs. He was treated with topical antibiotics using sterile techniques but did not improve. The lesions in his mouth made it impossible for him to feed, and he became anemic and hypoproteinemic. One month later he was diagnosed with epidermolysis bullosa and started on vitamin E, 600 international units orally, later increased to 800 international units. At age four months, 200 milligrams of ascorbic acid was added, and at age six months he was given iron supplementation and the vitamin E was increased to 1,000 international units. There was no response. He was then admitted to the hospital suffering from stomatitis, and again in April 1973, for gastroenteritis and pneumonia. By then he had multiple lesions, denuded areas on his legs, no nails, adhesions between his fingers and toes. On top of this he was constantly constipated. His mother had to remove his stools manually daily, and in 1986 he was admitted to the hospital to have his stools removed. In 1980 his parents took him to West Germany for two and one-half months to be treated by a biochemist, who was using special skin salves and other treatment with some success. He was placed on a vegetarian diet supplemented with a moderate vitamin program (doses unknown). This regimen was helpful. They went back to Germany once more for ten days and would have gone again, but they could no longer afford to do so.

The bullous lesions continued to erupt. He had lost all of his fingers and toes. An attempt had been made to separate them surgically in Italy with no success. When he came to see me, he told me that food did not taste normal and he was still severely constipated. To test his sense of taste for a possible zinc deficiency, I gave him a teaspoon of a special zinc sulfate solution. He found it tasted like stale water, not bitter as it would to normal individuals. I could not order a blood test for zinc since all his superficial veins were gone and it would have required a cut down. Zinc deficiency will cause dwarfism, retarded wound healing, and loss of taste. The classic response to chronic zinc deficiency is acrodermatitis enteropathica (AE). AE babies develop infections around their body orifices.

I advised that CC start on the following supplements: niacinamide, 500 milligrams twice daily; ascorbic acid, 500 milligrams three times daily (1,500 milligrams, about 100 times the RDA); pyridoxine, 100 milligrams twice daily; cod liver oil, one-half teaspoon daily; ten drops twice daily of a solution of zinc sulfate 10 percent with manganese chloride ½ percent; plus 1 teaspoon of linseed oil daily to increase his intake of omega-3 essential fatty acids.

Two weeks later he was much improved. His mood remained normal, but his parents were much more cheerful. In that brief period, he had grown half an inch in height, his skin appeared much healthier, and the lesions occurred about one-third as frequently. Those that did develop healed much more quickly. He had gained two pounds. He was no longer constipated and was able to have normal bowel movements for the first time in his life.

This patient's rapid response does not prove it was due entirely to the administration of the zinc. I suspect that zinc was the main therapeutic variable, but the other nutrients must also have played an important part.

I spoke to his pediatrician on October 17, 1991. She had just seen him a week before. She told me that his skin condition was stable, but that he had started to show emotional problems as he matured. CC called me on October 24, 1991. He said that his skin condition was stable even though he had remained on the total nutrient approach for only one year. Since then, he had minor skin eruptions in the spring and in the fall. He had grown about three to four inches and had gained fifteen pounds. His mood was level, and he was cheerful. However, he was experiencing constipation again. He died in November 1998 from a bowel obstruction.

ERECTILE DYSFUNCTION

Can niacin help erectile dysfunction (ED)? The most accurate answer may be "Yes," "No," and "Maybe."

A qualified "Yes," because niacin normalizes blood lipids. One may expect niacin's long-term circulatory benefits to include facilitating a male's erection, which is dependent on blood supply to the penis. Niacinamide will not achieve this.

A qualified "No," because vasodilation produced by ED drugs is longer-lasting than that produced by niacin. An example of this is the niacin flush itself, commonly ending in half an hour or so.

And "Maybe," because while improved mood tends to increase sexual interest, a sense of calmness from a goodly dose of niacin may actually diminish passion. There is also the unavoidable additional likelihood that if people think what they have taken will improve sex, it probably will.

Sildenafil (a common generic version of the better-known Viagra) is prescribed for pulmonary hypertension. It is a vasodilator. So is niacin, but I (AWS) am unaware that niacin has ever been accepted as a treatment for hypertension. But it is plausible. Some package inserts for prescription, extended-release niacin state that niacin may cause temporary hypotension [low blood pressure]. "From a chronic standpoint, larger studies, such as the Coronary Drug Project, suggest that niacin may lower BP when administered over a longer period of time."

Niacin and its flush have been employed by people with Raynaud's syndrome. The vasodilation effect has been reported to be sufficient to noticeably help, and the warming sensation of the flush is welcomed by people with cold extremities. It is about dose: enough niacin must be taken to get the flush. This varies greatly from person to person. Remember that vasodilation occurs only with niacin. Niacinamide will not work, and inositol nicotinate probably will not work.

Erectile Dysfunction and Niacin

by W. Todd Penberthy, PhD, and Andrew W. Saul, PhD

There is solid evidence that niacin on its own can help effectively treat erectile dysfunction.[115] Niacin's long-term circulatory benefits may include facilitating a male's erection, which is dependent on blood supply to the penis, because niacin normalizes blood lipids. Niacinamide will not achieve this.[116]

It's important to appreciate that an ED diagnosis likely denotes greater significance than just the loss of ability to have satisfactory sex. In fact, ED is considered to be one the earliest presentations prognostic of atherosclerotic cardiovascular disease—the most common age-related cause of death.[117] Hyperlipidemia, hypercholesterolemia, tobacco abuse, diabetes, or coronary artery disease are common risk factors present in ED.[118]

Fortunately, pennies a day of over-the-counter high-dose niacin is established as an effective treatment for directly addressing atherosclerosis, hyperlipidemia, hypercholesterolemia, and coronary disease, and niacin has been used safely and effectively for over 60 years in clinical medicine.[119-121] Generally, the higher the dose of niacin, the more effective it is.[122] It is always best to take it with food and not in a fasted state.

Similar to popular ED drugs, niacin is also a vasodilator, but the vasodilation induced by ED drugs may be longer-lasting. For example, the niacin flush itself commonly ends within half an hour or so. Still, it is not entirely known whether the flush pathway is the primary mechanism of action for how niacin works to provide benefits for ED patients as there are many therapeutic mechanisms for high-dose niacin treatment.

In short, the engorgement of the penis relies on a healthy circulation, and niacin directly addresses these concerns in a safe fashion.

The biochemistry of a male erection initiates from a cascade of nerve signals starting in the brain and running the length of the spinal cord down to the penis. In response to these signals, nerves within a spongy vasculature (corpus cavernosom) release nitric oxide gas molecules that drive production of cyclic guanosine monophosphate (cGMP) that ultimately exerts the relaxing expansive effect characteristic of an erection.

However, a permanent erection is of course unacceptable, so nature provided the phosphodiesterase type 5 (PDE5) enzyme to break down the CGMP and accordingly pharmaceutical companies developed drugs like Viagra to inhibit PDE5 to keep the cGMP levels elevated with stimulation of erection as desired. While Viagra is the most used approach, penile injections of prostaglandin (PGE1) mimetics were used prior to the introduction of Viagra and have been considered the gold standard for directly addressing ED, albeit with more side effects.[123] Niacin treatment increases nitric oxide synthase production and niacin causes a massive release of prostaglandins including PGE2 in the flush, but it is unknown whether niacin boosts PGE1 as well.

eNOS: Endothelial nitric oxide synthase, an enzyme that helps to make nitric oxide (NO)

PDE5: Phosphodiesterase type 5 (PDE5) breaks down cGMP (below)

cGMP: Cyclic guanosine monophosphate is involved in producing more NO

IIEF: International Index of Erectile Function, an accepted standard for measuring ED outcomes.

There is evidence that niacin alone does work for ED. The first niacin-only for treating ED study was "Effect of Niacin on Erectile Function in Men Suffering Erectile Dysfunction and Dyslipidemia."[115] The authors wrote:

[W]hen patients were stratified according to the baseline severity of ED, the patients with moderate and severe ED who received niacin showed a significant improvement in IIEF-Q3 scores and IIEF-Q4 scores compared with baseline values, but not for the placebo group. The improvement in IIEF-EF domain score for severe ED patients in the niacin group were 5.28 (p≤0.001) as compared to 2.65 (p < 0.04) for placebo respectively.

The results had high statistical significance (meaning they were almost certainly not due to chance). The authors concluded that *"Niacin alone can improve the erectile function in patients suffering from moderate to severe ED and dyslipidemia."*

Sildenafil (a common generic version of the better-known Viagra) is prescribed for pulmonary hypertension. It is a vasodilator. While niacin has not been commonly recognized as a treatment for hypertension, it can assist in lowering blood pressure. However, the effect of niacin is much more continuous than sildenafil, with a far greater number of clinically proven benefits than the PDE5 inhibitors. While PDE5 inhibitors work ultimately by increasing nitric oxide, niacin is also known to increase nitric oxide.

This makes perfect sense, given that increased circulation is the very basis of the male erection, and any dyslipidemia-associated blockage can be expected to interfere with this process.

Severe ED most commonly involves poor circulation that can be effectively treated with high-dose niacin therapy. This comes with the side benefit of possibly saving your life from a cardiovascular event. Reduction in mortality by the most common cause of death has been proven for niacin in RCTs even nine years after cessation of treatment (2.4 grams per day), but not for Viagra/sildenafil except in neonates, but not adults with pulmonary hypertension.[124–126]

One study has examined the PDE5 inhibitor vardenafil, with or without niacin, with propionyl-1-carnitine and 1-arginine (NCA). Treatment with NCA alone increased IEFF5 by 2 points, vardenafil increased it by 4 points, NCA plus vardenafil increased it by 5 points, and placebo exerted no change at all.[127]

In addition to ED, sildenafil (Viagra) is used for pulmonary hypertension, high altitude edema, and Raynaud's phenomena. We personally know people whose Raynaud's disappeared after two weeks of treatment with high-dose niacin. The vasodilation effect has been reported to be sufficient to noticeably help, and the warming sensation of the flush is welcomed by people with cold extremities. It is about dose: enough niacin must be taken to get the flush. This varies greatly from person to person. Remember that vasodilation occurs with standard niacin but not with other niacin forms. Niacinamide will not work, and inositol niacinate probably will not work. For comfort, niacin should be taken with food and not in a fasted state.

To the amazement of physicians and patients, high doses of niacin routinely correct dyslipidemia. Higher doses generally confer the greatest effect. This includes high-dose niacin-mediated routine correction of elevated total cholesterol, triglycerides, VLDL, and LDL, while simultaneously boosting HDL ("good cholesterol") more than any known pharmaceutical.

It should also be noted that there are many different marketed laboratory tests for assessing the lipid contributions to the risk of atherosclerotic cardiovascular disease. Among the most significant contributors, prognostic of future cardiovascular events is high Lp(a) and fibrinogen.[128,129] Niacin lowers Lp(a) and fibrinogen.[115,119,129] By contrast, statins in fact raise Lp(a), which is completely undesirable, and they are well known to have many side effects, including some that can be serious. Still, statins are commonly used and continue to be explored in new clinical trials given the great profit incentive.

PDE5 inhibitors (sildenafil/Viagra, vardenafil, tadalafil, and avanafil) do not directly cause penile erections but instead affect the response to sexual stimulation. Sildenafil was the first to be approved and is most effective in men with mild-to-moderate ED. Sexual stimulation is necessary to activate the response. The side effects of sildenafil include headache, flushing, indigestion, nasal congestion, and impaired vision, including photophobia and blurred vision. By comparison, niacin has been around much longer than sildenafil/Viagra. Since the 1930s, niacin has been examined in many more trials than sildenafil/Viagra, which was first marketed for ED in 1998.

Niacin's dyslipidemia-correcting benefits are highly dose-dependent, with plain old original immediate release niacin exerting the greater benefits than timed release.[122] These studies have clearly shown that correction of dyslipidemic measures of HDL cholesterol, triglycerides, total cholesterol, and LDL-C are greater when administering the high dose of 3 grams per day as compared to 2 grams, 1 gram, or 500 milligrams per day.

Niacin requirements and dosing is highly individual. Some individuals are more sensitive than others to the niacin flush response. First, one should always take high-dose niacin with food and not in a fasted state; secondly, the more one takes a high dose of niacin, the more one can tolerate it. So, one may start their "high dose" at 50 milligrams three times a day and go for one to two weeks before increasing this to higher doses. Ideally an individual can eventually comfortably take 500 milligrams or up to 2 grams (2,000 milligrams) per administration taken once or twice a day. Some are very sensitive to even 50 milligrams, while others can take 2 grams and notice nothing. Generally, the latter is not a good sign.

To prevent ED, it will likely be most effective to correct deficiencies in ED-associated biochemical pathways, including the levels of niacin and arginine, because these pathways depend on niacin and arginine for nitric oxide production. Further, the simple fact that niacin costs less than three percent of the cost of ED drugs is in itself reason to investigate further.

Additionally, the amino acid **arginine** has its own special benefits in improving blood flow, benefiting persons with angina[130] and even perhaps those with erectile dysfunction.[131]

FATIGUE

Diagnosing fatigue is very difficult, as being tired accompanies almost every known affliction from which so many of us suffer. Fatigue is a universal response to being sick, and is advantageous from an evolutionary point of view. It is a warning and forces us to decrease our activity so the body can devote more energy to healing itself. Fatigue is common in all nutritional diseases including starvation, deficiency, and dependencies; with all infections; with lack of rest and sleep; with diseases such as diabetes, multiple sclerosis (MS), and muscle disease; with chronic pain; with diagnosable cancer; and even in manic patients who do not appear to be tired but will admit they are. Fatigue is common to mood disorders and schizophrenia, and of course is made much worse by the modern antipsychotic drugs. I think the term fatigue should be reserved only for patients with no identified causes for their symptoms and suggest they be diagnosed with idiopathic fatigue (IF).

There is a cause for chronic fatigue in every sufferer that has to be identified. One of the major causes of idiopathic fatigue has been ignored. This is the hypothesis developed by the New Zealand biologist Les Simpson. Maupin's brief review of Simpson's research is excellent.[132] Simpson showed that impaired blood flow was a major factor in many chronic diseases which create chronic fatigue. Decreased blood viscosity and decreased capillary blood flow are involved. Since becoming aware of his work, I have found that his therapeutic program using essential fatty acids and large doses of vitamin B_{12}, to which I have added niacin, is very effective in treating many cases of IF. If the diameters of the capillaries are too small, they cannot deliver enough blood to the tissues. Associated reasons are the size and shape of the red blood cells, which slows down their movement through the capillaries. Red blood cells do not flow through these small vessels; they crawl or wiggle through. This makes sense, as this process facilitates the transfer of gases from the inner lining of the capillaries to the red blood cells. In abnormal conditions the cells may be too large, as in pernicious anemia, or they may be misshapen, and they may be too rigid. They must be flexible in order to transverse the capillaries. Simpson demonstrated these changes in many studies in chronic diseases such as MS.

Niacin and Fatigue

Ed Boyle, one of the first physicians to take our niacin findings seriously, discovered there were empty capillaries in the retina of some patients. He became interested in the sludging (clumping) of red blood cells, which made it difficult for them to traverse the capillaries. Red blood cells have to go through the capillaries individually, not holding hands with their neighbors. He thought that these cells had lost some of their surface electronegative charge and were no longer able to repel each other. Based on Boyle's theory I developed the following program for IF:

- Large doses of parenteral vitamin B_{12} (1 to 5 milligrams of hydroxocobalamin), up to several times each week, and gradually decreasing the frequency as the patient improved. This vitamin would decrease the size of the red cells.

- Essential fatty acids to increase the flexibility of the red cell surface membrane. Boyle used evening primrose oil; I use the fish oils, which are richer in omega-3 essential fatty acids.

- Niacin—up to 1 gram three times daily (that is, up to 3,000 milligrams total), after each of three meals. This breaks up the clumps of red cells by keeping them from sticking to each other. It also dilates the capillaries (via the flush or vasodilatation) and allows more blood to traverse them. There is an additional advantage. Simpson points out that when plasma cholesterol levels are raised, there is an increase in the cholesterol content of the red cell membrane. This change results in the red cells becoming less pliable, which reduces capillary blood flow.[133,134] Increased cholesterol levels are associated with increased blood viscosity.

This program increases the flow of blood to the tissues of the body by dilating the capillaries; decreasing the size of the larger red blood cells, making them more flexible; breaking up and preventing sludging of the cells; and decreasing viscosity. The results have been spectacular. It is possible to spot a person whose blood is sludged by their appearance. They are obese, very pale, sweaty, and short of breath. Often after the first dose of niacin their normal color returns. Patients find this program easy to follow. Perhaps this type of IF should be called blood rheology fatigue.

The above program is the specific treatment for rheology fatigue, but it is not the ideal treatment for IF. The best treatment for IF is the program that works so well for the pandeficiency syndrome (see chapter 7). The ideal program includes finding and dealing with the cause or causes of the fatigue. Nutritionally, it includes good nutrition free of the sugars, sweeteners, and foods that one is allergic to. It also includes vitamin C, selenium, essential fatty acids, vitamin D (especially in northern countries), calcium and magnesium, and quite often zinc. A female patient of mine with chronic fatigue and fibromyalgia along with depression, anxiety, and fear started on this program. By the end of the second year, she was normal and delighted with how well she was feeling. She had been started on vitamin D, 6,000 international units daily, but only after she increased the dose to 10,000 international units did her fibromyalgia suddenly clear. After a while she went back to 6,000 international units, and the pain did not return.

HARTNUP DISEASE

Hartnup disease is due to a hereditary inability to absorb tryptophan and some other amino acids. It is an uncommon condition that results in a skin rash and some brain abnormalities. Either niacin or niacinamide will provide relief from skin and neurological symptoms of this fairly rare, inherited disorder. Supplementation is essential, as dietary quantities of niacin are insufficient and ineffective.[135] Dosage recommendations vary; somewhere in the vicinity of 300 milligrams or more per day is probably optimum.

HUNTINGTON'S DISEASE

Huntington's disease is a mixture of schizophrenic symptoms and neurological signs and symptoms. It is quite rare. I (AH) have seen two cases, and they both recovered on a combination of niacin, which protects them from the psychosis, and vitamin E, which protects them against the physical symptoms. This is a series of only two patients, with a 100 percent success rate. Dr. Tenna wrote to me that she had three patients doing quite well. "The niacin is the key to energy, it seems. Even the sibling who is most affected is responding to activated B$_3$, B vitamins, coenzyme Q$_{10}$ (CoQ$_{10}$), and folate (5 milligrams three times daily)."

MIGRAINE HEADACHE

There has been interest in using niacin to treat and prevent migraine headaches since 1951.[136] Recently, the Mayo Clinic Division of Pain Management in Scottsdale, Arizona, described one patient's experience:

> [The patient's] migraine headaches responded dramatically to sustained-release niacin as preventive treatment. Niacin is not generally considered to be effective for migraine prevention. However, low plasma levels of serotonin have been implicated in migraine pathogenesis, and niacin may act as a negative feedback regulator on the kynurenine pathway to shunt tryptophan into the serotonin pathway, thus increasing plasma serotonin levels. Sustained-release niacin merits further study as a potentially useful preventive therapy for migraine headache.[137]

A 2005 review of nine articles investigating niacin therapy for migraine stated:

> Intravenous and oral niacin has been employed in the treatment of acute and chronic migraine and tension-type headaches, but its use has not become part of contemporary medicine, nor have there been randomized controlled trials further assessing this novel treatment. . . . Hypothetical reasons for niacin's effectiveness include its vasodilatory properties, and its ability to improve mitochondrial energy metabolism. . . . Although niacin's mechanisms of action have not been substantiated from controlled clinical trials, this agent may have beneficial effects upon migraine and tension-type headaches.[138]

MULTIPLE SCLEROSIS

New research confirms that niacinamide, also known as vitamin B_3, is a key to the successful treatment of multiple sclerosis (MS) and other nerve diseases. Niacinamide, say researchers at Harvard Medical School, "profoundly prevents the degeneration of demyelinated axons and improves the behavioral deficits."[139] Kaneko and coworkers found that nicotinamide, by increasing NAD levels in the nervous system, was therapeutic against MS in the mouse model. It prevented further degeneration of axons and inflammation of the axons and loss of myelin. A Reuters News report added:

> Dr. Abram Hoffer, who was not involved in the research and is in practice in Saskatoon, Saskatchewan, has treated over sixty MS patients over the years with large oral doses of vitamin B₃ ranging from 3 to 6 grams per day. "In most cases, when the treatment was started early, early results were very good," he said.[140]

This is very good news, but it is not at all new news. Over sixty years ago, Canadian physician H.T. Mount began treating multiple sclerosis patients with intravenous B₁ (thiamine) plus intramuscular liver extract, which provides other B vitamins. He followed the progress of these patients for up to twenty-seven years. The results were excellent and were described in a paper published in the *Canadian Medical Association Journal* in 1973.[141]

Mount was not alone. Forty years ago, Frederick Robert Klenner, MD, of North Carolina, was using vitamins B₃ and B₁, along with the rest of the B-complex vitamins, vitamins C and E, and other nutrients including magnesium, calcium, and zinc to arrest and reverse multiple sclerosis.[142,143] Klenner's complete treatment program was originally published as "Treating Multiple Sclerosis Nutritionally," in *Cancer Control Journal*.[144]

Dr. Mount and Dr. Klenner were persuaded by their clinical observations that multiple sclerosis, myasthenia gravis, and many other neurological disorders were primarily due to nerve cells being starved of nutrients. Each physician tested this theory by giving his patients large, orthomolecular quantities of nutrients. Their successful cures over decades of medical practice proved that their theory was correct. B-complex vitamins, including thiamine as well as niacinamide, are absolutely vital for nerve cell health. Where pathology already exists, unusually large quantities of vitamins are needed to repair damaged nerve cells.

Dr. Klenner used a combination of B-complex vitamins given by injection and orally to treat, and cure, many patients with MS. I (AH) have used a modification of the Klenner program, as many patients found it too difficult to obtain Dr. Klenner's preferred parenteral (intravenous) administration of vitamins. It is an effective treatment.

One man has gone public with his success story. Peter Leeds was diagnosed with multiple sclerosis in 2004. In October 2005, Dr. Hoffer put him on a high-protein but dairy-free diet, and had him take vitamin supplements including niacin, the rest of the B-complex, vitamins C and D, zinc, and salmon oil. One year later, he was "very much better. The only thing left is some slight numbness in his fingers, but there is a major improvement. In fact, he had several MRIs, and the second one showed a major deteriorating spot in his brain that is now almost gone, which was very surprising to the neurologist."[145]

And here is a November 2008 report from a client placed on treatment several years ago. He had the classical clinical and pathological changes in his brain and his prognosis was not good. "I just got the results of my latest MRI on Wednesday. It showed no progression of the disease since the previous MRIs of two years ago. The MS specialist was pretty pleased, and says I'm doing something right." He recovered after about one and a half years of treatment. The neurologist found him normal. The brain scan was normal. His doctor said that had he not seen the brain scan at first, he would not have diagnosed him as having multiple sclerosis. Then, having pronounced him well, he asked the former patient whether he would participate in testing a new drug for treating MS! Pharmaceutical hope springs eternal.

Niacin for Multiple Sclerosis

by W. Todd Penberthy

While large-scale RCTs exploring niacin as a treatment of clinical MS remains tragically unconsidered since Mount and Klenner's work, basic multiple sclerosis research continues perennially to produce positive results. This ignoring of niacin for MS by RCTs may perhaps only be explained by the average cost required for performing RCTs, which costs tens of millions of dollars. Meanwhile, basic research continues to impress with countless regular publications demonstrating its efficacy in every animal model of MS, preserving nerves before or after initiating the pathogenesis.

Wee Yong's work showing increasing myelination is amazing. He is also doing clinical trials exploring niacin for treating glioblastoma right now! He has over 200 publications to his name.

Wee Yong gives me hope that someone will reach a greater audience toward eventually understanding that niacin is a basic part of the human body machine divine, exceptionally perfectly suited for addressing MS.

He has published niacin clinical research in the highest-impact journals, and only within the past month have we connected by email. I sent him my IDO (indoleamine 2,3-dioxygenase) manuscript (largely inspired by my interactions with Hoffer and my proudest research accomplishment). It is an advanced concept, the idea of anatomically localized pellagra that can be complementarily addressed with high-dose niacin therapy. He will get it. Let's hope the greater medical community follows suit.[146]

NEPHRITIS

In the United States, only one in ten patients who need kidney transplants gets one. There are too few kidneys available, and the operation is expensive (over $100,000). Each year, some 30,000 transplants are done in the United States; about 100,000 persons are on waiting lists. In 2005, 341,000 Americans were on dialysis. Dialysis costs approximately $50,000 per year. But there is a potential solution. If diseased kidneys were cured, there would be no need for dialysis and transplants.

Kidney tissue is protected by niacinamide.[147] It protected rats against the diabetogenic effect of the antibiotic streptozotocin. Clinically, niacin has been used to successfully treat patients with severe glomerulonephritis, a condition that impairs normal kidney function and results in tissue swelling, high blood pressure, and blood in the urine. One of my (AH) patients was being readied for dialysis. Her nephrologist had advised her she would die if she refused to undergo this procedure. She started on niacin 3,000 milligrams per day and is still well, twenty-five years later.

Condorelli[148] listed a large number of cardiovascular problems he treated with niacin, including nephritis. About forty years ago a woman told me she had just been diagnosed with kidney failure. She would have to start dialysis immediately in preparation for a kidney transplant when one became available. Kidney dialysis had just been introduced to Saskatoon, and she was very worried. While she was telling me this, I remembered the Italian studies, and suggested she discuss them with her doctor. I advised that it could do no harm and might help. She discussed the studies with her doctor, who thought the idea was hilarious. But it was no laughing matter for her. She rejected his advice and started niacin on her own. Thirty years later, when we were having dinner in Victoria, her husband reminded me of this. She had recovered and remained well on niacin, three grams daily. Her recovery broke the rule that there was no treatment for nephritis.

Later Dr. Max Vogel, an orthomolecular physician in Calgary, told me about a similar case. A twelve-year-old girl with glomerulonephritis was given niacin by her father, a teacher. When no treatment was offered to her, he researched as much as he could and discovered this vitamin. She recovered. He then had Dr. Vogel examine her. He confirmed that she had been sick and was now well. So now we have two cases out of two self-treated with niacin. As far as I know, no one else has tried this.

Two recoveries may not be very convincing to physicians raised on double-blind studies, but it is convincing to me and suggests that there must be other patients with nephritis who could also benefit from this program. It is surely beyond all reason to conclude that these two recoveries, directly and indirectly known to me, would be the only cases on Earth. If one crow is white, it surely raises the odds that there are other crows that are white. In the same way, if one or two patients recover from a disease for which there is no treatment, it surely means there are other patients who will display similar results. But if no one looks into this, we will not know what proportion of the one-half million North Americans headed for kidney transplants can be helped. Think of the enormous savings to patients, families, and society if only one in a hundred were healed! But there is no incentive for Big Pharma to research this, as vitamin-based cures do not bring in billions of dollars in profit. The kidney transplant industry would be devastated if each patient has an average expenditure of only about $200 per year. Treating only ten patients successfully would save over a million dollars in treatment and maintenance costs—and given the 100 percent recovery experienced by our two patients, it is highly likely that the number of people who do get well would be much greater than ten.

Reversing Chronic Kidney Disease with Niacin and Sodium Bicarbonate

Review and Commentary by

Stephen McConnell and W. Todd Penberthy

This story began with initial discovery, motivated by necessity. It would lead a few years later to reproducible documented reversal of chronic kidney disease (CKD) stages 1 or 2. Success was achieved using 3 to 5 cents per day of 100 to 500 milligrams niacin three times a day, along with 1.0 to 1.8 grams of sodium bicarbonate (baking soda, 600 milligrams at lunch and 1.2 grams before bed) with or without approximately 2 grams per day elemental calcium, as calcium carbonate.

Excellent results from the use of niacin to treat CKD have now been documented for more than 25 case-studies. This approach is well supported by continuous basic and clinical research, including dozens of clinical trials that provide substantial evidence for the use of niacin and sodium bicarbonate. These approaches directly address the needs of the typical CKD patient. Unfortunately, this approach is rarely implemented in the clinical setting.

CKD commonly progresses with age as it is observed in 68 percent of Americans over the age of 60.[149] Patients with CKD usually experience progressive loss of kidney function moving toward an increasing risk of end-stage renal disease (ESRD). CKD is the 9th leading cause of death in the US.[150] Fortunately, there are several simple approaches including the addition of modest doses of niacin (immediate release- or IR-niacin) that can reverse CKD in many patients as described here.

Approximately 786,000 people per year in the United States progress to ESRD (stage 5 CKD), which is generally considered an irreversible condition. Most of these become completely dependent on regular trips to dialysis. Estimation of the stages of CKD is based on (GFR) glomerular filtration rates starting with less than 60 milliliters per 1.7 square meters, for 3 months, as definitive of initial

CKD diagnosis. Unfortunately, a creatinine derived GFR (crGFR) is only as reliable as the serum creatinine measure. Use of this creatinine-based test has a "blind-area" in the earlier stages, and frequently leads to an under-estimation of the true risk.

Stages of CKD

1. Mild kidney damage, eGFR 90 or higher
2. Mild loss of kidney function, eGFR 60 to 89
3. Moderate loss of kidney function
   a. eGFR 45 to 59
   b. eGFR 30 to 44
4. Severe loss of kidney function, eGFR 15 to 29
5. Kidney failure or close to failure, eGFR less than 15

Niacin for CKD

Supplementation with daily low-dose niacin reliably reverses a large amount of the functional loss. This simple treatment is effective and critically important. Mortality rates with CKD are striking, as the five-year survival rate for patients doing long-term dialysis is 35 percent compared to 25 percent in those with diabetes [T2DM] in the United States.[151]

Routinely, the first treatment approaches utilized for CKD patients, in the later stages, generally targets control of dysglycemia and reduction of hyperphosphatemia according to KDIGO guidelines.[152] Fortunately, there is an ever-increasing abundance of data revealing that simple niacin treatment is a profoundly effective treatment for reducing hyperphosphatemia—and that is just the beginning. In basic research the evidence in favor of niacin for CKD has continuously accumulated. Clinical research proves that the niacin stimulated pathways involving increased NAD synthesis, PCSK9 inhibition, sodium transporter effects, PPAR gamma activation, and more, are exceptionally well-suited to addressing CKD, multimorbidity, and ultimately all-cause mortality.[153-189]

The clinical and financial impact of CKD when it progresses to end-stage renal disease (dialysis-dependence; ESRD) is profound. Clinically, CKD progression quickly leads to lifelong dialysis with co-morbid life-threatening cardiovascular disease. Financially, the out-of-pocket cost of CKD is greater than cancer and stroke with ESRD dialysis costing $30.9 billion per year in 2013, or approximately 7.1 percent of total Medicare costs.[190] Medicare spends approximately $250,000 per year for every CKD patient, *prior to* the transition to ESRD and dialysis. Annual costs per dialysis patient can range from $720,000 to $2.2 million per year.[191] These problems and their associated costs can be reduced by using 5 cents per day of niacin.

Originally, I (SM) was formally trained to operate a heart-lung machine, maintain full life-support and anesthesia, in the operating room monitoring patients undergoing open-heart surgery. Much later, I transitioned to working as a field scientist, MSL (Medical Science Liaison) in the advanced laboratory diagnostics industry. My primary clinical focus since that time has mainly been lipidology. Because of my initial education/training, addressing cardiovascular disease, I now focus on prevention: lipidology. This training gave me an appreciation for nicotinic acid (niacin, vitamin B_3).

I have now personally observed more than 25 documented cases of individuals having their CKD progression not only halted but reversed with the addition of 3 to 5 cents worth of niacin per day (with 1.8 to 2.4 grams per day sodium bicarbonate with/without 250 to 500 milligrams per day calcium carbonate).

A Family Story

While I (SM) was learning lipidology in the period between 2002 to 2007, my father suddenly went to the ER late one Sunday night and my mother called me hysterically: "I took your father to the ER and now they are scheduling him for placement of stents." I was concerned, as any son would be, but also as a scientist because I felt I may have "failed him," somehow: If only what I had learned, I had learned sooner.

My father was 81 at the time and he had been jumping rope for 30 minutes, twice daily. His body had a deceptively healthy look, and his triglycerides were low, but when we put it all together, he was "Pattern-B"—insulin resistant. He had always been a "stodgy," stubborn, stoic World War II veteran. He was very introverted and typically had a limited range of emotions: rage, laughter, and silence. Later, I would find out he had Asperger's.

When I received the advanced laboratory data, it showed that he had low HDL2 and high ApoB. This is far more specific and confers much greater risk vs. an elevated LDL-C. Most importantly, this revealed he was insulin resistant (pre-diabetic). At the time, I really didn't fully understand this. Even today, most clinicians really do not, due to continued reliance on using only tests for FBG and HbA1c. Ultimately, my father survived that, and we continued to institute aggressive medical management: A hard lesson learned.

My father and my mother traveled everywhere together. They commuted, seasonally to Florida each winter, to escape the cold weather in northwest Pennsylvania. On New Year's Day, about six months after his myocardial infarction and stent-placement procedure, I received a call from my mother: "Your father is in the hospital! They're going to have to do open-heart surgery!"

They needed to do an aortic-annuloplasty (aortic heart valve repair) in addition to a quintuple CABG (5 bypass grafts). I thought to myself, "this is getting worse and worse." Having had previous personal experience working with thoracic surgeons during open-heart operations, I didn't want the procedure to begin until my brother and I were able to be present. Fortunately, the young thoracic surgeon and the techniques planned were excellent.

Later, in the spring, they returned home to Erie, Pennsylvania, for the follow-up visit. Dr. Dave (the physician who asked me to set-up my first lipid clinic) said, "Hey, I got some bad news for you. Your dad has renal insufficiency." I said, "Oh my God, he's in renal failure. What stage is he?" He did not know. That was a flag. Most clinicians don't know what stage their CKD patients are because the lab doesn't do calculations and the creatinine measure is not reliable or accurate. The creatinine measure has very little accuracy until after the CKD has "hit" stage 3B, and beyond.[192,193] So, a lot of these patients along the CKD disease continuum, through each progressive stage, appear to have less risk vs. the "true" risk that is present. It's better to test a urine sample and see how much protein is recovered, and run a Cystatin-C and a crGFR to calculate a more accurate value. At that time, I only knew he was in failure, but when I did the crGFR calculation, I could see that he was well into the latter portion, of CKD-stage 4.

Around that time, I had been putting together a new treatment algorithm with substantial literature support, data, on CKD. I was lucky to have been mentored by Dr. William F. Finn.[194] Even if a patient has not already been scheduled for dialysis, he explained, and especially if they are currently on dialysis, you must *get the serum phosphorus down*. Excessive phosphorus is toxic to the kidneys as well as virtually every organ system and the entire body.[195,196] Phosphorus is a primary initiator of vascular calcification, among several other pathologies. If the kidneys start to lose a certain fraction of their normal function, the body can no longer efficiently clear phosphorus. When phosphorus serum levels reach abnormal levels, then you begin to saturate the tissues. Then phosphorus binds to calcium, and it's the phosphorus, not the calcium, that starts the pathology leading to calcium phosphate stones.

Niacin Helps Get the Phosphorus Down

Even after you bring serum phosphate down you still have it in the tissues. The only biomarker available in a clinical setting, Fibroblast Growth Factor-23 (FGF-23), reflects the pathology behind long-term exposure to elevated phosphorus. FGF-23 can be decreased, simply by administering niacin.[162] However, the sodium phosphorus transporter works through a feedback mechanism to make more receptors to compensate.

So, calcium carbonate (from an antacid tablet) is commonly used first to bind the readily available intestinal phosphorus. This is among the cheapest and most effective phosphorus chelator approaches. Calcium carbonate should not be used above 2 grams per day elemental calcium, which is 40 percent of most of the formulations: Total 5 grams per day as calcium carbonate. This should be administered at mealtime. The idea is to "treat the meal," as there is generally very little phosphorus available to bind, outside of mealtime. When the kidney is in "failure," after meals, excess phosphorus remains uncleared and leads to deposition in the tissues: valve leaflets; at the endothelial barrier; arterial subendothelial space (Mönckeberg's medial calcification: arteriosclerosis).[197] When sodium bicarbonate (baking soda) is administered, based on the landmark study,[198,199] the transition from stages 3 and 4 to stage 5/ESRD/Dialysis, can be reduced by about 80 percent, with just 1.8 grams sodium bicarbonate, alone. Mealtime dosing twice a day (600 milligrams at lunch, and 1,200 milligrams at dinner; for a total of 1.8 grams total per day) optimizes the therapy.

In that study, the fraction of people that went to dialysis by the end of two years was roughly 35 percent on placebo, but the fraction that went to dialysis with the modest dose of sodium bicarbonate was reduced roughly 80 percent.[198] However, the concerns about sodium intake are frequently expressed. The literature is quite clear on this. The chloride salt of sodium is the issue, not the bicarbonate salt of sodium. This a key point. We just need to do a better job of identifying them early on. Do not assume the patient is stage 1 or 2 if the creatinine indicated that. We need better, more reliable biomarkers (example: Cystatin-C) and should insist the insurance companies reimburse for it.

This approach worked amazingly well for my father, because he reversed his CKD by more than two stages! I calculated it incrementally based on where he was at each stage. He was nearing end-stage renal disease (stage 5) and he reverted back to stage 2, which was a virtual miracle at that time! I had never heard of or seen anything similar.

Niacin interested me when I came across a company that was working on a new chelator for phosphorus. I had already seen some literature on an extended-release niacin (ER-niacin) study showing a phosphorus-lowering effect and IR-Niacin having an antiproteinuric effect. Niacin was so effective that it moved the GFR up enough to reverse the baseline status by a full stage, even at very low doses. This seemed to be the plausible explanation for this net result.

Niacin (as well as no-flush niacinamide/nicotinamide) inhibits the sodium phosphate transporter. There are at least twenty peer-reviewed publications demonstrating this.[153–189,200–207] What was discovered was, if you want to control phosphorus, niacin is one of the most effective methods and its efficacy is not affected by timing relative to meals. As little as 100milligrams of niacin will effectively reduce the serum phosphorus.

Some studies refer to this niacin-mediated effect as the "phosphorus fix." The additional CKD benefits of niacin include the antiproteinuric, as well. If you compare a blood test vs. urine test, then the urine is probably a much more reliable indicator, because when the basement membrane is damaged, filtration is impaired such that the basement membrane between the podocyte processes no longer conserves plasma proteins and the amount lost, "leaked," is present in the urine. The appearance of albumin (protein) in the urine is a "flag" that loss of serum protein is due to impaired renal function. Often, this is one of the earliest markers. Blood biomarkers have some variables that could result in misclassification of CKD stages. Protein leaking from the kidneys is a direct correlate to the podocyte/basement-membrane damage. This is the gold-standard measure of endothelial function. I always like to use at least one blood marker (ideally CystatinC) in addition to the urine test, to facilitate extrapolating, "pinpointing" the true stage at baseline and where they are at follow-up.

I believe niacin is probably one of the best treatment options for a variety of chronic conditions/pathologies. CKD is a complex disease state. At its "core," it is a vascular disease, but *if* you "hit all the right buttons," it is clearly possible to "drive" CKD backwards.

With stage-5 CKD, a.k.a. end-stage renal disease (ESRD), the scarcity of donor organs is a primary challenge. The reality is usually that dialysis will be required for the rest of the patient's life. That is a powerful motivator to the patient to consider niacin.

Ultimately my father's CKD reversed from stage 4 to stage 2. When the sum of all the data is considered, connecting-the-dots with all the biomarkers, he was close to end-stage renal disease as he was scheduled to have a first encounter with a nephrologist. So, he was likely headed to dialysis, sooner rather than later.

The Current State of CKD Treatment and the Importance of Addressing Multimorbidity

In regard to prevention, many physicians choose not to believe there is any way to prevent or reverse CKD. Unfortunately, most patients end up on dialysis, or at the very least their CKD continues to get worse.

Too often, a less than adequate job of correctly identifying pre-diabetes is implemented, early on in the CKD disease state. It is vitally important to have a method of measuring the glucose post-prandial glucose (PPG) level at 1 hour and 2 hours post-glucose challenge (OGTT). Currently, this is the gold standard test for assessing pre-diabetes. There are blood biomarkers that have a *very* high level of precision determining the 1-hour PPG: 1,5-AG and AHB (*Alpha-HydroxyButyrate*).

Measures of fasting insulin, fasting glucose, and HbA1c can miss an unacceptably large number of pre-diabetics. The OGTT test will reliably capture a pre-diabetes diagnosis. HOMA-IR; homeostasis model assessment as an index of insulin resistance) is an effective method to calculate and evaluate insulin resistance using conventional reference lab biomarkers: insulin levels, fasting glucose levels, and A1C.[208,209] If you have these three, you can then calculate the HOMA-IR. This enables accurate documentation and validates spending the modest expense to do the proper tests.

As much as 70 percent of adults over the age of 30 do not have normal postprandial glucose (PPG). It's that bad! They say it's only 30 percent or 40 percent, but that's likely based on poor statistics. In fact, during every year in the last several decades, the percentage of individuals over the age of 30 with obesity has risen. The antiquated Frederickson classification was based on cholesterol/triglyceride parameters, but we are presently in the "particle age" of clinical lipidemia assessment. Like the Frederickson classification for lipid disorder sub-types (which was largely based on cholesterol measurements), current methods to assess the presence and severity of insulin resistance (pre-diabetes) are essentially obsolete.

Another aspect to consider is multiple comorbidities. Modern medicine currently generally takes the approach of treating one condition at a time, but there are nearly always multiple disease symptoms present that are tightly associated and anything that can ultimately address this is going to result in the most effective therapies, ideally prior to the fulminant disease.

The Academy of Medical Sciences declared in 2018 that multimorbidity is the number one top priority in health care research.[210] Estimates for a cure of cancer reveal that this would only increase lifespan by a mere three years on average because the associated co-morbidities were not addressed.[211] Niacin, however, addresses so many common denominators for disparate diseases that the impact of niacin treatment for CKD/ESRD is likely to benefit many more indications, especially the number one killer, cardiovascular disease.

At the end of the day, it is the effect on all-cause mortality that matters the most for any treatment. After the termination of the Coronary Drug Project-CDP trial, it was determined that all-cause mortality was reduced by 11 percent, nine years after stopping niacin treatment (average dose 2.4 grams per day).[212] This may be a feat unparalleled in proven clinical medicine. By contrast, statin all-cause mortality data has yielded mixed results.

Conclusion

In over 25 documented individual cases of CKD stages 2 through 4, after initiation of a combination-therapy of supplements based on GFR, including 500 milligrams three times a day IR-Niacin, over a three-month period, it was possible to improve their disease by at least one stage.

In basic and clinical research, the evidence in favor of niacin for CKD is strong. Clinical research proves that the niacin is exceptionally well-suited to treatment and prevention of CKD, multimorbidity, and ultimately all-cause mortality.

Sampathkumar explained the current CKD treatment with niacin situation best:

> Pharmaceutical industry driven large-scale studies are unlikely to be undertaken given the low-cost of niacin. David is up against the formidable Goliath of players promoting

costly non-calcium containing phosphorus binders. It is time that international bodies like Kidney Disease, Improving Global Outcomes (KDIGO) take a call on usefulness of niacin as a low-cost, effective, and low pill burden agent for phosphorus reduction in CKD with multiple pleotropic benefits.[177]

Recommended Doses to Address Chronic Kidney Disease

- Low-dose immediate release-niacin, 100 to 500 milligrams, 1 to 3 times per day. No-flush niacin or niacinamide will have equal efficacy on lowering phosphorus levels, but negligible cardiovascular benefits compared with standard niacin.
- Sodium bicarbonate (baking soda) 1.8 grams per day ($1/3$ at lunch and $2/3$ at dinner).
- Calcium carbonate antacid pills (400 to 1,000 milligrams elemental calcium or 2 to 4 gram antacid tablets) with food to bind phosphorus in food.
- Low-dose-thyroid supplementation (25 to 50 micrograms T4/ Levothyroxine or ½ grain of desiccated thyroid).
- Methyl folate (0.8 gram to 2 milligrams L-methylfolate).

Recommended Additional Monitoring

A full panel of metabolic parameters [baseline and 90-day follow-up] can also determine "collateral" benefit[s], especially related to cardiovascular health:

- Apo-B decreases
- Apo-AI increases (INTERHEART Study)
- Lp(a) mass decreases
- Lp-PLA2 decreases
- MPO/myeloperoxidase decreases
- AST/ALT/GGT hepatic parameters improved

- Symptomology/Signs-Symptoms: TIA; Chronic Angina; Claudication; Dyspnea upon Exertion.

The views of the authors, who are not physicians, are presented here for educational purposes. All readers are reminded to be sure to work with their health care provider(s) before commencing this or any nutrition-based approach.

OBESITY

Many traditional nutritionists, who are strongly opposed to orthomolecular therapy and practice, promote the simple view that obesity is due to the very simple rule: too many calories in and too few calories expended out. This has become the standard belief of all anti-obesity programs because it seems to make so much sense. However, according to Taube, his massive examination of the clinical literature provides little support for this idea. There is no relation between the amount of food consumed and the amount of exercise expended and the absence or presence of obesity. Many people are not obese no matter how little or how much they eat, and too many are too fat no matter how little they eat. The problem is not the total amount, but the kind of food consumed. According to Cleave, Yudkin, Taube, and many others, the main factor that creates obesity is the amount of sugar and refined carbohydrates that are eaten. Sugars and foods that rapidly release sugars into the blood are the villains.

It is true that if one eats too many calories there will be a much greater tendency to put on weight, but the real question is: Why do these people eat too much junk food?

I (AH) think they do this because they are sick. An example is the intolerable weight gain of patients who are treated with Zyprexa, an atypical antipsychotic drug. I have seen young patients gain sixty pounds in six months after being placed on this dangerous psychiatric drug. It increases appetite enormously. But this is a relatively rare situation. A more common reason for obesity is the modern high-tech diet, which is deficient in every nutrient but contains plenty of sugars and a high proportion of refined foods. This combination creates an appetite to eat more. I call this theory the Wald hypothesis. George Wald got the Nobel Prize for his work with vitamin A. He also showed that starving rats were more active (ran a lot more) than rats on a normal diet, but rats on a diet containing enough calories but not containing enough of the B vitamins also displayed increased running.[213] It makes sense that hunger will increase running (activity) in animals since that motivates them to seek food; to hunt. But it is surprising that depriving them of the B vitamins will do the same, unless one postulates that the animals experience the B-vitamin deficiency as equivalent to hunger and try to deal with it by increasing activity. Dr. William Kaufman discussed how niacin deficiency causes increased running in his 1949 book, *The Common Form of Joint Dysfunction*.[214] The diet too rich in sugars is also too deficient in B vitamins. Since during evolution animals who did not respond to hunger by searching for food would not be around today, activity became a natural genetic reflex. Thus, the modern diet activates people in much the same way.

There are three scenarios that relate insufficient nutrition to increased activity. The first is our modern high-tech diet, where no one starves, food is plentiful but deficient, and it is easily obtained. The hunger for nutrients (which the body identifies as food) increases appetite, leading to too much being eaten. As a result, people get fat, but they feel better because they are getting more of the B vitamins. People on a high-tech diet remain uncomfortable if they are forced to remain thin. In the second scenario there is not enough food. In this case, populations deficient in B vitamins will not be able to get the vitamins they need by eating more as there is no more to eat. These people will become lean and hyperactive until they are felled by starvation. In the third scenario, in children, the drive for the B vitamins increases activity and leads to the hyperactive syndrome and later to obesity.

The hypothesis that intake of calories from foods deficient in B vitamins increases activity, either by eating more or being more active, is easily tested. I have done so to a limited degree. I tried to help many obese patients with little success using any type of reducing diet. But they would lose weight with comfort when I advised them to go back to the stone-age diet, to take ample amounts of B vitamins, and to eat as little or as much as they wanted. This is not a reducing diet; it is a healthy lifestyle diet. That is the best approach to eliminating obesity.

PARKINSONISM

Epidemiological evidence shows that Parkinson's disease is precipitated by trigger factors that activate the disease. The only effective, palliative treatment is L-dopa. It became the treatment of choice even though the original double-blind trials were not promising. The original researchers did not use a high enough dose, which supported the view that a deficiency of l-dopamine was responsible for Parkinson's disease. Later it was found that part of the brain was deficient in coenzyme Q$_{10}$ and NAD. But unfortunately, l-dopamine will be oxidized into l-dopachrome, which is toxic. It kills neurons and creates psychotic symptoms and signs. Foster and Hoffer discussed the psychoto-mimetic effects of L-dopa. They were also provided an explanation of Oliver Sacks' findings on the remarkable transient effect of L-dopa on patients with encephalitis lethargica, as dramatized in the film *Awakenings* (more on this below). Such huge doses of L-dopa are certainly very toxic to the brain.

On August 31, 2008, *60 Minutes* reported about improvement in patients who suffered from minimally conscious states (MCS). These patients retain some awareness even though they appear to have no consciousness. The program described one of the patients, who miraculously awakened after ten years and asked about his family. One of his doctors believes that he awakened after he was given an anti-Parkinsonism drug. This probably was L-dopa, but was not named on the program. A few others responded to a sleeping pill which normally puts people to sleep. If one hypothesizes that MCS patients are like the patients described by Oliver Sacks, this suggests that they should be treated with L-dopa and niacin. Since these compounds are not covered by patents and drug companies will therefore avoid them like the plague, it is time that investigators free themselves of their emotional and financial attachment to Big Pharma.

> Dr. Hoffer has discovered that high doses of niacin are very helpful in preventing Parkinson's psychosis. His use of this vitamin is based on the adrenochrome hypothesis of schizophrenia which has been described previously. Birkmayer et al. also found that both oral and parenteral NADH were equally effective in Parkinson's disease. They treated 885 patients with one or other of these methods and found that only about 20 percent did not benefit. Younger patients,

who had not been symptomatic as long, responded better. To avoid damage in the stomach their oral preparation had to be stabilized. NADH in ordinary gelatin capsules was not effective, as had been found with NAD when treating schizophrenic patients.[215]

As Foster and Hoffer described in a 2004 *Medical Hypotheses* article, "The Two Faces of L-DOPA: Benefits and Adverse Side Effects in the Treatment of Encephalitis Lethargica, Parkinson's Disease, Multiple Sclerosis and Amyotrophic Lateral Sclerosis,"[216] three measures must be addressed when treating Parkinson's disease. These are: dealing with oxidative stress (decreasing it where possible) and using natural antioxidants; giving natural methyl acceptors (the most readily available of which is vitamin B3); and using high-dose antioxidants to mitigate the adverse toxic effects of L-dopa.

Sacks described treating twenty patients with L-dopa. The initial dose was 500 milligrams daily but, if required, was increased gradually to 6 grams. Many patients showed great early progress, which Sacks termed an "awakening." Unfortunately, this dramatic improvement in health began to reverse. Sacks' book *Awakenings* first appeared in 1973. By the time his revised 1982 edition was published, seventeen of his patients were dead, mainly from Parkinsonism, and all had relapsed. Sacks describes the experiences of an encephalitis lethargica patient receiving high-dose L-dopa as follows: "For the first time, then, the patient on L-dopa enjoys a perfection of being, an ease of movement and feeling and thought, a harmony of relation within and without. Then his happy state—his world—starts to crack, slip, break down, and crumble; he lapses from his happy state, and moves toward perversion and decay."[217] Foster and Hoffer suggested that the initial improvement arose from the beneficial effect of the L-dopa and the final deleterious effect from the formation of dopachrome. The side effects of L-dopa probably come from excess formation of dopachrome-caused psychosis. A deficiency of dopamine and of dopachrome could be a factor in allowing the amyloid fibrils to develop and increased dopachrome with adequate niacin would be therapeutic. The side effects can be avoided by giving these patients niacin in adequate doses.

It is also possible that L-dopa could be beneficial for Alzheimer's disease. I am not aware of any controlled trials treating Alzheimer's disease with L-dopa.

Foster and Hoffer[218] explain that hyperoxidation of dopamine and adrenaline is part of the cause of Parkinson's disease, multiple sclerosis, ALS, and schizophrenia. They recommend high-dose treatment with selenium, cysteine, tryptophan, and glutamine, because these nutrients are needed to make glutathione peroxidase in the body. They also recommend thiamine, riboflavin, niacin, and coenzyme Q_{10}, vitamin C, and vitamin E. Natural thyroid extract and EPA (eicosapentaenoic acid, an omega-3 fatty acid) may be beneficial, especially to schizophrenics.

PEMPHIGUS

Pemphigus is a rare autoimmune disease that causes blisters on the skin and mucous membranes. One person suffered so horribly from pemphigus that he discovered his own cure. He had been given the best palliative treatment available, which kept him alive until he was able to create the program that has made him well for the past ten years. This is such an important case history that I (AH) am reproducing the entire letter which was submitted to the *Journal of Orthomolecular Medicine* in 2008.

I came down with my first symptoms of pemphigus in November 1994, just two weeks before Thanksgiving. I didn't know it at the time, because it started out as a sore throat, but by Thanksgiving Day, my mouth had begun to fill with blisters and raw spots that were so widespread and painful that I was unable to eat anything solid.

After a biopsy and consultations with several specialists, I was diagnosed a month or so later with pemphigus vulgaris, a variation of pemphigus that mainly affects the mucous membranes. I came under the care of a dermatologist who would guide me through the next three years of my life, treating me for what turned out to be a very painful and stubborn disease. His first step was to put me on 20 milligrams of prednisone, and 100 milligrams of Dapsone, per day. That turned out to be much too conservative, and did nothing to relieve the pain or stop the blisters from spreading. It got to the point where I stopped eating solid food altogether, and could only tolerate bland, liquid formulas, soups, baby food, and occasionally, a cup of yogurt.

By the end of March 1995, my body and mind were so exhausted from dealing with the pain, going without food, and being unable to sleep, that I was losing hope of ever getting back to normal again. I had become delusional, thinking that my body was filled with poisons or toxins that needed to be eliminated, and I tried fasting as a last resort. That only made things worse. I had already lost forty-one pounds, and was so malnourished I could barely get out of bed, and spent the better part of the next two weeks curled up in a fetal position, trying to get comfortable, and getting up only to go to the bathroom, take a shower, or to join my family at night. There were brief moments, lying alone, when I felt as if I was leaving my body. I had a near-death experience as a child, and again as a young adult, so I knew that feeling. I was letting go, and drifting into another world, and I didn't care. In fact, I think I would have welcomed the relief from the pain, and the sense of peace that was coming over me.

My wife had become so alarmed at my condition that she and my sister contacted the dermatologist and insisted that I be hospitalized. He hadn't seen me for over a month, and wasn't aware of how far I had slipped. He agreed to admit me to the dermatology unit at Yale-New Haven Hospital, where I was put on 80 milligrams of prednisone, 100 milligrams of Imuran, Percodan and a time-release morphine capsule, MS Contin, for pain. Because these drugs can cause debilitating side effects in themselves, I was also put on Compazine for nausea, Carafate to prevent stomach ulcers, an antibacterial rinse, stool softeners and laxatives to prevent constipation, and told to "swish and spit" with Lidocaine before each meal. Within three days, I was strong enough to go home, hopeful that my life would turn around again, but it would be several years before I was finally able to get control of my symptoms and enter into what is now a ten-year remission.

After I was released from the hospital, my treatment plan called for me to continue taking prednisone, at 80 milligrams, until new blisters stopped forming, and then to taper it down very slowly, in increments of 10 to 20 milligrams every other month. Each time I tried, I flared up again. Over the next two years, I was not able to get below 20 milligrams, and it seemed like I was always in pain, and still having difficulty eating and sleeping. The side effects of the drugs had begun to take their toll, and it felt as if I had lost my "sixth sense," and didn't know how to take what people were saying. I didn't understand the subtleties of what was being said, and had lost my ability to read between the lines, or to intuitively know when people were joking, for example, or when they were serious. I became depressed and angry, and during the worst moments, considered my situation hopeless and not worth living for. But there were also times when the higher doses of prednisone would have the opposite effect, and I would feel elated, and extremely happy with my life and my surroundings, even though the burning sensation inside my mouth was a constant reminder that I was still very sick.

Back in the '70s, I had worked as a clinical psychologist in an adolescent treatment program. My specialty was childhood schizophrenia, and I became very interested in the theories of Dr. Abram Hoffer, and Dr. Humphry Osmond, two psychiatrists who were experimenting with the use of vitamin B_3 to treat schizophrenia.

When we are faced with a stressful situation, adrenaline is released, causing a "fight or flight" response. The source of the stress does not have to be a physical danger. It can be something as simple as a heavy work schedule, lack of sleep, or anything that involves fears. It can become "chronic stress" when it occurs on a daily basis. Over the years, chronic stress can lead to an automatic response beyond your control, and serious psychological and physical disorders can occur. When faced with a stressful situation, you either fight back, identify the source of the stress, and stand up to it, turn inward, run away, or put off dealing with it to another day. Whatever the response, it is almost always accompanied by the sudden or prolonged release of adrenaline. In the case of schizophrenics, the adrenaline released under stress converts to adrenochrome, which is known to cause hallucinations. Since schizophrenia is considered to be a perceptual disorder, in that the schizophrenic "sees things" that are not there (hallucinations), and believes things that are not true (delusions), Hoffer and Osmond searched for a natural compound that would interfere with the production of adrenochrome. Dr. Hoffer, who was not only trained in psychiatry but as a biochemist, knew that niacinamide is capable of blocking the conversion of adrenaline to adrenochrome. He and Dr. Osmond began administering large doses of B_3 to their patients in Saskatchewan, with great success.

I was surprised to find that one of the treatment programs for pemphigus also involves the use of niacinamide. Usually, 500 to 1,000 milligrams of niacinamide is prescribed, three times a day, along with an antibiotic from the tetracycline family. It is always the amide form of niacin that is used. Since pemphigus is often referred to as "a stress-related" illness, could it be that the release of adrenaline in our situation is also converted to adrenochrome, or a similar compound, causing the immune system to "see things," and to attack healthy tissues and cells?

By 1997, after two years of living with pemphigus, I was determined to get back on my feet again, and willing to try *anything*. I knew that I needed prednisone and Imuran, and followed my doctor's orders to a "T," but I was also hoping to find something to add to my routine that might improve my overall health, and help to put this disease behind me. I remembered what I had learned as a psychologist, and how I had experimented with Hoffer and Osmond's vitamins myself, twenty-five years earlier. I had taken up to 1,000 milligrams of niacinamide, the same amount of C, 100 milligrams of B_1, 100 milligrams of B_6, and 200 international units of E, three times a day for years, just to see how it would affect me. In general, I felt much stronger and more energetic on the vitamins than I did when I would go off of them, but the major benefit, as far as I could tell, was that I seemed to think more clearly, as if the oxygen I was breathing was going straight to my brain. If I hadn't experimented on my own, back in the '70s, I might not have thought to go back on the vitamins when I had pemphigus. Knowing they couldn't hurt me, and were not contraindicated by either prednisone or Imuran, I started taking large doses of niacinamide again, along with C and the other vitamins, and waited for a miracle.

After several months, I did feel stronger again, and my appetite came back, but my blisters were no better than when I had started, and I wasn't feeling the kind of changes I had expected. I began to research the healing process in general, and discovered that zinc was used by many burn units across the country to treat severe burn injuries, and also to speed the healing of open wounds. It seemed to me that the blisters in my mouth were very much like burns (it was the same kind of pain), and were definitely open wounds that never seemed to heal. Adding zinc to my vitamin routine seemed like a logical approach to treating pemphigus, so I bought a bottle of zinc picolinate (22 milligrams) and began experimenting again.

When I was younger, I was in the habit of writing in a journal, so by the end of 1997, I ended up with a very detailed account of my experience with pemphigus up to that point. I had written about the usual things, how I was feeling, what was going on around me, and my thoughts about life in general, but I had also listed all of my medications, and any changes that my doctor made to my overall treatment plan, as well as how I was feeling and whether or not I was improving from day-to-day. In the process of trying to find something that worked, I bounced back and forth between adding zinc to my diet, taking the vitamins just by themselves, or going without anything at all, but I always noted these changes as well. It wasn't until I started reading back through my journals that I saw a definite pattern: when I had added zinc at 22 milligrams to my diet consistently for three to four weeks, my notes were always upbeat and positive. All of the improvements seemed to come after taking the vitamins and zinc together, so I decided to stick to that routine. After three months, I could see the sores in my mouth beginning to heal. I would examine them with a flashlight as often as possible, and noticed that they were surrounded by a ring of white tissue that seemed to be closing in on them. As the weeks went by, the redness at the center of each lesion eventually gave way, and only the white tissue remained. Within a week, it would turn a healthy pink. I was also aware that pemphigus was on its way out of my body, following the same path it had taken, but in reverse. In other words, the most recent sores were the first to heal, followed by the older lesions. By the end of the next three months, everything seemed to be under control again. Not coincidentally, I had also managed to taper down to 5 milligrams of prednisone, and went off of it completely in January 1998. I have not had a single blister since then, except for a brief flare-up in February of that year that lasted less than three weeks, and after ten years of relatively perfect health, I consider myself cured. I don't think it was merely the supplements, but on a biological level, I think they helped me to relax and to be able to better cope with having a major illness, and the everyday ups and downs of life that all people experience. From there, I was able to make some major changes in my life, end a very stressful relationship, and move further away from what I saw as the causes of my illness—without the need for supplements or medications of any sort.

POST-TRAUMATIC STRESS DISORDER

Serious though it certainly is, I (AH) do not accept Post-Traumatic Stress Disorder (PTSD) as a legitimate psychiatric disorder. In common with all psychiatric disorders, it is merely a description of what happens to some people who have been subjected to enormous stress for a specified period of time. The Canadian Hong Kong veterans discussed earlier in this book could be diagnosed as PTSD. Treatment of PTSD must remove the biochemical disturbances caused by the stress. Orthomolecular treatment is the best for this condition. One of the major nutrients needed by these patients is niacin. The veterans were made niacin dependent by their experiences. The stress caused sustained cellular damage that resulted in a sustained much-greater-than-average need for niacin. Like with diabetes: some of the cells are gone, and for the rest of his or her life, a type 1 diabetic must have insulin.

RAYNAUD'S DISEASE

Raynaud's disease causes extremities of the body to feel numb and cold. The smaller arteries to the skin are narrowed, limiting blood circulation to these areas. Niacin may help people with Raynaud's disease because it dilates small blood vessels, increasing circulation and providing a sense of warmth in the extremities. To feel the warm flush, one needs to select niacin, not niacinamide or no-flush niacin (inositol hexaniacinate), and take a sufficient quantity. The amount will vary from person to person. Raynaud's is discussed in the Erectile Dysfunction section of this book.

SKIN CONDITIONS

Vitamins may be used to treat thermal burns, sunburns, wrinkles, pigmentation, scrapes, bug bites, and even bedsores. The benefits of niacin have been proven in numerous controlled clinical trials. The scientific literature contains at least twenty-nine reports published since 2003 that use niacin creams.[219–224]

Acne

It is interesting that skin and the brain are both derived from ectodermal germinal tissue. I suspect they have the same nutrient needs. Often the appearance of a young person's skin will reveal a good deal about his or her nutritional state. Skin diseases that are vitamin B$_3$ responsive include acne, pemphigus, and epidermolysis bullosa.

In our book, *Orthomolecular Medicine for Everyone*, we wrote:

Adolescent acne is one of the most common afflictions, but it is seldom the main complaint among the patients referred to me (AH). Rarely is it so severe that it is the primary concern. About thirty years ago, in Saskatoon, a sixteen-year-old boy was very depressed. His face was hideously covered with huge, irregular, red, oozing bumps and lumps, here and there infected. He told me he could no longer live with his face and that if my treatment did not help, he would kill himself. He told me this very calmly and seriously, saying that the acne had ruined his social life.

I started the boy on a sugar-free diet, eliminated all milk products, and added a daily supplement program of niacin (3,000 milligrams), ascorbic acid (3,000 milligrams), pyridoxine (250 milligrams), and zinc sulfate (220 milligrams). One month later, his face was better: the vivid reddening had begun to recede, his face was no longer infected, and his mood was better. He told me he was no longer considering suicide. After three months, his face was almost clear. He was cheerful and had begun to resume his social activities at school and elsewhere.[225]

While this is a dramatic example, there are very few failures. I also advise people not to scrub their faces vigorously and not to squeeze or play with their faces. I will describe a few cases from a very large number whose acne was their main complaint and was associated with depression and anxiety. Most adolescents have minor degrees of acne: a few pimples on their face, shoulders, and back. They do not present it as a problem, but when questioned they admit they are concerned. In every case, their acne cleared on orthomolecular treatment.

I consider acne a symptom of a serious nutritional deficiency that has made the skin more susceptible to infections. Antibiotics can reduce the ravages of the infection but make the deficiency in the skin worse by their effect on the bacterial flora of the gastrointestinal tract. I have not seen antibiotics to be useful, but that may be because the cases who have been helped will not see me. Only the total failures of standard treatment come for help.

Susan, a mother of three children, had suffered from severe facial acne from childhood, but she had become so skillful with makeup that I was unaware of it, even though I had known her for many years. Several years ago, she complained to me about her acne and asked if nutrition and vitamins could help. I placed her on an orthomolecular program. Within six months, she was clear of acne, even though she had not responded to any previous treatment recommended to her by general practitioners and dermatologists. She remained well, but then began to deviate from this program and the acne came back. On resuming the nutritional program, the acne cleared, and she has remained well.

Many years later Susan consulted with the Mayo Clinic in Rochester about another matter. They advised her to stop the niacin as it was very dangerous and would destroy the outer layers of her brain. (Doctors are so creative.) She did stop the niacin. Fortunately, her acne did not recur, as she was still following her nutritional program and avoided foods she was allergic to. Parsons and his colleagues at the Mayo Clinic had shown many years earlier how safe niacin was.

L.N., age 25, could not remember when she was free of acne. Tetracycline helped, but whenever she went off it the acne recurred. She had several features indicating pyridoxine deficiency, including white areas on her nails, stretch marks on her body, and severe premenstrual depression. She was placed on a sugar-free program with niacin (100 milligrams three times daily), ascorbic acid (1,000 milligrams three times a day), pyridoxine (250 milligrams per day), and zinc sulfate (110 milligrams per day). Three months later, there was no improvement, so the niacin dose was increased to 500 milligrams three times per day; ascorbic acid to 2 grams three times per day; pyridoxine remained at 250 milligrams; and zinc sulfate was increased to 220 milligrams per day. I advised her to discontinue birth control medication. The acne began to improve in one week, and nine months after starting the program, she was well, and she has remained so for seven years.

Most mild to severe acne will respond to a diet that eliminates sugar and the foods that they are allergic to, supplemented by vitamins B_3 and C, pyridoxine, and zinc. However, optimum amounts, determined by varying the dose and judging the response, must be used. No one need suffer with acne or be exposed to the harmful effects of chronic use of tetracycline.

My patients who recover from their psychiatric illnesses invariably note a great improvement in their skin, while acne sufferers lose their depression and anxiety as the acne clears. There is a relationship that must account for some of the correlation. Simply being freed of acne will remove depression and anxiety. However, I have seen many whose acne was under control with antibiotics who still remained emotionally disturbed. Orthomolecular treatment removed both the acne and the need for tetracycline and the depression. Severe to moderate acne and psychiatric symptoms are both the result of malnutrition.

Psoriasis

The antipsoriatic drug monomethylfumarate is a niacin receptor agonist. An agonist encourages a response; it is the opposite of an antagonist. So, this drug triggers a response from a cell's niacin receptors. This is a component of Fumaderm, used in Germany for treating psoriasis.[226] Fumarate esters are potent agonists of nicotinic acid receptors in the Langerhans cells of skin, more active than 1,500 other substances. Tang and his colleagues suggested that these findings indicate that niacin may be valuable for treating psoriasis and multiple sclerosis. Niacin is valuable for treating MS and has been used as a component of an anti-MS regimen for many years, but it has to be used with caution in dealing with psoriasis.

Many years ago I (AH) treated a male schizophrenic patient with niacin. When he came back for a review one month later, he was ecstatic. He told me that the psoriasis from which he had suffered, which covered his torso, was gone. He had not told me that he had had this skin disease. But the next patient I gave it to treat psoriasis became worse. After a few more trials it was clear that one could not treat patients with psoriasis safely with niacin. It might help but it might make them worse, and this became a contraindication. The flush is important in this situation. I tried the no-flush inositol derivative instead and while it had reduced effect, I was able to use it safely for patients who needed the niacin but also had psoriasis. Niacinamide did not have any impact on these skin lesions.

Skin Lesions

Skin lesions are the most prominent feature of typical pellagra. Pelle Agra means "dark skin" in Italian. It is usually correlated with exposure to sun, so pellagra in Siberia will not cause the same darkened symmetrical skin lesions found in pellagrins in Egypt. But other lesions are also found.

In September 2005, a sixty-year-old woman came to me (AH) complaining that she had been suffering from very serious skin lesions for the previous two-and-a-half years. Her skin was blistered and had sores that had been coming and going all over her body. At the onset they were more common around her hips but more recently they had settled around her neck, face, and upper chest. Often these lesions became infected. She had seen at least nine dermatologists. In addition, she was just getting over shingles. Most of the pain was gone but there was residual scarring. And she had some arthritic-type pain. She was very depressed, spent the whole day crying, and could not work. The consensus diagnosis after a clinical conference of many dermatologists was that she was doing this to herself; it was factitious. This diagnosis was based simply on the fact that nothing had been helpful to her, thus proving it was a psychiatric condition. Pellagra was the last thing in their minds. Perhaps they had never heard of it.

Some of the dermatologists suspected that she was bringing this on herself by scratching excessively. She was very disturbed by this suggestion, pointing out that these lesions occurred even on parts of her body that she could not reach. She denied scratching and only applied certain essential oils very lightly to her lesions. In April 2005 her general practitioner, who referred her to me, received the following letter after she had been seen at a clinic:

> There was consensus of opinion, agreeing with my clinical impression of a compulsive disorder manifesting as multiple neurotic excoriations. In fact, the lesions are more of a picked or pinched nature rather the frank excoriations. No one felt that any further skin biopsies or other investigations were warranted. In addition, no one felt that this was a manifestation of a paraneoplastic syndrome, as I understand that she had had abdominal or pelvic ultrasound. Her husband J. was in attendance today and I reviewed the summary and discussed the fact that there is a vicious cycle of picking at the skin and the importance of trying to break this cycle. I have also started her on Luvox 50 milligrams for the first week and 100 milligrams thereafter.

Her referring doctors noted on his referral application to me, "Numerous dermatologists feel this is a self-induced rash from excoriation. I have difficulty with this."

She was aware that she was allergic to many foods and was on a dairy-free diet, as dairy products caused gas, bloating, and cramps. A rice diet for two weeks was not helpful.

The patient was a research chemist for twenty-five years and a very good observer and reporter. Serious efforts were made to help her beginning in 2003. Her medication history is very complex. Here is her account of the medication she was prescribed:

- December 2003: Antibiotics, prednisone, and methamethasone, hydroval, and fucidinII.
- January to April 2004: 1 percent HC+glycerine glaxal base, bactroban/desonide.
- May 2004: Suspected pemphigus. Biopsy report inconclusive.

- July 2004: Doxepine 10 milligrams, Noritate cream, severe Migraine on doxepin. Prednisone added. This made the lesions worse, and infections developed. Sores still present after three months.
- September 2004: Severe, painful lesions. Synthroid given.
- November 2004: Seroquel 25 milligrams. Appeared better on prednisone, dose increased to 50 milligrams.
- December 2004: More lesions, prednisone tapered off. Paxil started.
- January 2005: Celexa 20 milligrams started.
- March 2005: Discontinued Celexa.
- April 2005: Severe pain in three lesions on infected left inside ankle. Itching over whole body. Started tetracycline and Atarax. Now had been seen by eight dermatologists. Some were concerned the lesions were self-inflicted.
- May 2005: Completed two weeks of tetracycline. Lesions no better. All painful and wet.
- June 2005: Started oxycodone 5 milligrams for pain.
- July 2005: Started clindamycin 300 milligrams three times daily.
- August 2005: Severe post-shingles pain in left buttock, spreading to side of thigh and leg. Given Neurontin 100 milligrams and increased to 300 milligrams.
- September 2005: Some lesions were healing; but in many areas they kept repeating: on ears, side, and back of neck, upper and lower back. Very dense around spine and thighs. Also lesions and large bumps in hair.

In addition to the prescribed medications, she had been taking a large number of vitamin tablets, each containing very little vitamin.

When she came to me in September 2005, I started her on niacinamide 500 milligrams three times a day, ascorbic acid 500 milligrams three times a day, L-lysine 2 grams three times a day, zinc citrate 50 milligrams once daily; and B_{12} injections 1 milligram daily, until the pain was gone.

Many physicians offer their patients large numbers of vitamin pills that contain little more of the supplement than can be found in food. These very seldom do any good. It is important to use only those few vitamins that the patients need and to allow the remainder to be obtained from their food. I used niacinamide because this patient's lesions reminded me of the lesions of pellagra. Pellagra is so rare that very few dermatologists ever think of it.

This was the second patient I encountered with pellagrous skin lesions. That first patient had seen twelve dermatologists, all over North America, with no relief. As soon as she walked into my examination room, I saw the typical pellagrous lesion. A few months later, with the addition of vitamin B3, she was well.

I did not give my present patient niacin because I felt that the flush would be too uncomfortable for her. I gave her ascorbic acid because I give it to everyone. Humans cannot make this vitamin, nor can they get enough from food. We all suffer from what Irwin Stone called hypoascorbemia, a genetic disease that prevents us from converting glucose into vitamin C, as happens in almost all other animals. The combination of the amino acid L-lysine, ascorbic acid, and injections of B12 is a very effective treatment for the pain of shingles and seldom fails to help within a few days. I added zinc as this mineral is very essential for the integrity of the skin.

By November of 2005 this patient, who had suffered for over two years, was free of pain. The lesions were healing. She was free of all medication except the Synthroid and was getting on very well, except for one episode when she was exposed to a room that had been recently cleaned with cleaning fluid. That made the lesions temporarily worse. She was very cheerful and pleased, and felt for the first time that the problem was being solved. I increased her nicotinamide to 1 gram three times a day. Her husband was delighted. He looked on this improvement as a miracle.

TRIGEMINAL NEURALGIA

Hoffer and Walker wrote:

> Trigeminal neuralgia (tic douloureux) is a disease which causes severe lancinating pain lasting several seconds to several minutes, which may be repeated many times for many months. It is often set off by touching a trigger point, or by an activity such as chewing or brushing one's teeth. The usual treatment consists of drugs such as Tegretol, Baclofen, Phenytoin, and antidepressants, and has

included surgery to sever the fifth nerve. But there is an alternative which has worked very well for four of my patients who followed it.

September 15, 1992, a woman born in 1915 told me that she had been awakened one night in 1978, screaming from pain on the right side of her face. She suffered over six episodes of severe pain. She was diagnosed tic douloureux. Since then she had not been free of pain. In addition, over the previous year she also developed severe pain in her jaw diagnosed arthritis.

I advised her to take niacin 500 milligrams after each meal, ascorbic acid 1,000 milligrams after each meal, B-complex 50s once a day, vitamin E 800 international units daily, vitamin B_{12} sublingually 2 milligrams per day, and folic acid 5 milligrams twice a day.

One week later she was free of pain. September 20, 1994, she called me to discuss something not related to this problem. I asked her about the pain. She replied it was a miracle, and she had not suffered any further pain.[227]

Niacin was a component of the treatment program for my four cases of trigeminal neuralgia, but I also advised them to take vitamin B_{12} by injection, ascorbic acid, and more lately the amino acid L-lysine. I have seen no failures with this program.

CHAPTER 13

Niacin for COVID: How Niacin, Niacinamide, and NAD Can Help with Long COVID-19

BY W. TODD PENBERTHY, PHD

Just 1,000 milligrams per day of niacinamide, which costs about 5 cents, has been shown to clearly reduce mortality in patients with COVID-19-related acute kidney injury (AKI) by 25 percent.[1] Investigators observed that "niacinamide administered for the prevention of COVID-19-related AKI progression was safe and associated with reduced estimated risk of death or the need for renal replacement therapy compared with historical controls. The association was strongest in severe AKI."

Given that niacinamide and/or niacin (vitamin B_3) are routinely dosed at much higher levels, typically involving 1,000 mg taken 3x/d (T.I.D.) and also that these higher levels provide greater benefits, it is likely that even greater COVID-19 benefits may occur when using these higher niacin/niacinamide doses after regular administration for patients with COVID-19.[2]

HIGHER NEEDS ADDRESSED BY HIGHER DOSES

I personally take 2,000 mg T.I.D., totaling 6,000 mg/day niacin—and my lipids are always perfect and also my liver enzymes are fine. In fact, niacin is now known to reduce fatty liver and it is under development to treat non-alcoholic fatty liver disease.[3,4] So do not be misled by the myth that niacin is toxic to the liver. This was only shown for timed release formulations and not for the most common form, the less expensive immediate release form.[5]

As Stephen McConnell and I detailed in a previous orthomolecular publication, 500 mg of niacin 3x daily (T.I.D.) can effectively reverse the stages of chronic kidney disease, especially when used together with sodium bicarbonate (baking soda).[6] This activity has been proven in multiple clinical trials and in case studies. Still, the use of these common pennies-a-day agents is unfortunately not common in nephrology practice as somehow myths persist that it must be more complicated.

Without equivocation, the benefits of high doses of vitamin B3 as niacinamide or niacin for treating both COVID-19 and CKD are now proven. Moreover, these are safe therapeutics that have been used for over 50 years with unparalleled safety. In fact, niacin is so important to basic human health that the U.S. government mandated fortification of processed flour and rice in the 1940s, saving countless thousands of lives.[7]

NETWORK PHARMACOLOGY POINTS TO NIACIN

In the emerging field of network pharmacology, the benefit of treating multi-morbidity with niacin has been identified as exceptionally promising. The network pharmacology and bioinformatics screen was performed with criteria set to identify small molecules that may have favorable anti-viral, anti-inflammatory, and immunomodulatory activities. Niacin treatment was prominently identified based on five core desirable targets and the expression of 14 genes that it favorably modified.[8] The investigators concluded that niacin may provide therapeutic benefit as a treatment for patients with COVID-19 based on favorable effects on important signaling pathways controlling outcome, thus paving the way for clinical trials.

COVID-19 BASICS & NAD

Viral infectious diseases like coronavirus disease 2019 (COVID-19), caused by severe acute respiratory syndrome coronavirus 2 (SARS-CoV-2), stimulate an immune response that can have a disastrous effect when uncontrolled, leading to deadly cytokine storms. Ultimately this process actively depletes NAD (nicotinamide adenine dinucleotide) in infected cells. Accordingly, many NAD precursors have been tested to combat this virus-caused deficiency of the essential NAD molecule.[9]

Risk factors for increased susceptibility to COVID-19 are age, insulin resistance, and diabetes. Low NAD concentrations are commonly observed with aging and in diabetes. Depletion of NAD has been reported in severe COVID-19 patients. Moreover, the expression of genes controlling NAD biosynthesis from precursors (vitamin B_3s) are known to be changed after infection with SARS-CoV-2.[10] Many cellular enzymes utilize NAD in their biochemical reactions. When these enzymes are modulated with drugs, NAD can control the immune responses, so investigators conclude that boosting NAD is "an actionable component." Pennies-a-day niacin administered in divided doses may serve best to prevent catastrophic NAD deficiency.

STANDARD MEDICAL PRACTICE AND THE LACK OF TRIALS EXAMINING THE BASICS

Unfortunately, in standard of care medicine there is often little scientific consideration of the possibility that we simply need more of what keeps most of us from even succumbing to COVID-19 sickness in the first place. Adequate amounts of essential nutrients and sufficient high-quality sleep can enable the body to recover from virus-induced deficiencies of essential molecules and prevent death due to sepsis.

The majority of COVID-19 clinical drug trials are primarily profit-driven and involve patentable xenobiotic small molecules or biologics, with relatively little systemic investigation of the basics that are responsible for keeping the non-COVID-19-succumbing population resistant to developing disease.

With only a few exceptions, patients are served best if we start by following the acronym K.I.S.S. ("keep it simple, stupid"), making certain that all biochemical pathways are replete with all requisite co-factors and essential molecules. By following a basic K.I.S.S. orthomolecular approach, we are assisting all the steps in any given biochemical pathway needed to optimally fight pathogens in a manner consistent with a healthy functioning immune system. Monotherapeutic approaches are needed for making advances in basic science, but they rarely benefit patients, and are of ethical concern in clinical trial settings. Again, it is best to make sure adequate levels of all essential nutrients are present so multi-step biochemical pathways can function through to completion.

VITAMIN B₃ TO NAD

Niacin and niacinamide are precursors for the NAD molecule, which is required for over 400 different gene functions, many of which are essential for keeping the cell alive.[11] Genetic polymorphisms within the NAD-binding domain confer different vitamin B_3 dependencies. Some individuals have genes that endow a lower than usual binding affinity for the enzyme binding to the NAD molecule. Accordingly, these individuals need higher amounts of vitamin B_3 to achieve the higher levels of NAD required to achieve competent gene function.[12]

MECHANISMS OF DEPLETION

Vitamin B_3 is unique and our knowledge of it distinguished compared to the other vitamins in the amount of relevant scientific research. Perhaps more is known about the molecular details of protein degradations actively causing acute and chronic depletion of NAD levels from vitamin B_3 than for any other vitamin. In contrast, the consequences of vitamin B_1 (thiamine) deficiency and the mechanisms thereof are woefully understudied. Much more attention should be devoted to these questions especially given that deficiencies of vitamin B_1 clearly cause a clinical presentation that resembles Alzheimer's disease, a condition for which we have almost no effective treatment.

One function of NAD is to serve as a substrate in the poly ADP-ribose polymerase (PARP) reaction, which is involved in many essential cell functions including repair of DNA in response to DNA damage. However, hyper-activation of PARP1 rapidly depletes NAD, leading to catastrophic cell death. It has long been known that PARP1 hyper-activated cell death due to ischemic shock, DNA damage, or other stimuli can be prevented by pre-incubation or supplementation with vitamin B_3 as NAD or niacin or niacinamide. This effect is particularly dramatic in neurons which are energetically demanding. SARS-CoV-2 has been shown experimentally to upregulate PARP enzymes, which degrade NAD.[10] Again, the most rational intervention would be to increase NAD+ supply. This may be accomplished inexpensively by supplemental niacin or niacinamide.

Knowledge of the mechanisms causing active depletion of NAD and even genetically inherited greater dependence on NAD is increasingly garnered as research on NAD biology advances. COVID-19 is a disease condition in which known pathways are activated to cause a greater requirement for vitamin B_3. However, many other pathways requiring high levels of vitamin B_3 are also known.

Three major mechanisms causing NAD depletion are well understood. Firstly, depletion of NAD is likely most acutely caused by hyper-activation of poly ADP-ribose polymerase (PARP1) enzyme, which can rapidly cause depletion of NAD in the PAR polymerization reaction, ultimately leading to quick cell death. PARP1 activity is stimulated by DNA damage. Many other stresses and under defined conditions cell death can be prevented by either increasing NAD levels or by inhibiting the PARP1 enzyme.

Secondly, a slower decrease in NAD levels is likely caused by persistent activation of the enzyme indoleamine 2,3-dioxygenase (IDO), which depletes the source of de novo NAD biosynthesis. IDO enzyme activity is elevated in COVID-19, sepsis, and severe inflammatory response syndrome with higher values predicting mortality.[13,14] IDO is also excessively and persistently activated in autoimmune diseases and cancer—and for these many IDO-targeted therapeutics are under development.[15] This pathway likely may be involved in some of the symptoms of long COVID-19.

Thirdly, NAD is depleted via activation of CD38 enzyme expressed on many white blood cells. Therefore, CD38 is likely to be exceptionally significant in the context of infectious disease and so investigators have been targeting it as a potential approach to treat a variety of conditions.

GENETIC ASPECT OF GREATER DEPENDENCY

Everyone has their own unique needs for vitamin B_3 and, by extension, the NAD needed to enable approximately 400 gene functions. Some individuals need much greater doses of vitamin B_3 to achieve the higher levels of NAD required to achieve competent gene function.[12] These individuals are said to have a greater "dependency on vitamin B_3" in order to avoid symptoms of deficiency. This biochemical aspect of genetics is an advanced concept—at the peak of western biomedical scientific achievements—but it is not generally taught in medical schools with only a few exceptions, such as with glucose-6-phosphate dehydrogenase.

However, with advances in genetics and associated biochemistry, more examples of the variety of vitamin B_3 dependencies are regularly discovered. One of the most impressive and important to consider is the mitochondrial aldehyde dehydrogenase (ALDH2) enzyme, which functions to remove toxic acetaldehyde after drinking alcohol. As many as 50 percent of the Asian population have the Glu487→Lys variant, which confers a roughly 150-fold reduced affinity for NAD. Accordingly, the ALDH2 Glu487→Lys variant enzyme requires much higher NAD concentrations to function at a healthy level and ultimately prevent hyper-sensitivity to drinking alcohol.

Abram Hoffer, MD, PhD, treated thousands of patients with schizophrenia by using high doses of niacin in over 40 years of clinical practice (1950s–1990s). Hoffer finally settled on the observation that some patients required as much as 18,000 mg of niacin a day to avoid schizophrenic symptoms.[16] He described this genetic response as an inter-individual dependence. This dose of 18,000 mg for good health is more than one-thousand-fold higher than the RDA of 16 mg for adult males. Accordingly, we can expect that these inter-individual variations may play prominent roles in controlling COVID-19 susceptibility.

Not surprisingly, schizophrenia has been determined to be the second highest risk factor for dying of COVID-19, just after age.[17,18] Again, the evidence strongly supports that high doses of niacin should be administered after a COVID-19 or related diagnosis. It is safe and may be the difference that saves lives.

SARS-COV-2 COVID-19 BASICS, PATHOGENESIS

One of the potential catastrophic activities initiated by SARS-CoV-2 infection is a cytokine storm. The levels of circulating proinflammatory factors IL-1, IL-6, and TNFα are strongly associated with mortality in COVID-19 patients. Niacin (pennies-a-day doses) is well known to reduce IL-6 and TNF alpha. Meanwhile, IL-6 antibodies costing thousands of dollars are being tested for use against COVID-19.[19]

A great amount of focus has been devoted to the NAD precursors nicotinamide mononucleotide (NMN) and/or nicotinamide riboside (NR) in many clinical trials owing to their potential for return on financial investments. However, the truth is that in the rare occasions that plain old niacin or niacinamide (both discovered in the 1930s) are tested alongside these precursors, these older largely non-patentable forms of NAD precursor often give superior results.

In my own experience directing research comparing all NAD precursors, I observed the most impressive ischemic stress-associated zebrafish embryo lifesaving activities using preincubations with niacin as compared to NMN, NR, tryptophan, quinolinic acid, or NAD itself (unpublished experimental observations). These various molecules cross the intestinal mucosa. Their molecular sizes, cell-specific transporters, ability to cross the blood-brain barrier, and more are all factors controlling their ultimate activities in addressing disease that must be empirically compared and tested. Biochemical evolutionary studies of niacin suggest that it is among the oldest of all NAD precursors.

Between 1945 and 1961 several studies found vitamin B$_3$ to be useful in the treatment of TB of the lung, but this potential role was superseded by modern antibiotics. More recently it has been investigated and found to be promising for the treatment of HIV. A recent paper stated, "This small molecule could emerge at the beginning of the twenty-first century either as a therapeutic agent in itself or as the lead compound for a new class of agents with activity against both TB and HIV."[20]

Metabolic analysis of SARS-CoV-2 of COVID-19 patients determined that there is a tryptophan deficiency caused by infection with a correlative increase in pathogenic interleukin-6 (IL-6) levels.[21] Decreased tryptophan causes decreased NAD biosynthesis with concomitant NAD deficiency. High-dose niacin supplementation can correct this NAD+ deficiency and the multitude of associated clinical presentations. Chronic fatigue syndrome may be an IDO trap, the result of constant NAD deficiency causing symptoms similar to long COVID-19 that are likely to be preventable with regular high doses of niacin taken in divided doses.[22]

NIACIN ADDRESSING SPECIFIC ASPECTS OF COVID PATHOGENESIS

Investigators based in South Africa reviewed changes of macrophages in the context of sepsis with consideration of COVID-19 and pointed out the important role of the immunosuppressive molecule IDO in depleting vitamin B_3-derived NAD, concluding, "We strongly suggest that vitamin B_3 be investigated as a therapy for sepsis, including that caused by COVID-19, ideally as a single agent at high dose rather than within a multivitamin," which is likely to be insufficient.[13]

Hallmark features of pathological SARS-CoV-2 infection are marked elevations in pro-inflammatory cytokines and chemokines-including, most notably, interleukin-6 (IL-6), in addition to interleukin-1β (IL-1β), tumor necrosis factor-α (TNF-α), and monocyte chemoattractant protein-1 (MCP-1). Thus, a commonly proposed effective treatment of COVID-19 is targeting the blockade of IL-6, through inhibition of its most prominent transcription factor, nuclear factor kappa B (NF-κB).[23]

Sufficient doses of niacin have consistently been shown to markedly reduce production of pro-inflammatory cytokines (IL-6, TNF-α, MCP-1) in human monocytes, and can substantially inhibit TNF-α-induced NF-κB activation along with MCP-1 secretion in cultured human aortic endothelial cells. Niacin also suppresses TNF-α and IL-6 expressions through down-regulation of the NF-κB pathway.[24] Since vitamin B_3 is highly lung protective, it should be used as soon as coughing begins.

Physicians in India have recommended "the mass scale distribution and use of nicotinamide (NAM) supplementation to decrease COVID-19 prevalence," based on recent Phase II clinical studies observing that nicotinamide supplementation with the standard of care demonstrably reduced COVID-19 patient recovery time by nearly 30 percent compared to standard of care alone.[25]

In a mouse model COVID-19 study, injected NAD kept them alive.[26] Investigators examining the effect of treatment with NAD+ found that the pneumonia phenotypes, including excessive inflammatory cell infiltration and embolization in SARS-CoV-2 infected lungs, were significantly rescued by boosting NAD+ levels. Most notably, cell death was suppressed by greater than 65 percent with NAD+ supplementation!

Niacin attenuates lung inflammation and improves survival during sepsis by down-regulating the nuclear factor-κB pathway. A pilot phase of the COVID-19 trial showed an effect of nicotinamide on the time to complete resolution of COVID-19 symptoms.

Landmark clinical trials completed recently in Finland proved that niacin cures systemic NAD deficiency, reduces fatty liver, and also improves muscle performance.[27] Why this study isn't yet common knowledge in clinical practice may be due to the unfortunate excessive distraction of life in 2022. However, the results of this Finnish study were unparalleled in their positive outcome—the data supporting once again that more research needs to be focused on better determining the full range of clinical indications that respond favorably to high doses of niacin, e.g., 1,000 mg taken 2-3x/d.

CONCLUSION AND DOSES

The ideal niacin dosage varies depending on an individual's genetics and their infections and/or stresses. Ultimately, perhaps the best gauge of the most effective niacin dosage regimen may involve the flush response. The niacin-eliciting flush pathway is known to be independent of the NAD biosynthetic pathway in our understanding thus far, and the niacin dose that just causes flushing is currently known to be exceptionally therapeutic for several indications. Still, some will flush with as little as 50 mg while others still do not even experience a flush after taking 4,000 mg at one time! The latter situation is expected to involve an individual with other health problems.

A simple straightforward recommendation is to take whatever dosage of niacin that elicits a flush response, starting with low doses and increasing gradually over several days to weeks until a flush appears. Remember that 1,000 mg taken 3 times a day in the plain old immediate release form has been successfully used in medical practice for over fifty years. It reproducibly corrects the lipodystrophic profile favorably, to reduce cardiovascular events and is expected to provide benefits in the context of COVID-19—and much more!

Viral Illnesses

Niacin and other B vitamins have supportive value in the treatment of viral illnesses as serious as AIDS (acquired immune deficiency syndrome). Their role may extend to having actual antiviral properties of their own. For example, thiamine (vitamin B_1) seems to have benefits for persons with chronic hepatitis B infection.[28] Additionally, a form of thiamine known as thiamine disulfide may be important for AIDS chemotherapy.[29]

Niacin deficiency is a hindrance to recovery from serious viral infection. According to Murray, "findings consistent with niacin depletion have been described in patients with AIDS. There are also clinical and laboratory data to support the potential benefit of niacin in HIV infection."[30]

Niacin would likely work best in concert with other nutrients. A 1993 Johns Hopkins study of 281 HIV-positive men showed that those taking larger-than-RDA quantities of multiple vitamin supplements had only about one-half as many new AIDS outbreaks as those not taking supplements. This important seven-year-long study has received very little publicity. That is odd, since a 50 percent reduction in AIDS cases just from vitamins should be front-page news. The real wonder is that the dosages that achieved this success were fairly small: only about five times the US RDA of the B-vitamins, vitamin C, and beta-carotene. The authors concluded that, "The highest levels of total intake (from food and supplements) of vitamins C and B_1 and niacin were associated with a significantly decreased progression rate to AIDS (as were) vitamin A, niacin, and zinc."[31]

A 2004 Harvard study by Fawzi and colleagues also found that vitamins slow the progression to AIDS by 50 percent. In addition, vitamin supplementation cut AIDS deaths by 27 percent. The authors wrote, "Multivitamins also resulted in significantly higher CD4+ and CD8+ cell counts and significantly lower viral loads. . . . Multivitamin supplements delay the progression of HIV disease."[32]

Vitamins tend to work synergistically with each other and with other nutrients, including amino acids and minerals. *What Really Causes*

AIDS[33] provides an original theory for the nutrition-based treatment of AIDS. Harry D. Foster noted highly significant nutrient deficiencies in AIDS patients, which would be more correct to describe as nutrient dependencies. The human immunodeficiency virus (HIV) is something of a biochemical parasite, which seems to fatally drain nutrients from people who are already malnourished. Dr. Foster's treatment protocol consists of supplementation with the trace mineral selenium, plus the amino acids: cysteine, glutamine, and tryptophan.[34] This approach has been successfully clinically tested in South Africa, Zambia, and Uganda.[35]

CHAPTER 14

Niacin:
Why the Original Megavitamin Is
More Important Than Ever

BY RICHARD A. PASSWATER, PHD

T his chapter is a condensation of six interviews that appeared in *Whole-Foods* magazine during 2017 (February, March, May, June, July, and September). They are reprinted with the kind permission of *WholeFoods*.

***

I believe that the first vitamins used clinically in "mega" doses were vitamins C and niacin (vitamin B₃). Megadoses of vitamin C were used intravenously by Dr. Fredrick R. Klenner of North Carolina to cure polio and other viruses. Megadoses of niacin were used by Dr. Abram Hoffer to successfully treat schizophrenia and many other diseases. Dr. Klenner's results were ignored, but the dramatic findings of Dr. Hoffer could not be ignored. It was his clinical results with niacin that launched the megavitamin revolution. Many thousands of people owe their regained normalcy to the pioneering studies of niacin and schizophrenia. Many have forgotten the profound health effects of niacin. Niacin plays a role in over 500 reactions in the body.

If you ever complained about my repetitious style of writing, blame it on Dr. Hoffer. In an August 1974 letter to me, he wrote "it is important to emphasize these points over and over because many psychiatrists appear not to be able to read." I have taken his point seriously through the years.

Dr. Andrew W. Saul has been an orthomolecular medical writer and lecturer for 40 years. Dr. Saul has taught clinical nutrition at New York Chiropractic College and its postgraduate continuing education programs. He was also on the faculty of the State University of New York for nine years. Two of those years were spent teaching for the university in both women's and men's penitentiaries ("and no," he says, "not as an inmate").

Dr. Saul is editor-in-chief of the *Orthomolecular Medicine News Service* and has published over 200 peer-reviewed articles. His bestselling book *Doctor Yourself* has been translated into eight languages.[1] He has written a dozen other books, four as co-author with Abram Hoffer, MD. Dr. Saul's educational website is www.DoctorYourself.com, the largest peer-reviewed, non-commercial natural healing resource on the Internet. He is a board member of the *Journal of Orthomolecular Medicine* and the Japanese College of Intravenous Therapy. Saul was inducted into the Orthomolecular Medicine Hall of Fame in 2013. He is featured in the documentaries *Food Matters* and *That Vitamin Movie*.

***

Richard Passwater: Dr. Saul, I first learned of your efforts to improve the health of people through your books with Dr. Abram Hoffer. Please tell our readers how you met Dr. Hoffer.

Andrew Saul: I first met Abram at a conference. We had corresponded for some time previously, and he greeted me like he'd always known me. Perhaps in a way he did. Later, when I was sitting next to Abram, I took some vitamin pills. Dr. Hoffer leaned over towards me and said, "You know, you're going to live a lot longer if you take those." As I paused and seriously considered that statement, he leaned over again and added, "If you don't, come back and see me."

I owe Abram a most sincere debt of thanks. I have found everything that he has written to be extremely accurate and unusually helpful. It is difficult for me to fully understand why orthomolecular medicine has been rejected so thoroughly by the medical profession. My experiences in employing niacin and other vitamins have been consistently successful. Dr. Hoffer has said that it takes about two generations before a truly new medical idea is accepted. Perhaps in the case of megavitamin therapy, just a tad longer than that.

Abram Hoffer's 500 scientific papers and twenty books have yet to convince everybody, but they have already changed the course of medicine for all time. Those who have seen the benefits continue to tell everybody. Such momentum is unstoppable.

Passwater: That is inspiring. Now let's look at niacin itself. Why do we need niacin?

Saul: Niacin is the best therapy in existence for normalizing blood lipids. It is the best therapy for schizophrenia. It is also the best therapy for ADHD, obsessive-compulsive disorder, anxiety, and bipolar disorder. Niacin as niacinamide is effective against both osteoarthritis and rheumatoid arthritis. Niacin works and niacin is safe. It is also very inexpensive.

Passwater: What is niacin? Originally, niacin was called vitamin B_3. Actually, a couple of compounds have vitamin B_3 activity. Why the various names, and what are the compounds that are active in the body?

Saul: Niacin is $C_6H_5NO_2$. As organic molecules go, it is quite small. It weighs considerably less than glucose, the simplest of sugars. In fact, niacin is the smallest of all vitamin molecules. Absorption is excellent.

Niacin can be made inside you from the amino acid tryptophan. However, the reduction is about 60:1, so this is an inefficient and probably impossible way to get therapeutic quantities of niacin. The three most common supplemental forms of B_3 are niacin, niacinamide, and inositol hexaniacinate. Niacin causes a flush; people taking it should be ready for that. Niacinamide and inositol hexaniacinate do not cause a flush.

Passwater: How much niacin do we need? What is the RDA and what is the optimal amount?

Saul: The RDA is under 20 milligrams per day. For prevention, we need at least 10 to 20 times that. In illness, orders of magnitude more.

Passwater: How much are people actually getting?

Saul: Maybe the RDA. Maybe.

Passwater: Hopefully you will be kind enough to discuss a full column on this subject in a later issue, but can you give our readers a quick overview of how niacin can help schizophrenics?

Saul: Schizophrenia is not caused by a drug deficiency. Schizophrenia is a niacin dependency. It takes a lot of niacin to do the job.

An example: Jim was schizophrenic and was totally unmanageable. At 21, he'd already been kicked out of the state mental hospital for being too violent. So, they sent him home to his parents, whom he threatened on a daily basis while punching holes in the living room walls. Jim slept one hour per night, and roamed the streets for the other seven.

Medical science had not helped him, so the family was motivated to try Dr. Hoffer's approach. At really large doses, niacin has a profound calming, sedating effect. He took 3,000 milligrams of niacin a day, divided into three 1,000 milligram doses.

The first night on the niacin, he slept 18 hours. Subsequently, he slept about seven hours each night.

Perhaps this was the most moving part of the story. His father told me that one day, for the first time in many years, Jim came down for breakfast. He walked into the dining room and said, "Good morning, Dad."

Even on the phone I could hear the tears in the man's voice. It was wonderful. And niacin is cheap, does not require a prescription, and is easy to monitor: if you flush, you took too much. Still sick, you took too little. No flush and no psychosis means you did it right.

Passwater: There is still more to the niacin story. Niacin can help people keep their cholesterol levels normal. Would you please give our readers a brief overview of niacin and blood cholesterol?

Saul: Niacin normalizes blood lipids. Inositol hexaniacinate works too, though not quite as well. Niacinamide will not, by the way. If you want to lower LDL, lower triglycerides, and raise HDL, niacin is the best way to do so. Some years back, the president of the American College of Cardiology said, in the *New York Times*, "Niacin is really it. Nothing else available is that effective."[2] That is still true. Niacin is better than the statin drugs, and is far safer.

Passwater: If niacin is so safe and effective, then why do I keep seeing articles written by physicians trying to discourage the use of megadoses of niacin to help regulate blood cholesterol levels?

Saul: A fundamental bias in both medicine and dietetics rises darkly from the swamp when you even hint of a therapeutic validity for megavitamin doses. Why such resistance to such a useful nutritional tool? Is it perhaps because niacin therapy is really, really cheap? Ask yourself these two questions: Who paid the authors of those articles? Who paid for the advertisements in the journals publishing those articles?

George Bernard Shaw observed, "The test to which all methods of treatment are finally brought is whether they are lucrative or not." There may not be millions to be made with niacin, but in the end, the economics will not matter. What really matters is who gets better. Abram was once criticized by another doctor who said to him, "I don't think it's really about niacin, Dr. Hoffer. Your success as a physician is due to your excellent bedside manner." Abram replied, "I am nice to all my patients. But only those taking niacin get better."

Passwater: While we are giving our readers a brief overview of the health effects of niacin, what other effects do you see as being important?

Saul: Niacin is therapeutic for an astonishing number of conditions. Again, because it is so important: For decades, orthomolecular physicians have successfully used niacin to normalize cholesterol levels. Niacin or niacinamide is the best therapy for psychosis, ADHD, obsessive-compulsive disorder, anxiety and bipolar disorder. Niacinamide reverses both osteoarthritis and rheumatoid arthritis. Not bad for one vitamin. Too good to be true? Medical doctors have documented these cures for decades.

***

Passwater: Would you please comment on the recent meta-analysis of niacin and schizophrenia by Firth et al. in February?[3]

Saul: First of all, the authors actually said something worthwhile: nutritional supplements may reduce psychiatric symptoms.

However, it is vastly better than this. A very large number of physician reports and clinical studies have already clearly shown that niacin and the other B-vitamins are effective against mental illness. The meta-analysis you refer to selected only 18 randomized controlled studies and a total of only 832 patients. Yet Dr. Abram Hoffer successfully treated many thousands of patients. The word "Hoffer" is not found, not even once, in this so-called meta-analysis. His work was ignored. What kind of an analysis is that? And, although the meta-analysis ignored thousands of cured people, it was still positive about vitamins.

Imagine if they had used niacin. What, you say: they did not even look at niacin? Right. Believe it or not, they completely omitted niacin. The word niacin is not mentioned even once in the entire published paper. Dr. Hoffer said that niacin is the specific cure for schizophrenia. Not other nutrients; niacin. The meta-analysis totally ignored the one vitamin that is known to work best. That is like a college course in Shakespeare omitting *Hamlet*.

I feel sorry for the families of schizophrenics who will be harmed by not knowing the truth.

Passwater: Let's go back to the beginning. How did Dr. Abram Hoffer discover that niacin had curative powers in schizophrenia? What was his "eureka" moment?

Saul: I have Dr. Hoffer's own words describing his first schizophrenic patient that he treated with niacin: "The first was a 12-year-old boy in 1960. To get the boy to take it, his father crushed the niacin tablet and spread it into a jam sandwich. That boy is now a research psychiatrist."

Passwater: How did Dr. Hoffer explain the results of niacin therapy in schizophrenia? Did he modify his theoretical explanations over time and are they accepted today?

Saul: To the very end of his life Abram maintained what he termed the adrenochrome hypothesis. There is, he said, a chemical found in quantity in the bodies of schizophrenic persons. It is an indole compound called adrenochrome. Adrenochrome (which is oxidized adrenaline) has an almost mescaline- or LSD-like effect on the body. That might well explain schizophrenic behavior. Niacin serves to reduce the body's production of this toxic material. And niacin or niacinamide work on and with the body's benzodiazepine receptors, similar to tranquilizers. But niacin is cheaper and safer. Far safer.

Passwater: In 1981, Dr. Hoffer explained the biochemistry involved with the adrenochrome hypothesis:

> Adrenaline is oxidized to adrenochrome in a two-step process. One electron is lost, forming a highly reactive free radical, an oxidized adrenaline. It is readily changed back to adrenaline. The reversible NAD↔NADH system is involved. If another electron is lost, adrenochrome is formed but this is a one-way process. Adrenochrome is not reduced back to adrenaline. This may be a mechanism at synapses in the brain by which the body regulates the reactions of the neurotransmitter amines. Trihydroxy dopamine (6 hydroxy dopamine or TOPA) is highly toxic to dopamine receptors, perhaps because of the formation of aminochrome at the receptor site thereby destroying it. Vitamin B_3 which controls formation of NAD is thus involved. With a relative deficiency of vitamin B_3 too much trihydroxy dopamine may be converted into its aminochrome.[4]

Did Dr. Hoffer publish his research in peer-reviewed journals?

Saul: Certainly . . . until they refused his work. That is why he created his own journal, now known as the *Journal of Orthomolecular Medicine.*

Even a basic working knowledge of niacin can profoundly change so many patients for the better. This vitamin becomes very interesting very quickly.

Passwater: How else is niacin involved in brain health? Does it help protect against Alzheimer's disease and other dementias?

Saul: Niacin, or niacinamide, most certainly helps protect against Alzheimer's. The *Orthomolecular Medicine News Service* published an interesting article on this, "Vitamins Help Prevent Alzheimer's Disease: News Media Ignores Supplement Benefits . . . Again."[5] Because the news media did ignore it.

B-complex vitamins are absolutely vital for nerve cell health. Where pathology already exists, unusually large quantities of vitamins are needed.

Niacin is valuable against multiple sclerosis. Niacinamide, said researchers at Harvard Medical School, "profoundly prevents the degeneration of demyelinated axons and improves the behavioral deficits." And this was published over ten years ago in the *Journal of Neuroscience*.[6]

This is good news, but it is a long way from being new news. Half a century ago, Frederick Robert Klenner, MD, of North Carolina, was using vitamins and other nutrients to arrest and even reverse multiple sclerosis.[7]

Passwater: Does niacin help cognitive function?

Saul: Yes, but the best bet in this case is the entire B-complex. Dr. Ruth Harrell showed the great positive effects of supplemental thiamine on learning . . . in the 1940s! Decades later, she and her colleagues demonstrated improvement in the IQ of Down Syndrome children. This was major research, published in the *Proceedings of the National Academy of Sciences*. It has been ignored.

Passwater: Memory?

Saul: Maybe, but I forget. Just kidding. Yes.

You can subscribe free of charge to the *Orthomolecular Medicine News Service*. The *OMNS*, in its nineteenth year of publication, is peer-reviewed and has no advertising.[8]

Passwater: Why are some people concerned about taking large amounts of niacin?

Saul: The two biggest concerns people have with niacin are the flush, and the possibility of elevation of liver enzymes. People who do not like the flush can simply use niacinamide, or inositol hexaniacinate. These two forms of niacin will not cause a flush in 99 percent of those taking them. A small elevation in liver enzymes indicates increased liver activity, not liver pathology. Dr. Hoffer emphasized this. So did Mayo Clinic niacin researcher William Parsons, MD.

***

(From "Joint Pain Relief and Arthritis." An interview with Andrew W. Saul, PhD. June 20, 2017.)

Now let's look at niacinamide's amazing benefit in relieving the pain of arthritis, and better still, in repairing the damage of osteoarthritis. Niacinamide is another form of vitamin B_3. Reversing arthritis with niacinamide is an amazing story.

Passwater: The incredible clinical results from more than 60 years show that niacinamide not only relieves the pain of arthritis, but over time, leads to repairing the joints. Since arthritis is an inflammatory condition, does niacinamide work by reducing inflammation?

Saul: Evidently it does. In 1996, a study on niacinamide and osteoarthritis was published in the journal *Inflammatory Research*.[9] The authors could have omitted the words "pilot study" from their title. Dr. William Kaufman had already published, 47 years earlier, his meticulous case notes for hundreds of patients, along with specific niacinamide dosage information applicable to both osteoarthritis and rheumatoid arthritis.

In addition, the doctor added some remarkably prescient observations on the antidepressant-antipsychotic properties of B_3. Dr. Kaufman, whom his widow has described as a conservative physician, was nevertheless the first to prescribe as much as 5,000 milligrams niacinamide daily, in many divided doses, to improve range of joint motion.[10]

Passwater: Do the findings apply to both osteoarthritis (OA) and rheumatoid arthritis (RA)?

Saul: Yes. Dr. Kaufman said: "The relationship between the continuous administration of adequate amounts of niacinamide and improvement in both hypertrophic arthritis and rheumatoid arthritis was originally reported in 1943." That was the year Dr. Kaufman's book *The Common Form of Niacinamide Deficiency Disease: Aniacinamidosis* was published.

Passwater: How was this discovered?

Saul: Observation. Dr. Kaufman paid attention to, and spent a large amount of office time with, each and every one of his patients. Dr. Abram Hoffer considered him a superb clinician.

Passwater: Dr. Kaufman detailed his clinical findings in his 1949 book, *The Common Form of Joint Dysfunction*. That book contains a lot of information on the proper protocol to use for niacinamide in treating arthritis, but since it's a 1949 book, it probably can't be found in bookstores.

Saul: The late Mrs. Charlotte Kaufman graciously gave me exclusive permission to post the entire text of this important book at my website, www.doctoryourself.com. It is all free access.

Passwater: Did Dr. Kaufman publish additional information on his clinical findings or practical use of niacinamide to treat arthritis?

Saul: Yes. For those who just cannot get enough of the work of this wonderful physician, a complete bibliography of Dr. Kaufman's work will be found at my website.[11]

Passwater: Have others confirmed Dr. Kaufman's clinical findings?

Saul: Certainly. Those who follow his protocol duplicate his success.

Passwater: Why don't more physicians treat their arthritic patients with niacinamide?

Saul: One cannot help but wonder why. Is it that vitamins only worked in 1949, and vitamins mysteriously lost their value? Or could it be that they are cheap and provide no profit incentive for large pharmaceutical companies? Or could it simply be that "megavitamin therapy" is never the answer to any medical school examination question?

Here is what medical schools should be teaching: Dr. Kaufman gave 250 milligrams of niacinamide every one-and-a-half hours for a daily total of ten doses. That is 2,500 milligrams a day, not at all more than many doctors today prescribe to lower serum cholesterol. The result was improved grip strength and joint mobility. Dr. Kaufman went on to treat close to one thousand patients with niacinamide plus the B-vitamins thiamine (B_1), riboflavin (B_2), pyridoxine (B_6) and pantothenic acid. It will not surprise you that he also gave large doses of vitamin C. What will surprise you is that he started using vitamins to successfully treat arthritis as early as 1935, and niacin in 1937, immediately after it was identified.

Passwater: Amazing! Is there a safety issue with niacinamide?

Saul: Yes. Firstly, high-dose niacinamide or niacin therapy may elevate liver enzymes. The elevation is fairly common and usually modest. This, says Mayo Clinic niacin researcher William Parsons, Jr., MD, is not a sign of liver pathology. It is, Dr. Parsons says, a sign of liver activity.

Secondly, very high doses of niacinamide, that is, over 3,000 milligrams per day, may cause nausea. This may be eliminated by taking some of the dose as niacin. Of course, niacin causes a flush, which is harmless but to be expected. Niacinamide does not cause a flush. Dr. Kaufman used niacinamide because he personally did not like the flush when he experienced it! Either form is effective; either form is vitamin B_3. Niacinamide is far safer than any drug. Any drug.

Passwater: In your book, you quote Dr. Kaufman saying "niacinamide has ungated entrance to the central nervous system. It has a strong affinity for the central nervous system's benzodiazepine receptors and causes a pleasant calmative effect." Dr. Saul, would you be kind enough to translate that into plain English for our readers who may not be medically trained?

Saul: It means that niacinamide calms you down, very much like a tranquilizer does. But there are no harmful side effects, and no addictive issues with niacinamide. In fact, niacin or niacinamide can be used to wean people off of tranquilizers. Niacin researcher Dr. W. Todd Penberthy and I reported on this in the *Orthomolecular Medicine News Service* in 2014.[12]

Passwater: Dr. Kaufman also noted that niacinamide increases muscle strength, decreases fatigability, and heals broken strands of DNA. Do you concur?

Saul: Yes. No pharmaceutical on the planet can do all that, and niacinamide is cheap. And safe. And non-prescription.

***

Most nutritionally informed people associate niacin with optimizing blood cholesterol levels. But there's still more to niacin's health benefits. We have discussed niacin's benefits for those with schizophrenia, relieving the pain of arthritis, and better still, in repairing the damage of osteoarthritis. This month, let's chat with Dr. Saul about one of his favorite topics, niacin and learning and behavioral disorders.

Dr. Saul has encountered learning- and behaviorally-impaired students at all educational levels, not only children, but also adults.

Saul: I will say straight away that you have to see this to believe it. Some health practitioners reject niacin therapy out of hand. They do not know what they are missing. Furthermore, the parents of mentally troubled children—psychiatrist Abram Hoffer called them "battered parents"—are being allowed to suffer unnecessarily. And finally, when we let malnourished children struggle along and endure malnutrition, our world suffers with them.

Passwater: Since niacin and other nutrients are important to learning, are most learning "disorders" really diseases as the pharmaceutical industry claims or are they primarily nutritional deficiencies or allergies?

Saul: Perhaps more than anything, they actually are vitamin deficiencies. Not simple nutrient deficiencies, for low doses will not work therapeutically.

Not druggable diseases, as drugs are not working either. ADHD is not caused by a deficiency of methylphenidate. More, more, and still more kids are on medication today. That may be good for pharma profits but it is clearly failure to control a disease. Not simple allergies, because avoiding this food and that pet and this other dust does nothing to remedy the underlying situation. I know a young woman who was tested and found to be allergic to 72 different substances. She started on vitamin therapy, was retested some weeks later, and was allergic to zero substances. This does not mean there are no such things as allergies. Put type B blood into a type A person and there is going to be big trouble. That is an allergy. With most behaviorally-challenged kids, nutrient deficiency is more probably the cause than allergy.

Passwater: Are learning and behavioral disorders increasing or is it just a matter of increased recognition?

Saul: Both are increasing sharply. In 1990, some 750,000 American children were on ADHD medication. The number in 2012 was well over four million. And now, ADHD is diagnosed in about 11 percent of all children, and it's approaching 20 percent of teenage boys. Plus, as Dr. Hoffer has pointed out, there are all manner and all number of collateral syndromes and disorders. Yet, Dr. Hoffer said, "No matter which terms are used to classify these children, they are all recommended for treatment with drug therapy." So virtually none of those many, many children are ever put on niacinamide . . . unless the parents go and do it themselves.

Passwater: Can you share a case history of a child who was given the chance with niacinamide?

Saul: Yes. I knew a 10-year-old boy who was having considerable school and behavior problems. Interestingly enough, the child was already on physician-prescribed little bits of niacin, with a total daily dose of less than 150 milligrams. Not a bad beginning, since the RDA is under 20 milligrams per day. But it wasn't enough to be effective, and the boy was slated for the Ritalin-for-lunch bunch. So, the family went to Dr. Hoffer's suggested level of 500 milligrams of niacinamide, three times daily (1,500 milligrams total).

Niacinamide is a comfortable, flush-free form of vitamin B$_3$. That dose made a noticeable difference. At an even higher dose, divided all throughout the day, the boy's improvement was simply spectacular. Phone calls and notes from the school immediately went from negative to positive.

Passwater: In your book with Drs. Hoffer and Foster, *Niacin: The Real Story*, you mention some 1940s era comments by Dr. William Kaufman on hyper-activity in niacin-deficient animals.

Saul: You can create behavioral-social problems in animals by way of their diet (see chapter 9, "Treating ADHD with Vitamin B$_3$ (Niacinamide)"). So accurately does Dr. Kaufman describe the problems of ADHD children it is difficult to believe vitamin B$_3$ has been thoroughly ignored for nearly 70 years. Dr. Kaufman also said that frequently divided doses are maximally effective. The precise amount of niacinamide that an ADHD child requires needs to be thoughtfully considered by parent and physician together.

Passwater: In *Niacin: The Real Story*, you presented a number of other case histories wherein niacin was used by Dr. Hoffer and others to eliminate hyperactivity. Was this serendipitous using the power of observation during regular treatments by good doctors or were they planned clinical trials?

Saul: Both. Dr. Hoffer practiced psychiatry for 55 years. He paid close attention to what worked for his patients. He also pioneered double-blind, placebo-controlled megavitamin research and treatment back in the early 1950s. For those who say there is insufficient scientific evidence to support megavitamin therapy for children's behavior disorders, I say they haven't been looking hard enough. The simple way to determine whether vitamins will help a child is to try them.

Passwater: Upon hearing this, people often will ask, "If this treatment is so good, how come my doctor doesn't know about it? How come it is not on the news?"

Saul: The answer has more to do with medical politics than with medical science. With attention deficit hyperactivity disorder, orthodox medicine seems unwilling even to admit nutrient deficiency as a causal factor, let alone a curative one. Such nutritional information as does make news generally stays far from the headlines, unless, of course, it is critical of vitamins. The most widely publicized vitamin therapy trials tend to be low-dose, worthless, negative, or all three. Mass media attention to a given nutritional research study appears to be inversely proportional to its curative value.

Therefore, the public and many physicians remain unaware of the power of simple and safe natural methods due to contradictory, inadequate, or just plain biased media reporting. When the press touts the supposed "dangers" of vitamins while simultaneously overlooking the very real dangers of having kids on long-term drug maintenance, it strains at a gnat and swallows a camel. The chief side effect of niacinamide is failure to take enough of it. The quantity of a nutrient that cures an illness indicates the patient's degree of need for the nutrient. This amount may be quite high. A dry sponge holds more milk. ADHD children need more niacinamide.

Passwater: Mainstream medicine teaches reliance on pharmaceuticals. Are they more effective?

Saul: No. Dr. Hoffer put it succinctly: "Drugs make a well person sick. Why would they make a sick person well?"

Passwater: Are pharmaceuticals safer than niacin?

Saul: No. There is no drug on the planet that is as safe as niacin and niacin-amide, which does not cause a flush.

Passwater: Years ago, the drug "Ritalin" was the drug of choice. I seem to remember that school kids were given their Ritalin at lunchtime by school officials. Is that an accurate memory?

Saul: It matches my experience exactly. I have taught every grade there is. My students have ranged from primary school, long ago, all the way to the doctoral level. This experience has helped me to understand the essential role nutrition plays in the education process. May you never have a class full of sugared-up, chemically-fed, vitamin-deficient students. And on top of that, we go and drug them as well.

Many, perhaps most, of the "difficult" pupils in schools today are not "bad" but nutritionally impaired. This has to adversely affect their school performance. What would be surprising would be if it did not.

Passwater: Yet, today, school personnel in many states can't even give students a vitamin pill at school unless they have a medical doctor's prescription. Is that accurate?

Saul: Children are not allowed to take vitamin tablets in school without a doctor's written permission, along with the approval of the school nurse who will implement it. So let's see to it. There is reason to suspect that Attention Deficit Disorder is really Vitamin Deficit Disorder. What is so difficult about giving schoolchildren a vitamin supplement to make up their deficit? Don't tell me that vitamins would be too dangerous, expensive, or impractical to administer in school. They give kids prescription drugs in schools everywhere, every day. Look up drug contraindications and side effects in the Physicians' Desk Reference (PDR). Such information covers columns of fine print, and you might not enjoy reading it. Now compare this to non-prescription vitamins taken safely by over 150 million Americans every day. Kids as young as age six line up daily, in school, for drugs. Let's line them up for vitamins instead.

***

Dr. Fred A. Kummerow's lifesaving nutritional efforts began with helping to wipe out the deadly pellagra epidemic in the United States. Thanks to researchers including Drs. Kummerow, Joseph Goldberger, and Conrad Elvehjem, pellagra is essentially non-existent today in the United States. Pellagra is a disease that was present before 1938 in the southeastern United States. It is a deficiency of niacin. The symptoms of pellagra are swelling of the lips and tongue and swelling of the arms to the point that the skin breaks open. When it reaches this stage, the people usually die.

When Professor Kummerow arrived at Clemson, South Carolina, in 1943, thousands of people were still dying of pellagra. Some
3,000 to 6,000 people were dying each year (about five per 100,000
population). He figured out how to put niacin in corn grits, a food
staple in the South. By 1945, there were only 12 deaths from pellagra,
and it is rare today. It's now more than 70 years later and pellagra is
extremely rare, so that's roughly 250,000 lives he saved from premature death.[13]

Saul: Niacin is so good for lowering cholesterol and preventing heart disease that some years ago the *New York Times* quoted the president of the
American College of Cardiology saying, "Niacin is really it. Nothing else
comes close." Then, and since then, drugs old and new simply do not work
as well as niacin.

I would like to add this straight away: people need to realize that for
really good health there is no magic bullet. To stop cardiovascular disease,
they're going to have to take a good, hard look at everything they are doing.
To merely substitute niacin for a statin drug is missing the point entirely.
You're also going to have to make lifestyle changes, which includes a proper
diet of whole, unprocessed foods, exercise, stress reduction, possibly medication, and, definitely, learning.

Passwater: How does niacin work to lower elevated cholesterol?

Saul: The short answer is, niacin reduces the body's production of VLDL
and LDL; niacin lowers triglycerides; and niacin greatly raises HDL. Niacin
also inhibits oxidative stress and vascular inflammation.

The long answer is complicated and only in recent years has the mechanism been understood in detail. According to Ganji, Kamanna, and
Kashyap, "the beneficial effect of niacin to reduce triglycerides and apo-
lipoprotein-B containing lipoproteins (e.g., VLDL and LDL) are mainly
through: a.) decreasing fatty acid mobilization from adipose tissue triglyceride stores, and b.) inhibiting hepatocyte diacylglycerol acyltransferase and
triglyceride synthesis leading to increased intracellular apo B degradation

and subsequent decreased secretion of VLDL and LDL particles. The mechanism of action of niacin to raise HDL is by decreasing the fractional catabolic rate of HDL-apo AI without affecting the synthetic rates. Additionally, niacin selectively increases the plasma levels of Lp-AI (HDL subfraction without apo AII), a cardioprotective subfraction of HDL in patients with low HDL."[14]

Well, you asked for it.

Passwater: What dosages are required to achieve this benefit?

Saul: Several thousand milligrams per day, in divided doses.

Passwater: Will that cause a "flush"?

Saul: You can count on it. If you want to flush in a hurry, chew the tablet and take it with something hot, on an empty stomach. I was giving a lecture once to some post-doctoral students, and at their insistence, demonstrated a niacin flush. I thought, "Well, okay," since I always have my vitamin bottle in my pocket. That's why when I walk down the halls, I would rattle and all the students knew it was me before I turned the corner. It was before lunch, so I had an empty stomach. I took about 1,500 milligrams of niacin, and I said, "Watch this."

Now they're all watching pretty intently. It was a small class, only about 30 people. There's one fellow at the back who whipped out a pair of opera glasses. Now this was really funny. It wasn't that big of a room, and he didn't do it to be a wise guy. But it was a very funny moment. He wanted to actually see precisely where and how I flushed.

The cheeks, the neck, and the upper arms tend to flush first. Then later on you might have a flush on your abdomen and perhaps your legs. If you'd had a big meal, the flush could be delayed for an hour or two, so long that you might have forgotten you took the niacin at all.

Well, they liked the niacin flush so much that one of their evaluations said, "The niacin flush was awesome. Do you do birthday parties?"

We got a big laugh out of that. The niacin flush is not a big deal. People need to understand that it is a distraction. Niacin happens to cause you to have a flush. It's like a little bit of an embarrassment. Ladies, it's a little bit like a hot flash, I'm reliably informed. It's a little bit like feeling embarrassed or like you were maybe out in the sun for that extra hour.

Passwater: Just what is this "flush" and is it dangerous?

Saul: It is a vasodilation. As the small blood vessels open up, more blood flows to the skin's surface. Dr. Hoffer described it as harmless, and with thousands of patients over 55 years of practice, he was qualified to say so. Most persons will itch and feel hot. In some people, such large doses of niacin may cause a temporary drop in blood pressure and feeling faint. All of those side effects may be avoided by taking readily available, over-the-counter flush-free forms of niacin.

Passwater: Niacinamide doesn't cause a flush. Does niacinamide lower blood cholesterol?

Saul: It does not. Niacinamide is useful for all other niacin matters except blood lipids.

Passwater: Are there non-flush forms of niacin that work without causing a flush?

Saul: Inositol hexaniacinate is a virtually no-flush form that works but is not as effective as plain flush niacin. There are proprietary (patented) forms of time- or sustained-release niacin that cause little or no flush. However, these forms seem to have the most side effects, the most common of which is elevated liver enzyme levels.

Passwater: What is the most effective way to take niacin?

Saul: Consistently; in divided doses; with meals.

Passwater: How was it discovered that niacin lowered high cholesterol? What is the history?

Saul: Dr. Hoffer's psychiatric research up in Saskatchewan, early in the 1950s, showed that niacin also lowered cholesterol, that is, it lowered the bad cholesterol—and actually raised good cholesterol. This work was picked up by Dr. William B. Parsons, Jr. at the Mayo Clinic. Dr. Parsons, America's number-one niacin researcher, wrote a very fine book on this titled *Cholesterol Control without Diet: The Niacin Solution.*

Passwater: People seem to be interested in LDL and HDL values. Does niacin help normalize both or just one?

Saul: Niacin lowers LDL significantly and raises HDL spectacularly. It also lowers triglycerides.

Passwater: How does niacin compare to cholesterol-lowering pharmaceuticals?

Saul: Niacin is more effective. It is far cheaper. And it is vastly safer.

Passwater: Isn't niacin the first choice of many physicians?

Saul: The smart ones, yes. I tell my readers, and your readers, that if your doctor is not yet employing vitamins for treatment, then you have an old-fashioned doctor.

Passwater: I bet that annoys Big Pharma.

Saul: Darn straight it does.

Passwater: Hasn't there been a coordinated effort by the pharmaceutical industry to discourage the use of niacin for cholesterol lowering?

Saul: Let's just say that there is no money in therapy with a cheap vitamin. Pharmaceutical profits are more important to stockholders than public health is.

Passwater: There are occasionally warnings about "elevated liver enzymes" when using niacin at such high doses. Let's look more closely at this group of enzymes measured in standard blood tests. What are these enzymes and what do they do in the liver?

Saul: Usually it's alanine transaminase (ALT), aspartate transaminase (AST), alkaline phosphatase (ALP), and gamma-glutamyl transpeptidase (GGT). Dr. Abram Hoffer and Dr. William Parsons, Jr., the two most important niacin researchers, both strongly maintained that the elevation is an indication of liver activity, not liver pathology. A moderate elevation is not cause for alarm. Interestingly, the Mayo Clinic agrees, saying at their website I accessed today that "Most of the time, elevated liver enzymes don't signal a chronic, serious liver problem."

Passwater: Why would physicians be so concerned if these liver enzymes were above "normal"?

Saul: If they are way above normal, they should be concerned. But, as Dr. Parsons and Dr. Hoffer both asserted, a moderate elevation is not cause for alarm. And these two doctors concur that physicians need to understand niacin in order to use it.

Passwater: What is really happening with these enzymes in the case of high niacin intake?

Saul: They indicate that you are alive and that your liver is working. Those are both desirable outcomes.

Passwater: It has been believed that niacin could cause a methyl deficiency in the body, because it is a methyl acceptor. What about that?

Saul: Methyl deficiency can cause fatty liver. But, said Dr. Hoffer and colleague Rudolf Altschul, MD, it does not happen with niacin. They checked that out over 50 years ago. Supplemental vitamin C is additional protection. Vincent Zannoni at the University of Michigan Medical School has shown that vitamin C protects the liver. Even doses as low as 500 milligrams daily help prevent fatty buildup and cirrhosis. And in 1986, the Associated Press reported that 5,000 milligrams of vitamin C per day appears to actually flush fats from the liver.[15]

Passwater: So, niacin, unlike pharmaceuticals, gives many health benefits including brain health, and arthritis, as well as helping to control cholesterol. How safe is niacin in the high dosages used for lowering cholesterol?

Saul: Very. Safer than any drug, and I mean any drug at all. And people on long-term niacin treatment should still monitor their liver enzymes. That is easy to do when blood is drawn at your next physical. Always insist on your personally receiving a complete copy of all your test results, not a summary or dumbed-down interpretation. Look at the numbers for yourself; the test scores will come along with a statement of what the normal range is. If the numbers are very high, the niacin needs to be decreased. And not everyone needs huge doses of niacin! Dr. Hoffer figured that a few hundred milligrams a day is good prevention for most people. The therapeutic dose, 3,000 milligrams per day or more, is for those who would otherwise be on an inherently more dangerous drug regimen. The standard is not perfection; the standard is the alternative.

Passwater: Does niacin have any other cardiovascular benefit? Can it help after someone has an acute coronary episode?

Saul: Evidently it can. In his memoirs, Dr. Hoffer tells of researchers that, over time, found far fewer deaths among niacin-treated patients. He said, "Niacin, unlike the cholesterol-lowering drugs, has the power to extend lifespan."

Passwater: Where can readers find more information on this topic?

Saul: Dr. Hoffer's books are so clear, so good at explaining niacin therapy that I urge people to read them for themselves. An internet search will bring up titles immediately.

***

An Australian dermatologist, Dr. Gary Halliday, and his team have published a review in *Photodermatology, Photoimmunology and Photomedicine* calling for clinical trials of niacinamide to prevent melanoma.[16] Dr. Halliday, professor of dermatology at the University of Sydney, and his team see niacinamide (vitamin B$_3$) as a low-cost way of preventing melanoma skin cancer. They point out that nicotinamide enhances DNA repair and reduces inflammation caused by ultraviolet radiation. The researchers point to the results from the clinical trial, which reduced the incidence of non-melanoma skin cancer in high-risk individuals, and said it would be worthwhile to determine whether it would also be useful for high-risk melanoma patients.

Passwater: We have seen reports before this study about niacin's protective effect against non-melanoma skin cancer. What is the most likely mechanism involved?

Saul: Niacin (or niacinamide, also called nicotinamide) reduces two key pathways to carcinogenesis: DNA damage and UV-induced immunosuppression.

Passwater: Figure 1 graphically depicts this from the excellent article in *Melanoma Letters*[17] by Drs. Diona Damian, Andrew Martin, and Gary Halliday, who are Australian researchers. By the way, this is an excellent article for researchers as well as the public.

Saul: Niacin's role is probably much the same for all sorts of cancers, whether modest or aggressive. Niacin helps your body repair DNA and actually fix mutations. The benefit would be for all forms of cancer in all persons. This is the very information that Dr. Abram Hoffer brought forward to the scientific community decades ago. He was ignored, and as you read these "new" reports, you will see that he is not mentioned. That's why we are doing this interview.

Passwater: Another recent study suggests that vitamin B$_3$ might help prevent certain kinds of complex birth defects. Vitamin B$_3$ can help compensate for defects in the body's ability to make a molecule, called nicotinamide adenine dinucleotide (NAD), which researchers have linked for the first time to healthy fetal development in humans. This raises the possibility that boosting levels of vitamin B₃ in pregnant women's diets might help lower overall rates of birth defects.

Dr. Sally Dunwoodie, a developmental geneticist at the Victor Chang Cardiac Research Institute in Sydney, Australia, and her colleagues studied the genes that influence fetal development. They found that genes related to the production of NAD, a niacin-dependent molecule crucial for energy storage and DNA synthesis in cells, had a role in heart development.

Dr. Dunwoodie has counted at least 95 genes that are involved in NAD levels, and believes it's possible that mutations in any of those could leave a developing fetus vulnerable to birth defects and that extra vitamin B₃ in a mother's diet might help compensate for any of the faulty genes.

Saul: And there it is again: Niacin's ability to prevent birth defects is because niacin actually repairs DNA damage. I think this basic, life-giving mechanism has many applications.

Antioxidant vitamins, notably vitamins C and E, have diverse therapeutic uses. Niacin has many uses. Water has many uses. Money has many uses. Niacin is biochemical money: you can do so much with it. But the key is the dose. If you take in only the ridiculously low U.S. RDA of about 16 milligrams of niacin per day, that's like trying to provide for your whole family on a minimum wage paycheck. That is virtually impossible. Then, the NIH actually says, "The Tolerable Upper Intake Level (UL) for niacin for adults is 35 milligrams per day, which was based on flushing as the critical adverse effect." That is comical reasoning. Why? Because it takes at least hundreds of milligrams of niacin daily, and often thousands of milligrams, to get results. And the public are being told to not exceed 35 milligrams because someone, somewhere might flush.

Few people flush at 35 milligrams. Some do, but very, very few. And the kicker is that if you take niacinamide or inositol hexaniacinate, you won't flush at all, even at vastly higher amounts. The government knows this. Researchers know this. And still that silly "Upper Limit" sits at 35 milligrams per day. At the very least, medical authorities in the government should point out that there is no flushing with these other forms of B₃. "Flush fear mongering" is keeping America chronically ill and chronically dependent on the medical system. A cynic might suspect collusion.

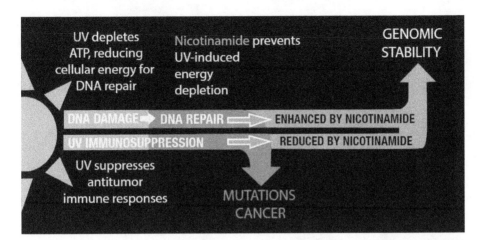

Figure 1. UV radiation both damages DNA and depletes cells of the energy required for efficient DNA repair, thus increasing the likelihood of genetic mutations that can lead to skin cancer. Unrepaired DNA photolesions are also a trigger for the immunosuppressive effects of sunlight. By preventing UV-induced energy crisis in skin cells, nicotinamide both enhances DNA repair and attenuates UV immunosuppression. Figure from Damian, Martin, and Halliday in *Melanoma Letters* (skincancer.org/publications/the-melanoma-letter /spring-2016-vol-34-no-1/nicotinamide).

Niacin is a small organic molecule and the very smallest of all the vitamins. It is C6H5NO2. That is considerably smaller than glucose, the simplest of sugars. Niacin weighs only 123 grams per mole; glucose weighs 180. Niacin is even smaller than vitamin C, ascorbic acid, which weighs 176. I think we would do better thinking of niacin as a food rather than as a micronutrient. Dr. Linus Pauling taught us that we need a lot of vitamin C, thousands of milligrams daily. Dr. Hoffer taught us that we need a lot of niacin, hundreds of milligrams daily. They are both absolutely correct.

Saul: Abram Hoffer began his education at a one-room schoolhouse, yet eventually earned PhD and MD degrees and wrote two dozen books and over 500 papers. Dr. Hoffer has changed medicine forever, and for the better. I urge everyone to read his books and learn how to get well and stay that way with fewer, or zero, pharmaceuticals. Dr. Hoffer said, "Drugs make a well person sick. Why would they make a sick person well?"

Passwater: If it wasn't for your follow-through, most of this information would now be lost. The Big Pharma-oriented medical profession has little interest in natural medicine. It seems that only the orthomolecular physicians are interested in Dr. Hoffer's teachings. How did you come to partner with Dr. Hoffer to keep his legacy going?

Saul: I met him at an Orthomolecular Medicine Today Conference in Toronto. I went over and introduced myself, and he very graciously greeted me as if we'd known each other forever. During the course of the conference, he personally introduced me to important orthomolecular doctors from all over the world. Subsequently I became a columnist and then contributing editor to the *Journal of Orthomolecular Medicine*, which Abram had founded along with Humphry Osmond, MD, way back in 1967. Now whenever I had a topic idea, Abram would invariably say to me, "How about you write a hard-hitting editorial on that for our journal?" So, I did, and he kept publishing them. Later, one of his books, *Orthomolecular Medicine for Physicians*, was in need of expansion and updating. Abram, knowing this full well, did not have the time to undertake the project and wondered who would co-author with him. I offered, he accepted, and we produced *Orthomolecular Medicine for Everyone* in 2008.

Passwater: What other books did you co-author with him?

Saul: One, and a very important one, is *The Vitamin Cure for Alcoholism*. Not everyone knows that Dr. Hoffer was Bill W.'s personal physician. Interesting story, that Bill W. cofounder of Alcoholics Anonymous, was unable to interest his own organization in niacin. Yet it was Dr. Hoffer and niacin that cured Bill W. of his long-standing, severe depression in a matter of weeks. Because Abram wished to write a history of hospitals, and I thought a how-to-survive-hospitals book could also be useful, we wrote *Hospitals and Health: Your Orthomolecular Guide to a Shorter, Safer Hospital Stay*. Our third author was Steve Hickey, PhD, a vitamin C expert, and my co-author for *Vitamin C: The Real Story*. Of course, there is *Niacin: The Real Story*, Abram's final book. Our co-author was Harold D. Foster, PhD, a very good friend, and colleague of Abram's. Additionally, there is also a lot of Dr. Hoffer in *The Orthomolecular Treatment of Chronic Disease*. These books are all in print, easy to find, and provide a strong grounding in just how orthomolecular treatments work.

Passwater: What is their importance? What do they teach?

Saul: In my opinion, all of Dr. Hoffer's work is important. These books teach how to live. Dr. Hoffer summarized this way: orthomolecular medicine consists of eating whole foods and taking some vitamins. That is one of the most powerful, practical, and deceptively simple maxims for life I have ever encountered. Years ago, in my first communication with Dr. Hoffer, I had told him that I had found by experience that everything he has written has proven to be true. And it has, to this day. I have been in the natural health arena for over 40 years now, and Abram Hoffer is one of a select group that I have found to be lifesavers. Others include Drs. Hugh Riordan, Robert F. Cathcart, Lendon Smith, Emanuel Cheraskin, Ruth Flynn Harrell, Frederick R. Klenner, and Linus Pauling.

Passwater: What are the most important teachings of Dr. Hoffer and yourself that are available on your website?

Saul: There are hundreds of articles at DoctorYourself.com, many by Dr. Hoffer and the other doctors I mentioned previously. Because health is such a large topic, perhaps doing a quick search at the site for the illness or nutrient you are most interested in is the best way to get started. One example would be Dr. Hoffer's comments on the DoctorYourself.com diabetes webpage, http://www.doctoryourself.com/diabetes.html, where he writes:

> I am very familiar with Type I (insulin dependent diabetes or juvenile diabetes), as two members of my family have it. Dr. Saul lists and describes both positive and negative factors in dealing with this condition. Thus, for Type I, we have on the positive side the B-complex vitamins, especially vitamin B_3, and vitamin C. The negative factors are diets which are too rich in free sugars and not rich enough in the complex carbohydrates. Negative factors also include milk, fluoride, coffee, and vaccinations. When it is started at an early age, niacinamide will prevent diabetes from developing

in many children born to families prone to the disease. I have also found niacin very helpful in preventing patients from suffering the long-term ravages of diabetes, which are not directly due to high blood sugars, but to the side effects involving the vascular system. Therefore, these patients are less apt to become blind and lose their legs. With medical supervision, it may be used safely in dealing with diabetics, but you will need to find a doctor who knows niacin. Type II Non-insulin dependent Diabetes Mellitus (NIDDM) is a very common condition. Positive factors listed are magnesium, exercise, weight control, chromium, fiber, vitamin E, vanadium, vitamin C, and complex carbohydrates. I have been using the positive factors for the past 40 years. When patients followed such a program, the results are very good.

Passwater: I was not too surprised to find that it was Dr. Hoffer who first got Dr. Pauling interested in orthomolecular therapy.

Saul: Indeed, it was. It started when Dr. Pauling saw a copy of Drs. Hoffer and Humphry Osmond's book *How to Live with Schizophrenia* on a friend's coffee table. Linus Pauling took the book home and stayed up all night reading it. Dr. Pauling decided then and there not to retire, but to investigate vitamin therapy. Now that was time well spent!

Passwater: Another clinician who was both a good friend of Dr. Hoffer and whose work has been largely ignored outside of orthomolecular medicine is Dr. Hugh D. Riordan. Many of our readers may be unfamiliar with Dr. Riordan's contributions. Please tell us about the relationship between Dr. Hoffer and Dr. Riordan and how our readers may obtain information about Dr. Riordan's discoveries.

Saul: Dr. Hoffer and Dr. Riordan were like-minded and true healers. Dr. Riordan was associate editor of the *Journal of Orthomolecular Medicine* when Dr. Hoffer was editor-in-chief, and I was assistant editor. Both men were brilliant, kind, and highly qualified physicians. Dr. Riordan and his team did very important pioneering work with intravenous vitamin C as early as the 1960s. Today, the Riordan Clinic in Wichita, KS, is probably the Western Hemisphere's leader in the field. In the Eastern Hemisphere, it would be Tokyo's Dr. Atsuo Yanagisawa and colleagues. Dr. Riordan also authored the three-part history *Medical Mavericks*. Hugh called me up just as he was finishing volume three. We had a delightful talk, and a few hours later, I got word that he had died suddenly. A real shock and a real loss to humanity.

Passwater: Just what is orthomolecular medicine?

Saul: Orthomolecular medicine is nutritional medicine. A simple internet search will bring up directories and doctors employing it. And, as Dr. Hoffer often said, if you cannot find such a physician, you need to learn for yourself. I am especially keen on this part, as I am not a physician. My website and my book *Doctor Yourself* are called that because we need to take responsibility for our own health. To do that we need education, not medication.

Passwater: You are the editor of the *Orthomolecular Medicine News Service*. What is the mission of the OMNS and how can readers find past releases?

Saul: Dr. Hoffer, Dr. Riordan, and I believed that people have had quite enough of biased, vitamin-bashing newspaper, magazine, and TV coverage. The OMNS is a wire-service style newsfeed direct to the public, as well as for those members of the press, radio, and TV news media that have the moxie to read it. Many of our readers are health practitioners. OMNS tells the truth that a biased, pharmaceutically-funded mass media routinely blacks out: vitamin therapy saves lives. The OMNS, begun in 2004, has a 64-member editorial board, and is peer reviewed.[18]

Conclusion

*Have no respect for the authority of others, for there
are always contrary authorities to be found.*
—BERTRAND RUSSELL

Niacin, and niacin deficiency, have always been with us. The niacin molecule itself was unknown before University of Wisconsin Professor Conrad Elvehjem identified it in 1937. One may marvel at how very far we have come in understanding it in fewer than ninety years. Yet, it is surprising how many physicians (not to mention pharmacists, nurses, dieticians, news reporters, and government policy makers) still insist that we don't need any more than 16 milligrams a day. (Okay, pregnant women are "allowed" a whopping 18 milligrams.) The RDA (Recommended Dietary Allowance) is one or even two orders of magnitude short of the optimal intake level for this very important nutrient. It is our contention that everyone needs at least several hundred milligrams of niacin every day. Diet cannot supply this amount. Most adults probably need closer to 1,600 to 1,800 milligrams per day to maintain good health, and require more for a therapeutic effect during illness. This is literally 100 times the RDA. Clearly, supplementation is essential.

Opposition to such dosage is strong. Hamstrung by an arbitrary but authoritative-sounding "Tolerable (or Safe) Upper Limit" of a ridiculous 35 milligrams per day, the vitamin-taking public has to overcome entrenched institutional bias. Long has it been said that "it's not what we don't know that harms us; it's what we do know that ain't so." Never have truer words been spoken.

Niacin dosage and niacin's utility are areas of medicine where we are far from agreement with authorities. This is odd, since high doses of niacin have been used to relieve arthritis since the 1930s. Dr. Hoffer and many medical colleagues used niacin to alleviate or even cure mental illness, including schizophrenia, confusion, and learning disorders, since the early 1950s. That high niacin doses are extremely effective in lowering cholesterol has been known nearly as long.

All this has led to something of a vitamin public relations problem. When vitamins are versatile, they are characterized as "faddish" and "cures in search of a disease." When pharmaceuticals are versatile, they are called "broad spectrum" and "wonder drugs." Such a double-standard needs to be exposed and opposed at every turn. We hope this book will help do so. It is high time.

Hyperactivity is not due to Ritalin deficiency, nor is high cholesterol due to a deficiency of statins, nor is arthritis caused by a deficiency of aspirin. But these seemingly unrelated health problems, and many others, may indeed be largely due to a common nutritional dependency. Treating accordingly was a good idea over half a century ago, and it is just as good an idea today.

The Introduction of Niacin as the First Successful Treatment for Cholesterol Control

BY WILLIAM B. PARSONS, JR., MD, FACP (1924–2010)

Reprinted with permission from the Journal of Orthomolecular Medicine[1]

My years of training in internal medicine were at the Mayo Clinic in Rochester, Minnesota. I was serving as first assistant on the Peripheral Vascular Service at St. Mary's Hospital for the summer quarter of 1955 when a series of incredible coincidences culminated in an event that changed my life. No one had any way of knowing at the time, but it also changed millions of lives around the world.

One morning, a knock interrupted our discussion in the conference room. Dr. Howard Rome, chief of the Section on Psychiatry at the Clinic, brought a surprising question: Would you be interested in hearing about a drug that reduces cholesterol levels? Skeptically (because there had been no successful drugs until then), we said that we would, of course, if there were such a drug. My mind quickly sorted through the short list of drugs that had been tried for this purpose. Thyroid had been tried but hadn't worked. Another agent that had also failed was a vegetable oil product, sitosterol, which one pharmaceutical company had marketed. I could think of no others.

The name of the drug surprised us, as Dr. Rome provided the few details he had. The preceding evening, he had had dinner with Dr. Abram Hoffer, a psychiatrist from Regina, Saskatchewan, who had been in Rochester to give a series of lectures on schizophrenia. For years, he told Dr. Rome, he had administered large doses of niacin (then often called nicotinic acid) to his schizophrenic patients, feeling that it had helped them. Learning of this, his former anatomy professor at University of Saskatchewan, Dr. Rudolf Altschul, had suggested that he measure cholesterol levels in patients receiving niacin. Altschul, who had done studies of atherosclerosis in cholesterol-fed rabbits, predicted that niacin would reduce cholesterol levels. When his prediction proved correct, the two teamed with laboratory director Dr. James Stephen to try the drug in other volunteers. Their brief observations showed that niacin did, in fact, reduce cholesterol levels in a short period of time.

EARLY NIACIN USE

Niacin was originally known as a member of the vitamin B complex, which prevents the vitamin deficiency disease pellagra in humans and black tongue in dogs. It was in all the pharmacology textbooks and well known to doctors. Niacin was notable mainly because its administration, usually in 50 milligrams to 100 milligrams doses, was rapidly followed by flushing of the skin (redness of the skin of the face and neck, sometimes the whole upper body), accompanied by a very warm feeling, often with itching. For this reason, in vitamin preparations the closely related compound niacinamide (nicotinamide) was used because it had the vitamin activity without the flush. At that time niacin had practically no use in medicine other than its vitamin activity.

Otolaryngologists sometimes recommended it for vertigo. Physicians sometimes hoped it might help patients who had experienced a thrombotic stroke. Mayo neurologists had studied this use, along with other agents alleged to dilate intracerebral blood vessels, but found that there was really no benefit. They acknowledged that the flush might make the family think that something was being done, although there was little that could be done for a stroke in those days. The fact that it was very safe seemed to justify its use, albeit as a placebo in those instances.

Niacin was made in 50 milligrams or 100 milligrams tablets. Our first thought was that the doses used by the Canadians, 1,000 milligrams three or four times a day, would cause greater, intolerable flushing. Dr. Rome hastened to assure us that, according to Dr. Hoffer, flushing usually subsided in about three to four days and was no worse than with small doses. The Canadians had also briefly tried giving niacinamide. Although it caused no flush, it had failed to reduce cholesterol levels. Dr. Rome really had no further details, just these few important facts Dr. Hoffer had shared with him. It was evident that the Canadian originators had not performed a systematic trial to begin developing a useful method of treatment. Their specialties—psychiatry, anatomy, laboratory science—were not conducive to a clinical trial. On rounds that morning, I told Dr. Allen that although it sounded like a strange idea, we could easily test the claim that large doses of niacin could reduce cholesterol. In those days we did not have today's vascular surgery, which can sometimes bypass occluded leg arteries. Therefore, we kept numerous patients in the hospital for weeks while we did everything medically possible to increase circulation, trying to heal ulcers on feet or legs. If our efforts failed and the leg became gangrenous, amputation was usually necessary, frequently above the knee. With so much at stake we often lavished weeks of hospital care, attempting to save a limb. One must remember that hospital charges at that time were reasonable.

NIACIN/CHOLESTEROL TRIALS

We customarily measured cholesterol and other blood lipids as part of our admission workup, even though we had no good method for improving abnormal lipids beyond altering diet. Then, as now, diet was a weak and often ineffective way to reduce elevated cholesterol levels. I told Dr. Allen that I could recheck lipids on five or six patients with hypercholesteremia, tell them about the new treatment, and see whether we could verify the Canadian observations. Dr. Allen gave his blessing and promptly forgot about it. I have always been grateful for his approval.

I found five patients on the service with high cholesterol levels and a vascular status that would keep them hospitalized for several weeks. That afternoon, at the bedside of each patient, I recited the fragmentary word-of-mouth report we had received and invited them to take part in a brief trial of a well-known drug, widely regarded as safe, to see whether it really did reduce cholesterol. I described the flush and assured them it would subside in a few days if our informant had been correct.

The patients agreed and began taking tablets (ten 100 milligrams tablets with each meal), after another baseline blood test. The flush lessened and disappeared in the first week, as predicted. So far, so good. After one week I repeated the lipid studies and could not believe the striking reductions in cholesterol, triglycerides, and total lipids. In disbelief, I waited for the second week's results (as good or better) before showing the results to the others on the service. The initial hospital trial continued for four weeks, by which time it was apparent that a longer, carefully planned study was the next step.

The Mayo Clinic has a section just for care of Rochester residents. One of the young consultants in that section was my close friend, Dr. Richard Achor. He and Dr. Kenneth Berge (whom I hadn't met until then because he joined the staff during my two-year absence) had a list of patients with hypercholesteremia, which they gave me to recruit volunteers. By telephone, I obtained eighteen participants for at least twelve weeks of study, using niacin in 1,000 milligrams doses with meals and measuring cholesterol weekly.

Laboratory scientist Dr. Bernard McKenzie brought a unique contribution to the study. His laboratory had been separating cholesterol fractions by electrophoresis, giving us a means of determining beta-lipoprotein cholesterol (now LDL cholesterol) and alpha1-lipoprotein cholesterol (now HDL cholesterol). Preliminary studies had shown that a high ratio of beta to alpha1 cholesterol often led to premature heart attacks. We incorporated his testing into our study.

The results were just as impressive as in the preliminary hospital observations. There were marked cholesterol reductions in the first week in many, if not most, participants. Not only that, but the cholesterol fraction was the site of major reduction, accompanied by an increase in the fraction.

My Mayo colleagues encouraged me to report this promising new treatment before leaving Rochester in April 1956 to practice with a Madison, Wisconsin, clinic. The paper I presented at a staff meeting was published in June in the *Proceedings of the Staff Meetings of the Mayo Clinic*,[2] the prestigious journal with worldwide circulation which since then has shortened its name to *Mayo Staff Proceedings*.

At the time I realized that I was reporting the first successful cholesterol-lowering drug in history. My enthusiasm was tempered by the knowledge that it would have to be studied in many persons for years just to show that it remained effective, that it was safe in prolonged use, and that reducing cholesterol would, as we hoped, reduce atherosclerosis, and prevent its disastrous complications.

The Mayo publication was important because it reported to its wide circulation the first systematic study, including the favorable results in the cholesterol fractions. Altschul, Hoffer, and Stephen had earlier published a letter to the editor of the *Archives of Biochemistry and Biophysics*[3] which might have been overlooked by clinical investigators and never implemented.

I first presented the updated Mayo report at the November 1956 meeting of the American Society for the Study of Arteriosclerosis, its first airing at a national meeting. (The ASSA later became the Council on Arteriosclerosis of the American Heart Association.) I first met Dr. Rudolf Altschul at the November 1957 meeting, saw him at many subsequent ASSA meetings he attended, and contributed a chapter to his book[4] on what was then known about niacin, which he was editing when he died in 1963. I also recall his talk at the 1957 or 1958 meeting about his rabbit work, in which he showed that niacin strikingly reduced the foam cell content of atherosclerotic plaques. This is now especially significant in view of emphasis in recent years on rupture-prone plaques as a cause of sudden arterial occlusion, even when the narrowing is no more than 50 percent of the arterial diameter.

I had never met Abram Hoffer when, in 1990, we had a momentous telephone conversation, which convinced me more than ever about my meant-to-be hypothesis. The story of how niacin came to be tested in hypercholesteremia was stranger than I had expected. In 1952 Hoffer had experienced some bleeding from the gums, for which he had taken vitamin C without benefit. He had already been using niacin for schizophrenic patients and decided to take 3 grams daily to see how the flush felt. His gums improved. He reasoned that niacin had promoted rapid healing in gums which had been affected by chronic malocclusion and, with age, had not been healing as well as in earlier years.

Dr. Hoffer's use of niacin in schizophrenia began in 1952, at which time he was using 3 to 6 grams per day, as well as niacinamide. He called his work the first double-blind psychiatric study ever performed. In the mid-1950s he lived and practiced in Regina. Dr. Altschul, who had been Hoffer's professor of anatomy in medical school at Saskatoon, had been doing oxidation experiments, exposing rabbits to ultraviolet light and to increased concentrations of oxygen in inspired air to see whether these measures would somehow alter cholesterol deposition in arteries.

On one occasion, Professor Altschul sought to arrange a trial in humans for his idea that exposure to ultraviolet light might reduce cholesterol levels. He contacted his former student, Abram Hoffer, who was Director of Research for the province, and asked for his help in setting up such a study at Saskatchewan Hospital, a 1,600-bed mental hospital in Wayburn. They planned a joint visit to the hospital for this purpose. Dr. Altschul took a train to Regina, and together they drove to Wayburn, seventy-one miles away.

During the drive they talked about their individual interests. Altschul expressed his opinion that atherosclerotic plaques developed because of injury to the intima. He went on to speculate that the intima was not healing fast enough. Hoffer suggested a trial of niacin, based on his personal experience with bleeding gums.

In our telephone conversation, Hoffer told me that when he made his suggestion, Dr. Altschul didn't know what niacin was! Having received large quantities of niacin and niacinamide for his work, Hoffer gave a pound of niacin powder (about 450 grams) to his former anatomy professor, who then fed it to rabbits whose blood cholesterol had been elevated to very high levels by dietary maneuvers well-known to animal researchers. How he knew how much niacin to use is among the bits of information still lacking, but apparently niacin reduced the blood cholesterol levels within days. Hoffer reported that Altschul then phoned him, excitedly shouting, "It works! It works!"

Until that September 1990 conversation, I had never known who Jim Stephen was. Hoffer explained that he was the chief pathologist and laboratory director at the hospital in Regina where Hoffer practiced.

With his permission, in 1954 Hoffer did a two-day study, giving niacin to about sixty patients who demonstrated a reduction in their cholesterol levels. Altschul, Hoffer, and Stephen then wrote their letter to the editor of *Archives of Biochemistry and Biophysics*.[5]

In our phone conversation, I picked up the story and told Hoffer of the chain of events which had brought his information to me and resulted in my decision to do further studies. He had never before heard the details. He had many complimentary comments about my research in the following years, correctly recognizing that it had provided the impetus that resulted in niacin's becoming a major cholesterol-control agent. We closed our telephone conversation with the mutual wish that we might someday get together to discuss our shared interests face-to-face.

In the fall of 1997, a medical association in Victoria to which Dr. Hoffer belongs invited me to speak to them and the public about my work with niacin and my book, *Cholesterol Control Without Diet! The Niacin Solution*.[6] This was the pilgrimage I had always envisioned to meet Dr. Hoffer. We used it for a dual purpose, which included beginning the promotion for the book. I finally met Abram Hoffer in person for the first time in the driveway of the Empress Hotel in Victoria, on November 11, 1998, more than forty-three years after my first use of niacin for hypercholesteremia. It was his eightieth birthday.

We reviewed the circumstances that had brought us together and all that niacin had come to mean to doctors and their patients around the world. We hoped that my book would teach patients the importance of niacin's distinctive advantages, not shared by any other cholesterol-control drugs, and also show doctors how to become proficient at using niacin.

I have always been happy to share with the Canadian originators whatever credit there may be for pioneering the use of niacin for cholesterol control and for its eventual reduction of heart attacks (24 percent), strokes (26 percent), cardiovascular surgery (46 percent), and deaths (11 percent, adding a mean of 1.63 years of life to men 30 to 65 years old with one or more preceding heart attacks).[7] Without their vision and Hoffer's taking their observations to the Mayo Clinic, I would not have been able to perform the first systematic study and follow it with further research in Madison, leading to the Coronary Drug Project's demonstration of niacin's preventive effects in cardiovascular disease.[8] Dr. Hoffer has correctly said that while pioneers in many fields argue about precedence, we are friends who readily acknowledge each other's roles in starting niacin research. Clearly, it was meant to be.

APPENDIX 2

The Historical Significance of 1940s Mandatory Niacin Enrichment: Niacin Rescues Cannibalistic Hamsters

BY W. TODD PENBERTHY, PHD

In an interesting recent research study, Tissier and colleagues at the Université de Strasbourg, France, identified wild hamsters that were eating primarily corn monoculture diets and exhibiting siblicide and maternal infanticide. Cannibalism was one of the theories for the decline of their population. Mother hamsters fed exclusively corn would take their pups, place them together with the stashes of corn they had stored in the cage, and start eating their young. Siblicide was also observed. Only 5 percent of the offspring of the females fed corn survived. The rest were eaten. The other group was fed a varied diet, and 80 percent of the babies survived. However, supplementation of corn diets with **just vitamin B$_3$ (niacin)** prevented the aggressive cannibalistic behavior.[1]

NIACIN FORTIFICATION

This recently published study raises the question of the historical significance of the timing of mandatory niacin fortification starting in 1942.[1,2] Mandatory fortification of the vitamin niacin in the United States was initiated at the precise moment when our society became aware of the need to rebuild. The historical tide began to change from "Let's see how many people we can kill with all these new ways to kill each other" to "I'm sorry, let's rebuild your country" and ultimately to "I want that Westy/Volkswagen camper!" today. *Was niacin fortification integral to rescuing an otherwise excessively violent world in the 1940s?*

The niacin-deficiency disease pellagra became more common after roller mills were used on an industrial scale in the United States starting in the 1880s. Although white flour had been available during the previous century, it was expensive and only available for the wealthy. Roller-milled wheat and corn were now inexpensive, and had a long shelf life. But this industrially processed corn was not correctly treated with alkali as practiced by the ancient Maya and Aztec people. Soon thereafter the masses enjoyed white flour and the new form of processed grits, but then came an epidemic of pellagra! Before the discovery of niacin, over 100,000 people died in the southern United States alone due to pellagra epidemics. Shortly after the discovery of niacin, scientists and medical professionals including Dr. Goldberger and Dr. Abram Hoffer helped to establish mandatory fortification in the 1940s.[3]

Modern hominy is created by soaking corn in alkali, as the ancients did in a process called nixtamalization. This allows niacin and tryptophan, its precursor, to be available for absorption in the gut. Although hominy grits are missing the bran and germ of the kernel that contain much of its vitamin content, they generally supply enough niacin to prevent pellagra in those who eat mainly corn.

Pellagra symptoms are conveniently remembered by the "4 D's": diarrhea, dementia, dermatitis, and death. Changes in behavior are difficult to measure, but mortality statistics for the United States suggest that pellagra was perhaps the most severe nutritional deficiency disease ever recorded in United States history.[2] With the fortification of niacin in white flour and bread, mortality rates were decreased by orders of magnitude in some states within a couple of years! *This underscores the critical sensitivity of all animals including humans to niacin deficiency.*

"Improperly cooked maize-based diets have been associated with higher rates of homicide, suicide, and cannibalism in humans," according to Gerard Baumgart, a scientist and expert on European hamsters. Epidemiological studies have confirmed this.[4]

PELLAGRA OR SCHIZOPHRENIA?

Nearly a decade after the initiation of niacin fortification in the 1940s, Dr. Hoffer noticed similarities between pellagra and the schizophrenic patients he was treating, so he considered that perhaps these individuals needed higher amounts of niacin. In the 1950s and later, Hoffer treated over ten thousand schizophrenics with high doses of niacin. He showed that many schizophrenics can be successfully treated with niacin administered in high doses divided throughout the day. In Hoffer's last book, *Psychiatry Yesterday and Today*, he said. "Schizophrenia is not a multivitamin deficiency disease. It is in fact the disease pellagra; a vitamin B_3-*dependency* disease. It will not be treated successfully no matter how many dozens of vitamin pills are given if these patients are not given the correct doses of this vitamin."[5] Hoffer and other practicing physicians have observed that high doses of niacin can work for the treatment of acute schizophrenia, but it is not as effective for longstanding cases.

Before niacin was discovered, there was a focus on corn and grits in particular because of their high correlative association with pellagra.[6,7] At the end of the 19th century, this intense focus developed into medical conferences organized to discover the cause of pellagra.

BUT CANNIBALISM?

On first thought, it seems incredible that a single vitamin can prevent a behavior as complex as cannibalism. How could niacin do this and exert so many other benefits? Niacin is converted to NAD (nicotinamide adenine dinucleotide) in the liver. NAD is involved in more reactions than any other vitamin-derived cofactor; over 400 different reactions (see database: https://www.cmescribe.com/vitamin-dependent-gene-databases/). NAD is required for basic bioenergetics (glycolysis and beta oxidation) and in P450 reactions like the phase I detoxification enzymes. Niacin is depleted by a wide variety of stresses (hyperglycemia, aerobic, ionizing radiation), pollutants, and more. Most practically, people with genetic polymorphisms in the DNA encoding for the NAD binding domain that result in reduced binding affinity for any of these greater than 400 different reactions can require higher amounts of niacin to prevent pathologies.[8] These people are niacin-dependent. Dr. Abram Hoffer observed this condition in many schizophrenic patients.

History and this study of hamsters suggest that aggressive, unempathetic behavior may be an indication for a need for higher levels of niacin in the diet that could be met by high-dose niacin therapy. With so many psychologically disturbed acts of violence occurring after years of trying to save individuals with pharmaceuticals, it may seem ironic that high doses of niacin have not been generally employed to help these individuals to sense the beauty of life more clearly.

HOW NIACIN IS USED AS THERAPY

Dr. Abram Hoffer's approach to niacin therapy involves administration of 1 gram (1,000 milligrams) taken three times a day. This high-dose niacin therapy has an exceptional safety profile. It has been used for over 60 years and is lacking serious adverse events, except for when using the slow-release types, which can cause hepatic toxicity.[9] The common type of plain niacin, inexpensive and available over the counter, is not slow-release. It is considered "immediate release." Therapy with plain niacin (also known as nicotinic acid) is far less expensive than pharmaceutical treatment.

When taking plain niacin for the first time, it is important to **start at low doses** because it gives a "niacin flush" on the skin. This is a vitamin that one will notice for sure. So, get to know the flush by first taking 100 milligrams of niacin (nicotinic acid form) and then gradually trying higher amounts up to 1,000 milligrams at a time until you notice the flush. A little flush is ideal for health. It raises HDL levels more than any pharmaceutical (including statins), lowers triglycerides, lowers VLDL, and has a better safety profile than statins.

NIACIN AND EYESIGHT

Cystoid macular edema has been observed, but only in rare instances, when daily niacin doses are over 3 grams (3,000 milligrams). If during high-dose niacin therapy you experience blurred vision, reduce or stop taking the niacin and see your medical doctor.

In a recent study, niacin (in the form of niacinamide) was shown to be effective in reducing (by more than 90 percent) the development of glaucoma in a strain of glaucoma-prone mice.[10] Glaucoma is a leading cause of blindness worldwide. It is thought to be caused by a sequence of pathological events including an increase in pressure inside the eye, which reduces the blood flow into the eye and damages the eye's energy metabolism. When compounded with improperly functioning mitochondria in retinal neurons the result is cell death and blindness.[11] A very high dose of niacinamide was therapeutic, especially in aged mice, and helped damaged mitochondria to support normal metabolism, allowing retinal neurons to survive.[10]

The concept of orthomolecular medicine was born and pioneered by Dr. Linus Pauling in the 1960s with the inspiration of Dr. Abram Hoffer. Under pathological conditions, our body naturally needs much more than average amounts of certain vital nutrients due to stress-mediated vitamin/mineral depletions. Historically, this first involved administration of high doses of the essential vitamins B_3 and C for the treatment of mental health disorders and cancer, respectively, but the full list of responsive indications is always expanding and depends on the individual's symptoms. As compared to pharmaceuticals, vitamins are exceptionally safe and have withstood the test of time.[12]

CONCLUSION

Some niacin researchers believe that many people with mental illness might be saved if more physicians can end their subscription to the mantra "let's develop foreign chemicals and drugs" as medicine and instead consider "maybe some people have subtle genetic differences that make them require higher amounts of niacin." This theory has already been proven for several niacin vitamin-responsive genetic conditions.[8,10]

APPENDIX 3

An Interview with
Abram Hoffer, MD, PhD

INTERVIEWED BY ANDREW W. SAUL IN 2008

Some years ago, as I sat at lunch with Dr. Abram Hoffer, I took some vitamin pills. Dr. Hoffer leaned toward me and said, "You know, you're going to live a lot longer if you take those."

As I looked at him, he added, "I guarantee it. If you don't, come back and tell me."

So says the founding father of orthomolecular medicine.

It was nearly sixty years ago when Abram Hoffer and his colleagues began curing schizophrenia with niacin. While some physicians are still waiting, those who have used niacin with patients and families know the immense practical value of what Dr. Hoffer discovered. Abram Hoffer's life has not merely changed the face of psychiatry; he has changed the course of medicine for all time. His thirty books, 600 scientific papers, and thousands of cured patients have yet to convince orthodox medicine. Dr. Hoffer has said that it takes about two generations before a truly new medical idea is accepted. Perhaps in the case of megavitamin therapy, maybe it is three generations. Great ideas in medicine, or anywhere else, are never self-evident. At least not until a brilliant mind like Dr. Hoffer's sees more than others have seen, and has the courage to speak out in the teeth of some often surprisingly bitter professional adversity. As a college lecturer, I learned some years ago that if you want to clear the department's lunchroom in a hurry, just say something positive about megavitamin therapy.

The day after I first met Dr. Hoffer, I sat in as he taped a television production about his work. He did the entire 43-minute video in one take. Over the years, I was honored to ultimately write four books with Abram, and work with him as Assistant Editor for the *Journal of Orthomolecular Medicine.*

Abram taught me much, as he taught so many. Among the lessons I had was this: a speaker at a medical conference made two factual errors about niacin. I was sitting next to Abram, and he was, to all appearances, dozing off. He was not. He gave me a nod, and during the question session, got up to take the microphone. He complimented the speaker on his presentation, mentioned a few additional things about niacin, made another supportive remark, and sat down. The speaker was delighted. And, the speaker never knew he had just been contradicted and corrected. This was Abram Hoffer.

At 91 years of age, Dr. Hoffer was widely and justly regarded as a living legacy. As I had conducted a series of interviews with some of the key figures in nutritional medicine for DoctorYourself.com, it seemed high time to interview him. Abram being in British Columbia and I in New York, we settled on email for our conversations. He was a prompt responder and enthusiastic. Hardly a day went by without an email from Abram, and typically there were several. They were both wide-ranging and frequent, answering my questions and then some.

My final email from Abram was a copy of his announcing to his colleagues the publication of one of our collaborative books, *The Vitamin Cure for Alcoholism.* It is based on Abram's experiences with one of his patients: Bill W., cofounder of Alcoholics Anonymous. We will begin there.

***

Andrew W. Saul: Dr. Hoffer, you cured AA founder Bill W. of his depression using niacin.

Dr. Abram Hoffer: His depression, yes, but I did not cure his alcoholism. He never did consider himself cured. He organized AA, and was able to establish fellowships that helped millions stay sober. However, it was the niacin that made him comfortable in his sobriety. It takes the entire nutritional approach, plus AA.

Saul: Tell us more about Bill W.

Hoffer: From the day he was freed of lifelong tension and insomnia by taking 3,000 milligrams of niacin daily, Bill Wilson became a powerful runner with us. Bill helped me organize the first Schizophrenics Anonymous group in Saskatoon, which was very successful. Bill introduced the orthomolecular concepts to a large number of AA members, especially in the United States. AA International did not approve of this. Bill made an immense contribution to orthomolecular medicine because he publicized the term "B₃" to replace the chemical names niacinamide or nicotinic acid. Had Bill W. lived another ten years, orthomolecular medicine would have been much further advanced than it is today.

Saul: And how do things stand today?

Hoffer: I have treated 5,000 schizophrenic patients with niacin. The first was a 12-year-old boy in 1960. To get the boy to take it, his father crushed the niacin tablet and spread it into a jam sandwich. That boy is now a research psychiatrist. The treatment that worked in 1960 is still working today. That treatment is called orthomolecular medicine. Orthomolecular medicine restores natural metabolism with nutrients, such as vitamins and minerals, in optimum quantities. This means much more than the RDA or DRI. To overturn decades of error on the part of governments and the professions will take a good deal of effort and patience. Linus Pauling often spoke vigorously against the RDA in general and was ignored. These old, erroneous standards are part of the vitamins-as-prevention paradigm and will not yield until this old and stale paradigm is fully replaced by the vitamins-as-treatment paradigm. Pauling took 18,000 milligrams of ascorbic acid daily, which was 300 times the RDA. He loved to tell his audiences why he took so much.

Saul: That's what I personally take. When people ask why, I tell them that Dr. Pauling did, and he had two more Nobels than I have. Dr. Hoffer, where has high-dose nutritional therapy been most successful?

Hoffer: It has been most successful for treating the walking wounded, that is, for those with arthritis, neurological conditions, and virtually all the psychiatric diseases. Orthomolecular medicine can be utilized within the whole field of medicine, even for patients whose primary treatment is surgery.

Saul: When were you convinced that orthomolecular medicine was the way to go?

Hoffer: By 1960 I was convinced. My conviction was reinforced by the hostility generated by the profession. I assumed that this hostile reaction was stimulated by our success. The same thing happened to the Shute brothers with vitamin E. New research exposes the weakness of current medical doctrine. Such a challenge is often answered only by hostility, as there is no evidence to otherwise disprove it.

Saul: Please tell the story of how Linus Pauling first learned of nutritional medicine.

Hoffer: Linus became aware of our work from two families I treated who got well and stayed well. By then my book, co-written with Dr. Humphry Osmond, called *How to Live with Schizophrenia* had been published, and one night Linus saw it on a friend's coffee table. He stayed up all night reading it. That book convinced him that here was some merit to the idea of vitamin therapy. Later he found no contrary evidence. Linus had the desirable personality characteristic that he tended to believe people if there was no logical reason for them to lie to him. For that reason, he did not accept the stories put out by the drug companies and the FDA. Pauling knew for whom they were working, and it was not for you or me.

Saul: What about niacin and cholesterol?

Hoffer: My colleagues and I demonstrated that niacin lowered total cholesterol in a 1954 study, and we should have been given an award. But, of course, niacin is not a drug and cannot be patented, and therefore our discovery remains mainly a major irritant to the drug companies who have not been able to discover anything as safe and as effective. It is remarkable that niacin is the best for blood lipid levels and also for the psychoses. Nature is not dumb.

Saul: What are the alleged "dangers" of niacin therapy?

Hoffer: Niacin is probably not quite as safe as water, but pretty close to it. Patients ask me, "How dangerous is niacin therapy?" I answer them, "You are going to live a lot longer. Is that a problem for you?"

Saul: Data compiled by the American Association of Poison Control Centers (AAPCC) indicates that, over the past 25 years, there have been a total of one or two deaths attributed to niacin. When I looked for evidence to substantiate even this very low number of alleged fatalities, it was absent or assumed.

Hoffer: There have been no deaths ever from niacin. The LD 50 (the dosage that would kill half of those taking it) for dogs is 6,000 milligrams per kilogram body weight. That is equivalent to half a pound of niacin per day for a human. No human takes 225,000 milligrams of niacin a day. They would be nauseous long before reaching a harmful dose. The top niacin dose ever was a 16-year-old schizophrenic girl who took 120 tablets (500 milligrams each) in one day. That is 60,000 milligrams of niacin. The "voices" she had been hearing were gone immediately. She then took 3,000 milligrams a day to maintain wellness.

Saul: If I do not press this point, a reader will: maintained high doses of niacin may raise liver function tests, and this is used as evidence of harm.

Hoffer: Niacin is not liver toxic. Niacin therapy increases liver function tests. But this elevation means that the liver is active. It does not indicate an underlying liver pathology. Dr. Bill Parsons discussed this extremely well in his book on niacin and cholesterol.[1] I personally have been on 1,500 to 6,000 milligrams daily since 1955. The biggest danger of taking niacin is that you live longer. One of my patients is 112. She does cross-country skiing and has been on niacin for 42 years. The fear doctors have of niacin is not based on data or facts and, like any myth, is very had to eradicate. So many patients are on niacin that by chance some will also have liver damage from other conditions such as alcoholism, hepatitis, and so on. Niacin does not make it any better nor worse.

Saul: What are the differences among the various forms of niacin?

Hoffer: Niacin and niacinamide are equally effective for schizophrenia, but higher doses of niacin can be tolerated without nausea. Inositol hexaniacinate (a no-flush form of niacin) works, too, but not quite as well. Only niacin or inositol hexaniacinate can lower cholesterol; niacinamide does not.

Saul: You have long been interested in nutrition as adjunctive therapy for cancer.

Hoffer: I have treated over 1,600 cancer patients, most of whom were given 12,000 milligrams per day or more of ascorbic acid, in combination with other nutrients. The results have been good and at least 40 percent of the 1,600 reached ten-year cure rates. A small number of patients who were on every attending physician's terminal and untreatable list were cured. Linus Pauling and I had examined the follow-up data and found that the significant prolongation of these patients' lives favors the use of the vitamins. We published this in our book *Healing Cancer: Complementary Vitamin and Drug Treatments.*[2]

Saul: Another of your close colleagues was Dr. Hugh Riordan (1932 to 2005), also an advocate of high-dose vitamin C therapy for cancer.

Hoffer: Hugh was such a great healer, a marvelous physician, afraid of no one and willing to do what had to be done to help his patients get well. I am so sorry he went too soon. He needed another five years at least so that he could enjoy the fruits of his labors. I do hope that Hugh did have the final vision, the eventual result of the work that he did. I am reminded of Moses who angered God because he struck the stone instead of pointing his staff at it in order to bring water for the complaining Israelites. God said, "You will never see the Promised Land." But at the end God relented and he showed Moses in a far vision the Promised Land. This is a remarkable little tale and

I have learned a lot from it. I learned to be very patient. The lesson is that no one should ever expect to get into the Promised Land because it will always recede from you. The noble objective is to strive to reach it knowing full well that it cannot be done.

Saul: I had just spoken with Hugh the very morning of the day he died.

Hoffer: The last time I felt so bereft and hopeless was when my wife Rose died three and a half years previously. Death is so sudden and so unexpected, especially to be struck down when one is so close to achieving so many great things. I do believe that the good Hugh did will live forever.

Saul: There seems to be a lot of bad press about vitamins, claiming evidence that they are not effective against disease.

Hoffer: The modern church of medicine does not relish alerting the press when the news is good about vitamins. There is no money in it and potentially a loss if vitamins displace drugs, as they should. I sometimes harbor a silent wish for all our critics: that is that they should never under any circumstances ever take any supplemental nutrients, and must be restricted to only eating modern high-tech food. Can you think of a more severe punishment?

Saul: Yet it turns out that most of the negative reports are based on research that used ineffectively low doses of vitamins.

Hoffer: I agree. I could also spend millions to prove that the small amounts of these nutrients will not prevent car accidents. Who is funding all these silly studies? No orthomolecular physician ever claimed that giving 200 international units of vitamin E and 500 milligrams of C cured anything. Perhaps you should write a paper with tongue in cheek in which you announce, ANTIBIOTICS DO NOT CURE INFECTION. Then, report somewhere hidden in the paper that you only gave them 200 or even 20,000 international units of a drug that requires doses of one million or more. Such reporting is a superb example of the cynical, expensive, and sleazy research so loved by Big Pharma. This is because it delays the real introduction of good medicine, in the same way that tobacco companies denied smoking causes cancer and we supposedly needed more and more and more research to prove anything. All this allows the companies millions to their coffers. Their defense is delay, delay, and delay. The only objective of Big Pharma is to make money, lots and lots of it. How dare we try to prevent them from doing so.

Saul: Vitamins have also been attacked with allegations that they are somehow actually dangerous.

Hoffer: I am really impressed with the concern some scientists share over those "dangerous" vitamins. I wish they were as worried over those dangerous poisons called drugs. Each bottle of pills should have a poison label with skull and bones, and the word "poison" in large letters.

Saul: It seems that lately, while advised to take more vitamin D, the public has been specifically warned off of vitamins E and C.

Hoffer: I am always amazed at the chicanery and slipperiness of vitamin critics. Perhaps they realize they are beginning to lose the public and they are flailing out in all directions. Almost all of my patients, whenever they read one of these screeds, laugh at it because they know firsthand how wrong it is. Half the population of Canada and the United States is taking vitamins. And, if it will help dispel the nonsense about any supposed "dangers" of vitamin E, here is the program I personally follow. I started years ago. But I also take several other antioxidants. A combination is better than any one alone. Currently I daily take 1,200 international units of vitamin E as succinate, the water-soluble form. For my patients I have gone as high as 4,000 international units as a treatment for Huntington disease and it has been very helpful. I cannot recall any adverse reactions even though thousands of my patients are also taking vitamin E. I do take the B vitamins, vitamin C of course, vitamin A, vitamin D, and other nutrient factors. I think this has been helpful in keeping me active at my present age.

Saul: How do we best tailor nutrient doses for our own unique needs?

Hoffer: Each person must take an individualized program which they can discover if they are lucky to have a competent orthomolecular doctor. If they do not, they can read the literature and work out for themselves what is best for them. I believe the public is hungry for information. As more and more drugs drop by the wayside, the professions are going to become more and more dependent on safe ways of helping people, and using drugs is not the way to do that. Using nutrients is.

Saul: When does orthomolecular medicine not work?

Hoffer: It usually does work. For schizophrenics, the natural recovery rate is 50 percent. With orthomolecular medicine, the recovery rate is 90 percent. With drugs, it is 10 percent. If you use just drugs, you won't get well. This is because mental illness is usually biochemical illness. Mental illness is a disorder of brain dysfunction. Schizophrenia is vitamin B_3 (niacin) dependency. Not a deficiency; a dependency. If schizophrenia strikes someone at age 25, he's finished. That is, if he's only given drugs. Patients are given drugs and released. The new mental hospital today is the streets.

Saul: You have been a sharp critic of Evidence Based Medicine.

Hoffer: One would be very polite to even describe EBM as pseudoscientific. The word "science" cannot be used anywhere close to what is happening with EBM. It has become the main weapon to prevent innovation. It must be sent back to its archaic roots. Instead, we once more have to learn to think rather than calculate.

Saul: And double-blind, placebo-controlled studies?

Hoffer: Double blinds are for the birds. I have been opposed to double-blinds for decades, even though my colleagues and I were the first psychiatrists to do them, starting in 1952. I consider them a license to kill. They are a dangerous fashion. There is no evidence that anecdotal information is any less accurate than clinical information. Devotees see everything filtered through their beliefs. If we abolish anecdotes, guess what will happen to medicine? It will die from sheer boredom.

Saul: You have actually described this as a paradigm war.[3]

Hoffer: Yes, and we are winning the paradigm war. Clinical research is continually a battle, pro and con. The reason is that probability theory is of no value whatever when dealing with people. This was pointed out very clearly by Lancelot Hogben over 50 years ago.[4] Clinical tests were developed for plants and for animals and the various factors were much more readily controlled.

Saul: Much medical knowledge has come from physician reports, which are neither double-blind nor placebo controlled. They are the valuable experiences of qualified observers. They are valid: just ask the patients that got better. Yet doctors' reports, as well as those of their patients, are typically marginalized as mere "anecdotes."

Hoffer: Where are the good old days, when honest physicians honestly reported what they saw in language that any doctor could understand?

Saul: What is the primary problem with modern medical research?

Hoffer: The problem is a monstrous cancer affecting all of us and it is called Big Pharma. It needs a combination of surgery, radiation, and chemotherapy. The medical profession has been reduced to the state of well-paid salaries for the drug companies and it is we who pay the bills. For example, Vioxx was promoted by one of the largest of advertising budgets and had characteristically high kill rates. Money, like water, will leak into every possible crevasse. We are literally inundated with this poisonous water coming from this industry. For too long has Big Pharma ruled the roost.

Saul: You are still a fighter, at nearly 92 years of age.

Hoffer: We have to continue our way without regard to the opposition. If not, we will soon be working for them.

Saul: Tell us about your roots.

Hoffer: I was born on a farm in southern Saskatchewan in 1917 in our first wooden house. My three older siblings were born in a sod shack. Public and high school education was completed in single room schools. I had little to do with selecting my parents, selecting Canada, being raised on a farm, learning how to live with yourself, and having to work hard physically. I was educated by and during the Great Depression. The Depression was so enormous that any recent so-called recession is laughable. I remember when the president of the University of Saskatchewan in 1938 circulated a memo to staff and students that they must use toilet paper sparingly. Some tried to split the rolls. That was a real depression.

Saul: Where does your drive today come from?

Hoffer: I have a secret which I cannot patent. I married Rose, had three marvelous children, made nutrition my career choice, and took niacin for the past fifty years.

My parents provided me with the love and security and the same type of toughness they had shown in coming to the Saskatchewan prairies in 1904 and preparing me for this run. And my wife Rose, who helped push me into medicine, and supported me during every phase of our run. Her parents Fannie and Frank Miller helped us out so that I could become a medical student from 1945 to 1949. Rose believed in fate. She often told me that I would get the Nobel Prize. I did not bank on it, even though Linus Pauling had nominated me.

Saul: Many honors have come your way. You won the Dr. Rogers Prize, have been inducted into the Orthomolecular Medicine Hall of Fame, and have won the Linus Pauling Functional Medicine Award, among others. Still, there is one distinction that not everyone is already aware of: Abram Hoffer is an honorary Maori Chief.

Hoffer: Many years ago, Rose and I were on a speaking tour. In New Zealand we were staying in a hotel where there were many guests. One afternoon, I was asked whether I would like to be made an honorary Maori Chief. When I discovered that all I had to do was to be there, I agreed. Later in the afternoon, in the large lobby with Rose and a swarm of hotel guests, the doorman, who was a Maori, started the solemn ceremony. I stood in front of him very respectfully. He began to talk to someone, silently, using his facial expressions and contortions. I was then told that he was cleansing me of any evil spirits. He did not tell me that he had seen any, and I was too cowardly to ask, but this was an important precaution as no one with evil spirits was going to be given that honor. After he had cleansed me, he stepped forward and threw a rather large, and, I hope, dull sword which fell in front of me. He must have had ample practice with this. Then he came forward and did something with it and lo and behold, I was a Chief. I have always taken this honor seriously, especially since I am free of all evil. Someone should tell the American Psychiatric Association.

Saul: You and the APA have not exactly seen eye to eye. Why?

Hoffer: In 1950, I became Director of Psychiatric Research for Saskatchewan's Department of Public Health. I was a founder of the Canadian Schizophrenia Foundation, now the International Schizophrenia Foundation. My main objective was to research the cause of this disease and to find a better treatment. This is now called "orthomolecular medicine," after Dr. Pauling published his seminal paper in *Science* in 1968. After the American Psychiatric Association called my good friend and colleague Humphry Osmond and me before their Committee on Ethics because of what I had published, they effectively killed interest in the use of vitamins for treating mental illness. The APA bears major responsibility for preventing the introduction of a treatment which would have saved millions of patients from the ravages of chronic schizophrenia. Just as the APA was once captured by psychoanalysis, it is now captured by pharmaceuticals. They are biased. No amount of evidence will persuade someone who is not listening.

Saul: And for those who are, you and I have two new books in the works.

Hoffer: Our publisher is a great gambler. At age 91, I cannot guarantee that I will be around by the fall of 2010. But let's go ahead anyway, and you youngsters can complete it if I move on to other fields of existence.

***

Abram Hoffer died May 27, 2009. Thanks to Dr. Hoffer, medicine will never be the same. That may be the best of legacies.

APPENDIX 4

A Special Interview with Andrew W. Saul

INTERVIEWED BY DR. JOSEPH MERCOLA

Dr. Joseph Mercola: Welcome, everyone. This is Dr. Mercola, and today I'm here with Dr. Andrew Saul, who we've had the pleasure of interviewing before. He's had over 35 years of experience in natural health education and is currently serving as editor-in-chief of the *Orthomolecular Medicine News Service*. He's authored over 175 publications and 11 books. He's been named as one of the seven health pioneers by *Psychology Today* and is featured in the movie *Food Matters*, which I'm sure many of you have seen. Welcome and thank you for joining us today, Dr. Saul.

Dr. Andrew Saul: Well, thank you for having me on your program to talk to your readers and your listeners.

JM: Yes. Today we're going to be exploring the topic of niacin. It is an interesting one. Well, it's a natural product, obviously. It's a vitamin supplement. As a result, it's relatively inexpensive and has relatively few side effects—certainly no lethal ones, as far as we know, which cannot be said, of course, for many of the drug approaches to our health care problems.

But it's one also that I had avoided for a while (and I think we'll get into that in a bit), because I thought there might have been better approaches. But I re-explored this when you wrote your recent book on niacin, which is really an excellent read. So, that's why we're having you on the program today to expand on that in more detail.

If you can tell us how you first came to embrace natural health education, and maybe share a highlight or two with us about how your colleagues and peers have responded to your approach to good health. Then we'll start to explore the use of niacin.

AS: Well, I would say that I started to have an interest in natural healing when I was an undergraduate. The more I looked into the possibility of a medical education, the less it appealed to me. And I wasn't sure exactly why at the time. But I started reading books, especially those recommended by some faculty who perhaps sensed that I was not quite sure what I wanted to do when I grew up. I read a number of books. I suppose it's almost like the index of books you really aren't supposed to read.

What made these books and research papers interesting is that they were authored by physicians and researchers with really good credentials and a lot of experience. They were all about high-dose nutrition therapy—all about high-dose vitamin therapy.

Now, I didn't understand why a person would go to medical school, or go through a traditional PhD program in one of the hard sciences, and then make such a sharp right-turn approach to a totally different field. Why would doctors do that? Why would doctors who put in all that time in training to learn about drugs and surgery more or less drop that in favor of nutrition? The only answer I could come up with was, "It had to be effective. It must be working for them, their families, and their patients."

Having read enough and then crowning this with reading Linus Pauling and Dr. Abram Hoffer, there was just no turning back.

When I had children, it immediately verified the truth to what Dr. Pauling and Dr. Hoffer had said in their books, that high-dosed nutrient therapy is safe and effective. When you have children, safe comes first. When we look into vitamin safety, we find out according to the American Association of Poison Control Centers, who collects data every year from 59 poison control centers coast to coast, that there have been 11 alleged deaths in the last 28 years.

However, none of them have been documented. There hasn't been a death from a vitamin, including niacin, in 28 years.

Now, when I eventually became a college faculty member (I taught for the State University of New York and also at New York Chiropractic College), I noticed that you could get into trouble for talking about high-dose nutrition therapy. It seemed odd to me. I thought academic freedom, exploration of new ideas, and bringing up unusual research and discussing it was all part and parcel of that life. Well, you just see what happens when you bring this up at your next faculty meeting.

Did you know that in 1935, professor of biochemistry Claus Jungeblut at Columbia University showed that vitamin C destroys polioviruses? Then he went on to show in a series of experiments—all in the late 1930s—that vitamin C reduced the symptoms of polio, prevented polio, and even giardia. Now that is a statement.

This got me into trouble. You can understand that it's so serious that my students were talking to their instructors about the things I was saying, which got me in trouble with the colleges.

An example of this would be: There was a young woman—a junior—and she wanted to do a paper on vitamin C and polio. She thought it was pretty interesting. I said, "Well, it's extremely controversial. You're going to have to really back this up with references." And since I had access to about 25 references about Jungeblut and others using vitamin C against polio ... This includes Dr. Frederick Robert Klenner, who in the 1940s actually presented at an American Association meeting his cases on curing polio with vitamin C. They asked him a few questions for 10 minutes, and then he was ignored. So, this young woman decided to pursue these references, read these papers, and she thought it was worth putting together a paper.

A faculty person who had her in one of his classes got wind of this and said to me—not knowing that I was assisting and providing her at least with some jumping-off points, some references to read—that this was absurd that she was doing this paper and would only described the student as a dial tone. This is the kind of hostility that you run into. I've talked to services and hospitals, and everything's going fine when I talk about nutrition and vitamins in general. But as soon as I mention niacin for schizophrenia, vitamin C for hepatitis, or vitamin E for heart disease, all hell breaks loose. This is what happens.

Dr. Hoffer had this for 55 years in medical practice. Linus Pauling got this. Dr. Pauling is the only person I know that has ever received two unshared Nobel prizes. I think he's the only one who's ever had that in history. Now, Pauling took 18,000 milligrams of vitamin C a day. Abram Hoffer took 3,000 or 4,000 milligrams of niacin every day. It's good enough for them; it's good enough for me.

When I applied vitamin therapy to my children, it was so effective preventively and therapeutically that I raised my kids all the way into college, and they never had a single dose of any antibiotic. Not one, not ever.

JM: It's certainly a good and ideal testimony to the effectiveness of the approach. You had mentioned Dr. Hoffer. He's since passed away a few years ago or a while ago, and maybe you can go into detail with that, as to what exactly he's well-known for. But he's really a pioneer in orthomolecular medicine. His last book was actually co-written with you, and this is really what we're here to discuss today. It's the use of niacin.

Maybe you can discuss Dr. Hoffer a bit, and how you came to collaborate with him and write this book. Then we'll start discussing that topic.

AS: Dr. Hoffer is probably the world authority on therapeutic use of niacin. He started doing tests, studies, and research into niacin back in the early 1950s. And by 1954, Abram Hoffer had performed the first double-blind, placebo-controlled nutrition studies in the history of psychiatry.

Now, the early '50s were an odd time. Drugs were on the move; more were coming along. But they hadn't developed to the point where they are today, to put it mildly.

There were drugs for psychiatric issues, but they were not the treatment of choice. There were still a lot of other types of therapy going on then. Dr. Hoffer looked at psychiatric problems as a biochemic problem. He tried using niacin, simply because they didn't have anything that really worked for schizophrenia, and high doses of niacin worked.

Now Dr. Hoffer had a PhD in biochemistry, and he specialized in cereal biochemistry, which means the study of the vitamins and nutrients in grain. He was also a medical doctor.

He was also a board-certified psychiatrist, and he was also head of psychiatry for one of the provinces in Canada. This is a person with a lot under the hood. Dr. Hoffer reasoned that schizophrenia had symptoms that were very similar to those of pellagra. Pellagra is extreme or total niacin deficiency. Pellagrins also—in addition to skin problems and many other things—have mental illness symptoms.

When vitamin B$_3$ or niacin was first added as an enrichment or as a fortification to flour, about half of the people in mental institutions went home. This is not a well-known fact. They were there not because they were mentally ill—because of genetic, environment, or social reasons—but because they were malnourished. Dr. Hoffer thought that was pretty important. He wondered about the half that didn't go home. What about the people that had a little bit of niacin, but didn't get better?

Like Linus Pauling would decades later, Dr. Hoffer thought that maybe they just need more. So, he started giving what at the time were preposterously high doses of niacin: 3,000 milligrams a day. And he was curing schizophrenia in 80 percent of the cases. This is astonishing. The cure rate for schizophrenia with drug therapy is not particularly good. Dr. Hoffer saw again and again that niacin worked. Then he studied it, did the placebo-controlled, double-blind test, and started writing paper after paper on this.

At that point, the American Psychiatric Association effectively blacklisted him. One of its officers, said Dr. Hoffer, told him back in the '60s that he would never be published in that journal again. Dr. Hoffer then formed, founded, and produced the *Journal of Orthomolecular Medicine*.[1]

Since Dr. Hoffer founded the *Journal* in 1967, there have been a very large number of studies that have confirmed niacin not only for treating schizophrenia, but also attention deficit disorder, psychosis in general, anxiety, depression, and obsessive-compulsive disorder. In addition to this, Dr. Hoffer's work early in the '50s showed as a side effect (I think "side benefit" might be a better phrase) that niacin lowered cholesterol—that is, it lowered the bad cholesterol—and actually raised HDL and dramatically lowered triglycerides.

This work was picked up by Dr. William Parsons Jr. at the Mayo Clinic. Dr. Parsons, America's number one niacin researcher, wrote a book on this a few years ago. Parsons mentioned that Hoffer was right, and then expanded it into a protocol that many physicians use to this day.

Niacin is so good for lowering cholesterol and preventing heart disease that the *New York Times* quoted the president of the American College of Cardiology saying, "Niacin is really it. Nothing else comes close." We can thank Dr. Hoffer and Dr. Parsons for this.

You can see why I wrote the book. This information is important. The number one killer of Americans is still cardiovascular disease. And it isn't just the number one killer of men: it's the number one killer of women, too. Women tend to get it later, but they still die from it. So, if niacin were not even used with psychiatry at all, it would still be valuable—and is valuable—for cardiovascular disease. But it's also very valuable in treating schizophrenia and other severe mental disease.

As if that's not enough, another friend of Dr. Hoffer's was Bill W. Bill W. was that Bill W., as in, "Hi, my name's Bill, and I'm an alcoholic," the co-founder of Alcoholics Anonymous. Bill W. became a patient of Dr. Hoffer in the early 1960s. Bill W. had severe depression. Abram Hoffer treated him with 3,000 milligrams of niacin a day. Bill W.'s depression was gone in a week. Bill W. was impressed, so he told his friends—about 30 of them—that they should try this. And they did. Ten of Bill W.'s friends got over their depression within a week just like he did. Another 10 got over their depression, but it took them about a month. And then another 10—one-third—didn't seem to have any benefit.

Bill W. concluded that niacin helps about two-thirds of alcoholics using it and wrote two papers, which he circulated on his own, at his own expense, to physicians and the membership of AA. In addition to this, another friend of Abram Hoffer's was William Kaufman. Dr. William Kaufman, back in the very late 1930s, was using niacin in a no-flush form, niacinamide, to treat common arthritis. Dr. Kaufman found that 250 milligrams of niacinamide six to 10 times a day improved range of motion and improved joint function in people who had arthritis so bad that they couldn't bend their arm. Kaufman wrote a book in 1949 called *The Common Form of Joint Dysfunction* explaining all these.

Now, you put all these together and I think the reason I wrote the book pretty much stands right up. Niacin is too good for too many things. Niacin has a public relations problem. The public is being told not to take it. And yet it's good for all of these things. We needed a book that would once and for all clarify what people and the physicians need to know about the safety and the effectiveness of niacin.

As I mentioned earlier, I was not particularly intrigued with the use of niacin to treat, optimize, or lower cholesterol for a number of reasons. One is that high cholesterol—I think—values are really not a big, massive problem that is purported to be by the media and many physicians.

Actually, it's a sign or indication that something else is going on. And that really, to address it with a pill—whether it's a statin or a supplement—may not be the wisest approach to treat the underlying cause, which is usually a disturbance of insulin physiology—it's insulin, leptin. And to address it at that level not only treats or optimizes the cholesterol level, but also treats other conditions that the dysfunctional insulin or leptin levels would create.

I wasn't that intrigued with it, because, you know, there are some very powerful strategies that normalize cholesterol in almost everyone. But I was really intrigued with the psychiatric components of it and the connection with that, especially because we don't really have any good models. I mean for cholesterol, we have a very effective nontoxic natural approach. But for psychiatric problems, other than these energy psychology techniques like EFT, there really isn't anything that works really well, consistently, and effectively.

But I think this is the aspect of the book that really most intrigued and appealed to me. It's the use of it in the psychiatric component.

Let's talk about that some more then.

JM: Yeah. Because it's just ... To me, it's fascinating. And really, it borders on criminal that this approach isn't being more widely utilized.

AS: Well, Dr. Hoffer would agree with you. And by the way, I also agree with you that focusing on lowering cholesterol is an inadequate way to approach cardiovascular disease. I'm not a believer in monotherapy. I think it requires a lifestyle to really get a healthy body. There's nothing profound in that. Everybody knows it. We're just not doing it.

JM: Yeah, let me ... I know you're going to talk about it. I just wanted to interject and add one point to that. That is really an artifact of the typical approach in America, which is the "magic pill therapy."

They wanted one pill of statin to solve their problem, using simple no-responsibility on their part. Then they tend to transfer this approach to natural approaches.

AS: That's right. To substitute niacin for statin or statin for niacin is missing the point entirely. People ask me all the time for courtside advice, and I tell them this: "You have to change your life."

You're going to have to make lifestyle changes, which include proper diet, whole foods, unprocessed foods, exercise, stress reduction, vitamin supplements, possibly medication, and definitely learning.

The only way we're going to get out of this is when people realize that there is no magic bullet, and just because it's not in the pharmacy, doesn't mean it's in the health food store either. What they're really going to have to do is take a good, hard look at the whole package of everything they're doing. Now with psychiatric cases, you can't really get people to do that. You can't say to somebody who's dreadfully depressed, "Cheer up!" or, you know, "Make lifestyle changes."

This is an emergency situation.

I worked with a fellow once, who was about 22. He was so violent. He had been kicked out of the New York State Hospital for the Insane. They sent him home (and you have to think about that for a minute). So, here's this kid home with his parents, and he's absolutely terrorizing them. He's punching holes in the living room wall. On a good day, his parents, he, and I got together, and they were understandably interested—desperate would be more accurate. We talked about Dr. Hoffer's protocol, which was about using 3,000 milligrams of niacin a day, along with at least 3,000 and preferably 10,000 milligrams of vitamin C. The fellow on this good day agreed to try it, and he actually did.

Now, the niacin was so effective that he saw the difference. He used to sleep one hour a night, and he'd wander the city streets the other eight. The first day he took niacin, he slept for 18 hours that night. After that, he slept seven hours a night like clockwork. The following Friday, I got a call from his father, who said this morning his son came down and for the first time said, "Good morning, Dad." So, here's the young fellow who saw crystal clear; it couldn't have been more plain. The niacin worked pretty much more accurately.

This is also the case with ADHD kids. I knew a neighbor who had a boy who was really, really in trouble—constantly in trouble at school, constantly in trouble at home. He was violent. This was really serious. This was more than ADHD. I'm calling it ADHD, because that's what the boy's doctors called it. But the fact is it was far beyond that. Nevertheless, they gave him one of the usual drugs for attention deficit disorder, and it made him worse. So now he was even more violent and even more psychotic. The parents were in a state, as you can imagine; the kid's only 13, everything's falling apart at home.

They learned about Dr. Hoffer's niacin approach. And because it was a child, they figured, "Well, we'll start him at a lower level." They gave him 1,500 milligrams a day of niacinamide. Now, niacinamide and niacin have the same psychiatric benefits. They both work. The difference is niacin will cause a flush in almost everyone who takes it in quantity, especially for the first couple of weeks. Niacinamide is the type of niacin used in almost every multivitamin preparation, because the manufacturers don't want people bringing the product back to the store where they bought it, saying, "This made my skin hot." Niacinamide works as well as niacin for mental illness.

The boy, who wasn't about to tolerate the flush, started taking 1,500 milligrams a day of niacinamide. The parents noticed an immediate improvement. Within days, the child was less angry. He was less troubled at school. He was less oppositional. He was less violent. They immediately figured that if a little helped, maybe more would help more. They wouldn't know unless they tried, and they had no other options. Again, medication was making him worse not better.

They took him totally off of his medication, and they increased his niacin to ultimately about 5,000 milligrams a day. They even got the boy's psychiatrist to prescribe niacin, so he could take it at school.

JM: Well, this is niacinamide, right?

AS: Niacinamide, correct. The school nurse was giving the boy niacinamide twice a day at school, as well as at home. All of a sudden, calls were coming from the teachers, saying, "The kid was just transformed. He was doing great. He was doing great. He was doing great." At home, everything was better.

This young teenager was taking nearly 5,000 milligrams a day of niacinamide. Now, this is an important caution for people thinking of doing this. Niacinamide has a disadvantage, and that is it's more likely to cause nausea at very high doses. And the boy did start getting nausea at around 5,000 milligrams a day. So, what they did was they cut back the niacinamide quantity and started giving him more niacin. He got used to the flush. Then he was able to take the full high dose.

There is yet another form of niacin called inositol hexaniacinate. This is the most popular no-flush niacin. Inositol hexaniacinate works almost as well as niacin or niacinamide. It has the advantage of not causing a flush, except with very rare exceptions. It's only slightly more expensive than niacin or niacinamide, which are both very cheap. And inositol hexaniacinate will still help with cholesterol, whereas niacinamide will not. Again, all three of them have psychiatric benefits.

JM: Yeah, it's just fascinating. You know, it seems to me it's almost an error in the diagnostic system that many of these people who have the diagnosis of schizophrenia or ADHD . . . really, the proper diagnosis should be niacin deficiency with schizophrenia or ADHD symptoms.

AS: Well, not only that. Dr. Hoffer took it one notch further. He said, "It is not a niacin deficiency. It is a niacin dependency." And I get more mail on this. People think, "There is a typo in your book. There is a typo on your website. You meant to say, 'niacin deficiency,' and you said, 'niacin dependency.' No, it's not a typo. Niacin dependency means a person needs more, and they need more all the time. Some people are dependent on insulin. My mother was grand mal epileptic. She was dependent on Dilantin; she took it for half a century.

Without it, she would have had seizures. With it, she did not. We all know about insulin, but we don't understand that orthomolecular medicine using niacin goes beyond mere deficiency.

Dr. Hoffer worked with prisoners of war—Canadians who were captured by the Japanese during the Second World War. Those who survived were in poor shape. They were malnourished. They were sick. They were weak. They were thin. What Dr. Hoffer noticed was that as they started getting some vitamin supplements and proper diet, and they recovered, they didn't recover completely. They still had an unusual amount of mental and emotional problems. We can understand that brutal captivity would be enough to mess anybody else.

But Dr. Hoffer couldn't change the past. What he wanted to know is: could better nutrition help them over what they've been through? Part of what they've been through had been emotional trauma. But part of what they've been through was protracted, long-term vitamin B deficiency.

He found that most of these prisoners did not respond to a low dose of niacin. The U.S. RDA is not even 20 milligrams of niacin a day. Dr. Hoffer was giving these men at least, 3,000, and in many cases 9,000 or 10,000 milligrams a day.

His cure rate was very high. Dr. Hoffer described and defined cure as "if the patient is paying taxes." How do you know if a mental patient is well? They're paying taxes. They're not in a mental hospital, or they're not in an assisted living facility on a pension. Rather, they're holding a job and paying taxes. Dr. Hoffer agrees with you that ignoring niacin therapy as thoroughly as it's been ignored by the American Psychiatric Association, other medical organizations, and our government is bordering on criminality.

JM: It really is. It's so tragic. Because these people, there's really not a lot of good options for them. And these drugs certainly don't treat or even control it in most of the cases.

AS: Well, Dr. Hoffer put it even further. He said literally, "The Quakers were getting a 50 percent cure rate with mental illness, simply by giving people with mental illness good food, compassionate care, a nice place to live, and being good to them." Fifty percent cure rate.

Orthomolecular niacin treatment gets a cure rate of about 80 percent. Dr. Hoffer said that drug therapy alone has a cure rate of 10 percent. He added to that, "Drugs make a well person sick. How can drugs make a sick person well?" He saw this over and over and over and over again. He treated thousands of patients for a practice of 55 years. When he retired, he said, "I think everybody should have a career change every 55 years."

Dr. Hoffer's experience was buttressed by Dr. Humphry Osmond and a number of other researchers who have confirmed in practice that niacin is the best therapy for many forms of mental illness. And not only that, drug therapy is making people worse. It's not just a matter of perfection. The standard care is not perfection. The standard is the alternative. People would be better off—in many forms of mental illness—if they had no medication.

But with niacin, we're not just negating, we're affirming. Niacin is a way that the person can tell within a few hours if it's going to help. If someone has anxiety, depression, psychosis, or schizophrenia, if they take high doses of niacin, they'll notice two things right away. The first is: they're going to flush like crazy. And the second is: they're going to feel better. Now, as far as the "flush like crazy" thing goes, people are more concerned with the niacin flush than they need to be. But if you just can't contain the idea of having a niacin flush, take inositol hexaniacinate, and that will work just fine.

Dr. Hoffer said, "The best cure for the niacin flush is more niacin." If you keep taking the niacin, the histamine flushes out of the body and the vasodilation stops. It takes, perhaps, a couple of weeks. Quite frankly, I didn't believe Dr. Hoffer at first when he said that. I was very cautious.

And I didn't like the flush. But I figured, "Well, this is the expert here. I've got the world authority telling me something; the least I can do is give it a whirl."

I started taking very high doses of niacin, and I flushed a great deal. I found that I kind of liked the feeling. Within a couple of weeks, I stopped flushing.

The second thing people worry about with niacin therapy is liver function tests. There's been a fair amount of literature saying that if you take a lot of niacin—specifically, a sustained-release niacin—you're going to have increases in liver function tests. Now common sense tells us that if you have unused high doses of niacin, we should be monitored.

JM: And this would be hepatitis, typically?

AS: It's a rattling of a hepatitis. Niacin usually uses one of those sustained-release forms of niacin. The other people that tend to have more trouble with liver function tests rising are folks that have a history of alcohol use. The liver, of course, is the detox gland, the big four-pound gland in the body. And that's the site where alcohol is detoxified, so we would expect activity.

Again, it's good to be tested. But interpretation of those tests is very, very important. How many people have gone to have their thyroid levels checked and been told they don't need thyroid, only to find out that they actually do, because the doctor didn't look at G3 and they spend all their time on the others?

JM: Yeah, I couldn't agree more. Thank you for explaining that important distinction. Now, these proprietary forms of niacin, would these be ones that have the inositol hexaniacinate? And another part of that question is, has niacin itself—without the sustained-release form—ever been documented to increase their enzymes?

AS: Dr. Hoffer said that plain old niacin has never killed anybody. We don't know how much it takes to kill a person. In dogs, it's 5,000 milligrams per kilogram body weight, which is actually quite a lot—kilogram being 2.2 pounds. That, of course, is a dog, and dogs are different. Cats, for instance, you can poison a cat on Tylenol at a very low level.

We know from Dr. Hoffer's experience, his many books (he wrote over 20), and his papers, which numbered into the hundreds, that he had two cases of jaundice in 55 years. And he treated thousands and thousands of patients. So, the risk is there. But everything carries a risk literally.

We have to be sure that we understand what the true risk is. You can do anything wrong. If a person were to go out and take a massive amount of niacin all of a sudden, they might have some strange findings. They might find their blood sugar going up. They might find that their blood pressure goes down. They might find that they'd throw up. They might find that they get beet red.

Well, this just means that people aren't informed. That's why we wrote the book. We don't want people going half-baked and taking huge amounts of niacin, just because somebody said it's the magic bullet, as you and I talked about earlier. There's no substitute for being informed. The more you know about niacin, the better it's going to work, and the healthier you're going to be.

Doctors are poorly informed about niacin therapy. In fact, as Dr. Hugh Riordan, out in Wichita, Kansas, says, "Orthomolecular is not the answer to any question asked at medical school."

The American Psychiatric Association has actively published, saying, "Do not take niacin. It's dangerous, and it won't work." Those statements are untrue. It is not dangerous, and it does work. You earlier asked how my colleagues responded to what I do, and I think I've given you a pretty good sense of that at this point.

But I don't care. The fact is that if we can help people by letting them know about Dr. Hoffer's work, that's the thing to do. And then folks are going to have to make up their own mind. But this is not about a belief. This is about observed clinical results. And nobody observed more clinical results in a lifetime with niacin and psychiatric problems than Abram Hoffer.

JM: There's great value to exploring other people's life's work, seeing what they've learned from that, and applying that to our own lives personally. But I'm still curious about the proprietary forms of niacin—the sustained-release niacin.

AS: There are several ways you can package niacin. We've talked about three. There is plain old niacin that quickly dissolves and causes flush in most people for a while. There's niacinamide, which is used in most supplements, and which never causes a flush, but has no lipid benefits. And then there's inositol hexaniacinate, which is the best of both worlds, slightly more expensive, not quite as effective.

There are also different types of niacin, such as sustained-release forms. A sustained-release tablet can be a matrix, kind of a concrete-like tablet that simply erodes gradually in the system.

When people are told not to take sustained-release tablets because some plumber found vitamin tablets undissolved underneath the toilet in some house, it's usually this type of tablet. An eroding matrix sustained-release tablet will not dissolve in the elderly, for instance. And they do tend to pass right through some folks.

You can crush the tablet and improve absorption, but of course, it's no longer sustained release.

The other way you can do it is to have a chemical form of release, like those time-release cold medicines that are advertised so frequently. These little individual sub-capsules, their little particles have different chemical codings, and they break down at a different rate. This is a more reliable way to get the product absorbed.

I cannot explain why sustained-release niacin causes so much trouble. Dr. Hoffer seemed to feel very strongly that all you really have to do is to sidestep the problem by taking regular niacin, which is so safe, but take it more frequently. He had his patients take it at least three times a day.

Remember, I mentioned Dr. William Kaufman. He treated arthritis with high doses of niacinamide. He found that a divided dose of 500 milligrams each for a total of 3,000 to 5,000 milligrams a day was effective. But he found that if you divided the doses into 250 milligrams per dose, it was almost as effective at half the total. So, dividing the dose is a good idea. And sustained release sounds like a good idea. But it doesn't play out that way.

JM: That's good to know. So, a simple way might be to avoid that for a number of reasons. One is it is a more pharmacological approach. It's also a lot more expensive, and there are unnecessary side effects that you can easily avoid. I'm wondering also if there's any concern for using the niacin in high dose. How much higher dose would you expect to receive if you're eating an optimized natural food approach? Typically, the concern would be that you would create other nutrient deficiencies because of an imbalance in the ratios of other B-vitamins. You mentioned earlier the benefit of taking them with larger doses of vitamin C. Are there any concerns in this area that you're seeing, or the literature has brought out, that you're creating other micronutrient deficiencies?

AS: The B-complex is not called the B-complex for nothing. These B-vitamins are related to each other, and, like a World Series baseball team, they work best together. Nobody ever won the series simply because they had a good pitcher and had nobody else out there. So, we need the whole team.

One example we have that does stand out is pyridoxine or vitamin B_6. It is well-known that really high doses of pyridoxine alone can cause an imbalance of other nutrients and some neurological side effects. For a while, vitamin B_6 was the big thing for treating carpal tunnel syndrome—and by the way, it is very effective for that. It's also very effective at relieving premenstrual tension symptoms.

The amount of vitamin B_6 is the issue. Some people were taking 2,000 to 4,000 milligrams a day of vitamin B_6. A few of them developed problems, and most of them were taking only B_6. But a much larger number of people were taking 500 milligrams a day of B_6 alone, and only one or two reported side effects. There had been no vitamin B_6 side effects documented below 200 milligrams. Now, 200 milligrams is 100 times the RDA for vitamin B_6.

We simply have to remember that although I'm shifting the balance point, there's still a balance point. Not everybody needs massive amounts of niacin. My view is you should take enough vitamin C, take enough niacin, or take enough vitamin B$_6$—take enough of a nutrient to be symptom-free, whatever the amount might be.

Dr. Richard Passwater introduced that to me when I was a very young man. Try the vitamin, add a modest dose, and see if it works. If it helps you, take a little more. If you feel better still, then you need more. If you don't notice any difference, or if you noticed something negative, back off. It seemed like common sense to me.

With niacin and all the B-vitamins, I think we should take them as a team. But you're going to need disproportionately more niacin. Oddly enough, if you look at the U.S. RDAs for the B-complex, niacin stands out. It's the highest—by weight—of any U.S. RDA. Thiamine is around a milligram and a half. Riboflavin is about the same. Pyridoxine is around 2 milligrams. Folate, B$_{12}$, these are measured in micrograms. Biotin is measured in micrograms. And then there's niacin—20 milligrams.

Now remember that a milligram is 1,000 micrograms. That's expressed as the cake mix analogy. Let's say your child is going to have a party, and you want to make a chocolate cake. Well, you don't have any mix, so you'll make it from scratch. You can't just take a pound of cocoa, put it in the oven, and call that a cake.

On the other hand, if you take all the ingredients but in the wrong quantity, that's not a cake either. Is a chocolate cake really a cup of sugar, a cup of salt, a cup of cocoa, a cup of flour, a cup of oil, and a cup of baking soda? It's not. There's a small amount of salt. There's a large amount of sugar. There's a medium amount of cocoa.

The RDAs basically indicate that niacin is needed out of proportion to all other vitamins in the body. The numbers themselves generated—and with the exception of vitamin C—RDAs are based on animal research.

Dr. Hoffer and I and others think that the niacin RDA is way too low. We think it should be at least 200 milligrams—10 times more than it is. And I think you could make a very strong argument for 500 milligrams of niacin a day. Now, the government doesn't like that idea.

JM: Can you get 500 milligrams in your diet?

AS: Couldn't possibly. As soon as we raised the RDAs to where they make people healthy, it exposes that our diet is incapable of making us healthy.

JM: Yeah. But that's sort of an ancestral argument against the use of niacin. Because it would seem that if our ancestors didn't have access to this level of a nutrient, then why do we need so much?

AS: Well, there are several differences between modern life and ancestral life. I think that all ages at all times have always been under terrible stress. I'm not sure if the stress of being attacked by wild animals is any lower than living in a noisy city with commutes every day to work. But I do think that we have several other factors that are unique.

First of all, our food has been heavily processed. If we get back to an ancestral type of eating, probably, our niacin intake would go up substantially. It would not get to 500 milligrams. But again, I'm not saying 500 is necessarily the number. I'd be very happy with 200. If people ate a really good diet where they had a lot of whole unprocessed foods that haven't had the niacin taken out, I think we would be able to push our niacin intake around 100 milligrams a day, possibly more. The other thing to remember is that we eat minus foods. We eat things that actually cause vitamin washout or philosophically create the need for more niacin. If you want to make somebody crazy, give him a lot of artificial color, preservatives, and sugar.

Now, Dr. Benjamin Feingold was saying this back in the 1970s. He was an allergist—board-certified allergist. Some people listened. A lot of people said he was nuts. The Feingold Association has been valiantly urging people to try his approach, since there's no downside to not eating "paint," which is what I call food colors. There's no downside to not eating sugar. You have nowhere to go but up. You save money, and you're going to feel better. The only question is: how much better are you going to feel?

The Feingold Program works on at least 50 percent of the children who do it. They avoid the colors and, of course, avoiding sugar is going to help, too. Anyone who's ever taught (and I'm one of these people, my background is in education, not medicine), we know that on the day after Halloween, you're going to have trouble. No matter if it's a six-year-old or a graduate student, they have all been eating the sugar and the artificial colors. These cause actual psychiatric changes in behavior.

You want to take a perfectly normal kid and make him crazy? Just feed him lots of artificial color and sugar, and you can do it. We know this, because if you do it to animals, they'll go nuts.

Dr. William Kaufman pointed this out in 1949. He noticed that if you give laboratory animals niacin, you'll get a phenomenon called "decreased running." When animals are upset, they don't just sit there and pout about it. They take action because they're desperate. When animals were troubled, they would be panicky.

When Kaufman looked at the research, he noticed that giving niacin caused them to calm down. I think that has a direct application to the classroom. It certainly [Laughs] wouldn't hurt to try. So, whether we add niacin or eliminate sugar, either way, we've effectively done the same thing.

This is why, as you and I said earlier, it has to be a holistic approach. Niacin is a big part of the solution. The best thing about niacin is that it is a fast-acting, safe, and inexpensive emergency measure. If someone is having a terrible day, if they take niacin, they will feel better in 20 minutes. If they chew the tablet and take it with hot tea, they'll feel better in five minutes.

JM: That's a great approach. Thank you for providing the insights that the Feingold approach or the avoidance of these artificial colors and sugars may actually have its mechanism of action that—not under direct toxicity, but indirect approach—would result in niacin deficiency or dependency, as you mentioned.

AS: Yeah, and there was confirming research in the last 10 years or so, mostly in Britain. First, they did a study in prisons. They took away the junk foods, and the violence rate went down by about half. That sounds pretty promising.

Then there was another study, an actual very carefully controlled crossover study with kids. They gave one group a combination of preservatives, colorings, and sugars that extremely closely resembles a highly caffeinated, yellow-colored soft drink that's marketed in America. And these kids went ballistic behaviorally. They measured this scientifically. Then they gave them a good diet, gave the other group that, and you can see what happened.

There is no question any longer. The old thought that food additives and sugar don't affect your child has been put to rest—admittedly not until the twenty-first century. But Dr. Feingold was right. And with all due respect to his memory, Dr. Frederick Stare of Harvard was wrong.

JM: Interesting. Just finishing up on the nutrient requirements that might be considered useful with the use of niacin, would you recommend that if someone is taking a therapeutic dose of niacin which can typically range up to 3,000 milligrams, that they also take a high-quality B-complex supplement?

AS: With each meal.

JM: With each meal?

AS: Yeah.

JM: What type of dosages? Because, you know, there's a large range.

AS: There's a very large range indeed. With vitamins, especially water-soluble vitamins, that means vitamin C and all the vitamin Bs, dividing the dose always works best. Remember, Dr. Kaufman found that 250 milligrams of niacinamide many times a day work as well as 500 milligrams of niacinamide many times a day. We often hear this: if you take vitamins, you'll just have expensive urine. Well, of course, if you take antibiotics, you will also have expensive urine. But that isn't much. The trick here with vitamins is that you need to divide the dose with the water-soluble vitamins, no matter which ones they are.

I recommend that people take a B-complex for breakfast, lunch, and dinner. If you're too energized at night, cut out the dinner one. Some people actually notice when they take B-vitamins—and even though vitamins don't give you energy, they release energy. You need B-vitamins for the Krebs cycle to work. Without that the whole thing crashes down, and you're sitting down there with beriberi or some similar disease with no energy and no strength.

Dividing the dose of B-complex means you really don't have to worry about how much you take. You could get a 25-milligram B-complex and take that breakfast, lunch, and dinner, and that's a total of 75 milligrams balanced. I don't like that word "balanced," because of the cake mix analogy we talked about. Dr. Roger Williams sets out some very good, reasonably low supplemental goals in his books. Dr. Williams, who discovered panto-thenic acid, was doing this before 1950. He estimates that people only need maybe three, four, or five times the RDA. In studies at Harvard on people with AIDS, they had a 27 percent reduction in deaths with AIDS patients who were taking about five times the U.S. RDA. It doesn't have to be a huge dose. It just has to be substantially more than the RDA. For most people, doctors in particular, five times the RDA is a walk on the wild side.

With niacin, there is a so-called theoretical phase-off or limit. The government has actually issued statements that suggest that you really shouldn't take any more than about 35 or 40 milligrams of niacin a day. The RDA is only a little under 20. You may have seen a recent paper that was published, which suggested that Americans are obese because they get 30 milligrams a day of niacin instead of 18.

This is how far the public is being hornswaggled. Common sense just goes right out the window when you talk about foods and supplements. It's time that we brought common sense back into it. My dad taught me when I was young, when you want to know something, go to the organ grinder, not the monkey.

I was very fortunate to have worked with Dr. Hoffer for the better part of a decade. I wish he was still with us, because I had a lot to learn, and he had a lot to teach. And I'd like to think it's a fitting tribute to the man that changed the treatment of psychiatry forever, even though the psychiatric profession doesn't realize it yet.

JM: Excellent. To the best of your knowledge—because I'd like to go into some of the practical details of how one would administer this if you're convinced or compelled to try for yourself or someone else—is there a company that produces a supplement that has a balance of these high-quality accessory B-complex supplements in addition to the niacin? So maybe a 250-milligram dose of niacin with far smaller amounts of the B-complex?

AS: Well, I normally don't make any statement about particular brands, because I have no financial connection with the health products industry, and this is an important factor in my approach with the public. However, it is very, very easy for anyone to go to a health food store or via the Internet and get a 50-milligram balanced B-complex. I don't think you can go far wrong with that.

And a 50-milligram balanced B-complex three times a day, you simply cannot make a case against that in terms of side effects or toxicity. In addition to that, you need additional niacin.

The amount of niacin will vary from person to person. It will not only vary from person to person based on their height, weight, lifestyle, and gender, but it will also vary based on whether they're sick or not, or whether it's a weekend or whether you're in a high-pressure meeting. We know that we need more of the B-vitamins, more people at different times.

I think the 50-milligram B-complex three times a day plus extra niacin, in my opinion, an extra 200 to 500 milligrams three times a day, would be a good place for most people. However, if you're not going to be happy with the flush, you have to make sure it's inositol hexaniacinate or niacinamide.

We have a very large margin of safety with vitamins. Dr. Hoffer had a patient, a teenager who was mentally ill. She was taking niacin, one day got mad at her parents, and downed the whole bottle. Now that might have been just an adolescent gesture of defiance or might have been some sort of a suicide attempt, but it didn't work the way she planned it. She was schizophrenic. She'd been hearing voices. This girl was really sick. She was about 16. She took an entire bottle. Dr. Hoffer said it was around 60,000 milligrams of niacin at once.

She had a side effect: the voices went away. After that, she just took normal amounts of niacin. You can do anything wrong. With niacin, the trick is to take enough to do the job for you.

In *Niacin: The Real Story*, we tried to present as much information as we could to help people and their doctors arrive at the amount they need in a commonsense, therapeutic-trial way. The first lesson in medical school I was taught a long, long time ago—before I had even considered going; I was still a boy—I heard it said that the first rule in medical school is, "Do no harm." But the second rule is, "Every case is different." One size doesn't fit all. One of the problems with the RDA is that it's nutritional communism. It's sort of like having a minimum wage and saying, "Everybody gets the minimum wage, but nobody can get any more than the minimum wage." It's really kind of silly.

We have doctors who have taken a stance like Dr. Hoffer, Dr. Kaufman, and Dr. Parsons. They have gone public, saying, "Niacin is a nutrient that some people are dependent on. And if they are dependent, they need thousands of milligrams a day."

In fact, Dr. Hoffer and Dr. Foster made a case that schizophrenia has genetic advantages. It has an evolutionary advantage. Dr. Hoffer noted that in all his thousands and thousands of patients that he treated for psychiatric problems with niacin, he had less than half a dozen that had cancer.

Well, he and Dr. Foster looked into this. They think that schizophrenia is a beneficial genetic trait. It makes people creative, and it also makes them more resistant to cancer. Whether this is true or not is a subject for smarter people than me.

But there is a real possibility that today, we are living at the moment where for the first time ever, we cannot merely say, "The pharmaceutical industry is too powerful. Its products are too dangerous, and they're not working." Instead, we can say, "We have a readily available nutrient that costs six dollars a bottle at a big-box discount store, and that will help you feel better in half an hour. It's safer, cheaper, and more effective than any drug." Of course, we've all been taught that that's impossible. But it is possible. Dr. Hoffer confirmed it decade after decade.

JM: Interesting. So, you've mentioned the 50-milligram B-complex, but earlier you said 25 might also work equally as well.

AS: Yes. If it came in a capsule, you better take the 50. If it comes in a tablet, I'd get a pill cutter and cut it in half. Dividing the dose is very important. Dr. Steve Hickey talks about this with vitamin C. He calls it dynamic flow. It's basically very, very, very frequent oral doses can get you blood levels of vitamins that are approaching intravenous levels.

JM: Interesting. In many areas in life, I believe this one's true. The devil's in the details. The use of this therapy would seem to be . . . You'll be taking a large number of pills, especially, when you get the B-complex and the niacin. And you're going to be out long-term, perhaps the rest of your life. From our perspective, it would seem it might, you know.

When we look at supplements (like what we do as a company, we sell them) we have some concerns about using magnesium stearate, which for those who are not familiar with it, is a flow agent that is traditionally viewed as relatively benign or innocuous. But there's some concern that it may contribute to developing these intestinal dysfunctions, which impair other nutrient absorption.

You know, my only caution for people considering this is to find a company—not all supplements are created equal. Finding a company that would be providing a supplement that didn't have this magnesium stearate. Or titanium dioxide would be another one. But that's typically a coloring agent not typically used in this type of circumstance.

AS: Right. And very frequently, if people can find a capsule, they'll notice there are fewer excipients than a gelatin capsule, because you don't have to glue and stamp this thing together. Excipients are necessary to make a tablet—or so the general idea in the industry goes—so we have to allow them.

Linus Pauling actually said decades ago that when you take vitamin C, you're better off taking it in pure crystals. Not everybody likes the taste. Not everybody is going to do it. Tablets do have their advantages. Get the best ones you can. Capsules can have fewer excipients in them. You can also take powders. But believe me, B-complex powder tastes vile.

When you open a bottle of B-complex vitamins and smell it, you'll have the same experience I had when I was a boy, and my family doctor prescribed a B-complex vitamin pill for me. My father (I still remember this) said, "Here." They called it a tonic, but it was a B-complex vitamin. He handed me this oblong-shaped tablet, and I said, "Is it a chewable?" My father said, "I don't know, vitamin C!"

I did that exactly once, and the taste was vile. There is something to be said for taking things in tablets and capsules. I want to emphasize that you don't have to become a chronic pill popper to do this right. You can get niacin in 500-milligram tablets; you quarter that thing. You have your dose four times a day, and that's just one tablet. If you take a B-complex capsule with each meal, that's only three more, so that's four. On top of that, you probably want to take some vitamin D. You can get that in capsules.

Niacin is so valuable that we need to get it into everybody. For those who cannot afford good-quality supplements, I emphasize that a bad-quality niacin supplement will still cure schizophrenia.

JM: For some with schizophrenia, I would agree, because of this issue with the manganese stearate and the biofilm. It's a matter of priority or a triage in things, so it becomes less of an issue.

AS: We do the best that we can. Dr. Rudolf Altschul said this years ago: "Spend as much money as you can on your health."

What I'm trying to do is make sure that we don't lose anybody on this. Because for those folks that are having trouble making ends meet—their house values have gone down, they lost their jobs, or who knows what else they're dealing with, their medical bills are higher, they're dealing with the elderly or who knows—they need to keep in mind that this is very simple. The niacin tablet, buy the big potency, break them into little pieces, take it all day, and that will cost you less than a nickel.

JM: Yeah, that's very cost-effective. For those who are interested in using this program, you've mentioned several times, and I think most people are aware anyway that there's niacin flush. So, can you describe sort of an optimized program to minimize this as a side effect, so that people will be more comfortable in engaging in this type of supplement protocol?

AS: That's an excellent question. Everybody who's listening or reading has that question right there, and they wanted you to ask it. There are many ways we can approach the flush. First of all, we can avoid the flush issue completely by getting niacinamide, or we can virtually avoid the flush completely by using inositol hexaniacinate. Once in a while, somebody flushes from that. But it's rare, about five percent.

Niacinamide, I don't know of anyone that's flushed from niacinamide. Problems with niacinamide: the nausea level is lower. With niacinamide, it's usually around 4,000 to 8,000 milligrams a day, where people might start feeling nauseous. With regular niacin, it's probably over 50,000 milligrams a day. That's two ways you can deal with it.

The third way you can deal with avoiding the flush is to go to your doctor and get a prescription for the various proprietary sustained-release niacins. We've already talked about that. They carry the greater safety risk.

The next way that people can avoid the niacin flush is to divide the dose. If you take 4,000 milligrams of niacin at once, you're going to flush for sure. But if you take 4,000 milligrams of niacin in eight 500-milligram doses, you'll probably flush less. The next way that you can do it is to have it with meals. With food, the dilution is better. Or you can take niacin with lots of liquid.

With liquid, the dilution is better. You can also take more vitamin C. Dr. Abram Hoffer said that more vitamin C reduces a niacin flush. His preferred way was to say to people, "Well, just buckle up and do it. Take the niacin. You're going to flush like crazy for a couple of weeks. Keep taking it, the flush will go away."

Then there's the way that I've mentioned to people for the last 35 years. This way worked for me personally and seems to be a good option. Here it is: start with an idiotically tiny amount of niacin. Now, what would be an idiotically tiny amount of niacin? The U.S. RDA, that would be an idiotically tiny amount of niacin.

Start with, say, 20 or 25 milligrams of niacin per meal. Some people will flush at that level. But probably it won't be you. Increase by another 25 milligrams each meal, each day. Each day, start out 25, 25, and 25, the next day, 50, 50, 50, next day, 75, 75, 75, next day, 100, 100, 100. This is a good way to determine what dose seems to work for you. In fact, some people go up even slower than that. They just go up 25 milligrams a day. You can gradually introduce it, and just see what happens. There is no need to have apprehension over using niacin.

Dr. William Parsons said, "In order for a doctor to use niacin, they have to understand niacin." Most doctors don't understand it. Quite a few use it and give it to people for cholesterol. But they don't really understand it. When you understand niacin, you realize that the flush is sort of an indicator—and it's a good indicator.

If you're flushing a lot, for instance, as Dr. Hoffer pointed out, it may indicate that you have a food allergy. If I eat certain foods, I have a different reaction to my regular dose of niacin. That isn't niacin's fault. It's because I ate the food that I shouldn't have eaten. Again, everybody's different. We don't know. We talk to 100 people; we're going to have 101 variables on this.

With niacin, if you want to flush, chew the tablet. If you want to flush, take it with something hot. If you want to flush, take it on an empty stomach.

JM: What dose are you taking a day, and how long have you taken it?

AS: That's a good question. Dr. Hoffer refused to answer that question. He would not tell people what he took, because he was concerned that they would go and do it. He felt that it was between them and their doctor.

Not being a physician, I have a slightly different viewpoint. I think telling people what I do is a valid way to get them thinking about what they might want to look into and ultimately decide on their own time. I take 1,000 milligrams of niacin three times a day, which is exactly what Dr. Hoffer gave most of his patients. In addition to that, I take additional niacin mid-afternoon and at bedtime, so I have probably around 4,000 milligrams of niacin a day. However, if I am under stress, I triple that amount. I would take about 12,000.

JM: Aside from your initial experience with the flush, you've never had it even in these high doses?

AS: Oh, I'm having a niacin flush right now. I took 1,000 milligrams about an hour and a half ago, and I'm having a very slight flush at this second. I figured you might enjoy that. I was giving a lecture once to some post-doctoral students, and at their insistence, demonstrated a niacin flush. I thought, "Well, okay."

Since I always have my vitamins bottle in my pocket (that's why when I walk down the halls, I would rattle and all the students knew it was me before I turn the corner), I took some niacin with some water. It was before lunch, so I had an empty stomach.

I took about 1,500 milligrams of niacin on an empty stomach, and I said, "Watch this." They're all watching pretty intently. It was a small class. There were only about 30 people. There's one fellow at the back who whipped out a pair of opera glasses. Now, this was really funny. It wasn't that big of a room, and he didn't do it to be a wise guy. But it was a very funny moment. He wanted to actually see precisely where and how I flushed.

Normally, you flush from the head down. The cheeks, the neck, the upper arms, they tend to flush first. Then later on you might have a flush on your abdomen and perhaps your legs. When I say, "later on," we're talking possibly in a matter of a minute or two, or we're talking—if you had a big meal—it could be hours. In fact, if you took niacin after Thanksgiving dinner, you literally might not flush for three or four hours, so long that you would have forgotten you took the niacin at all.

Well, they liked the niacin flush so much that one of the evaluations said, "The niacin flush was awesome. Do you do birthday parties?" We got a big laugh out of that. The niacin flush is not a big deal. People need to understand that it is a distraction. Niacin happens to cause you to have a flush. It's like a little bit of an embarrassment. Ladies, it's a little bit like a hot flash, I'm reliably informed. It's a little bit like feeling embarrassed or like you were maybe out in the sun for that extra hour.

A niacin flush—if you're doing it right—will last about 20 minutes. If you take enough niacin to flush for an hour or two and you have to lie down and feel nauseous, you did it wrong. You took too much. Don't do that. Well, how do you make sure you don't take too much? You gradually increase. Dr. Hoffer started people at 3,000 a day right off. But he was a physician, and he was working with them.

For people that are doing this on their own, they're going to have to be realistic. You really should work with a doctor. To do that, you're going to have to educate the doctor. For those who that are not going to go to that trouble and just take it on their own, I suggest that they start with very tiny amounts and gradually increase, observing what it does for them. Some days I have a flush, some days I don't. Now I live in upstate New York, and I don't have to tell you that a nice warm feeling in the extremities up here is a prized experience.

JM: You've presented in your book, and you discussed here some very compelling arguments for the use of niacin in psychiatric disorders like post-alcoholic depression and schizophrenia, and then, of course, as an adjunct optimizing cholesterol levels. And arthritis. I'm wondering if you could explain why you're using this if you're not treating those disorders.

AS: All right. That's an excellent question. I do eat a pretty good diet. I live in a built-up area and yet my entire backyard is a whole other world—a giant organic garden. I think everybody ought to do that. It saves you money. It's good for your health. It's good for your mind. It's just good for so many different things.

The reason I take a lot of niacin is that I—like you—have a schedule that can sometimes be very stressful. And if I'm travelling, I definitely need more niacin. I have several books in production right now. I'm the editor of the *Orthomolecular Medicine News Service.* I have the website, interviews, and a lot of media work. I find these things stressful. I always have. I enjoy public speaking, but quite frankly, I do feel some anxiety. Why do you think I took the niacin before doing your interview? That's one reason I take it. The other reason is a number of years ago, I had a test at my once-a-decade physical and it indicated that my blood lipid profile was not as good as it could be. The triglycerides were a little high. The LDL was a little high, and the HDL could have been higher. Well, I thought, "I think I'll take some niacin," because I was eating a good diet, exercising, and doing stress reduction but I still had those numbers. With the knowledge that we had 15 years ago, I decided to take some niacin and noticed the numbers have all improved.

The other reason I really like niacin is that it helps you sleep better. It is a wonderful sleep aid. People that have never tried it don't know what they're missing. If you can't sleep at night—or better yet, before you go to bed, take some niacin. I would say, that could be anywhere between 25 and 250 milligrams depending on who you are, what you ate, and how much you need. But take a small amount of niacin about a half-hour before going to bed. It definitely shortens the time it takes to go to sleep.

There are some writers such as Dr. Jonathan Prousky, who is editor-in-chief of the *Journal of Orthomolecular Medicine* and on the faculty of the College of Naturopathic Medicine in Toronto, who said that niacin actually works like a benzodiazepine. It works very similarly and works with the same receptors as this anti-anxiety drug.

Niacin is not just a quaint idea that Dr. Hoffer had in the early '50s. This is an extremely well-documented medical approach that doesn't involve medicine. It is so inexpensive and so varied in its application that it sounds too good to be true. We need to keep in mind that sometimes the greatest gains in health care come through the simplest methods. My grandmother said, "Chew your food." One cannot even begin to list the number of health problems that go away if you take her advice and stop bolting your food and chew it well. Vegetable juicing—we had Jack LaLanne , who was certainly big on vegetable juicing and who summed it up that if man made it, don't eat it.

Eat no junk. That's what Abram said to his patients who were teens and children. I still remember Abram leaning over. He would say to the child, "No junk." And Abram said to me, "There's not one kid that didn't know exactly what I meant." If we can get people to eat better, a lot less niacin is going to need to be consumed. But until we can get people to do what they really need to do, the very word "supplement" provides the answer.

JM: But you know my lifestyle is such that I feel pretty good. And most of my health parameters are optimized, so I don't perceive a need for myself. But I do think that many others would seem to certainly benefit from it, especially with this anti-anxiety and insomnia issue. Also, I'm wondering if you could touch a little bit about its use for arthritis. I'm assuming this is the degenerative arthritis. But maybe it might even have some useful utilities in rheumatory arthritis.

AS: All right. First of all, let's just take sleeping for a second. We now have recent studies. There's one that just came out in March of this year that indicates that people who take sleeping pills are five times more likely to die prematurely than those who don't. They found in this study that even 18 sleeping pills a year almost triples your risks of dying prematurely from something. So, just the fact that niacin helps you fall asleep at night in itself could save half a million premature deaths a year in America.

This study really makes us think. If just sleeping pills are making half-a-million people every year die early, niacin is good for many, many people and will save their life. We're not even talking cholesterol. We're not even talking psychiatric issues. When we bring in psychiatric issues and heart disease, now we're saving tens of thousands more.

Arthritis isn't killing too many people. But by golly, it is such a disabling, painful, and miserable condition. When we look at the work of Dr. William Kaufman, it's astonishing to think that this medical doctor, who also had a PhD, was practicing in Connecticut and getting such good results using niacinamide for osteoarthritis primarily back before World War II started, was getting mail delivered by the U.S. Postal Service, and on the envelope, it said, "Arthritis Doctor, Connecticut."

Dr. Kaufman kept careful records of his patients. He documented them in this book called *The Common Form of Joint Dysfunction*. I talked with his widow, Charlotte, who very kindly gave me permission to scan and post the entire book at my website for free access.

People don't have to go looking for a copy of this rare book, because it was privately printed and it's hard to come by. They can go to DoctorYourself .com, type in my search box "Kaufman," and they can read Dr. Kaufman's entire book, including his case histories on how he treated arthritis.

He had people that were unable to bend their legs or their arms or get out of a chair. Once they started taking niacinamide—250 or 500 milligrams five to possibly eight times a day—he noticed a profound gradual improvement. It normally took months. This is not an overnight sensation. Exactly why niacin helps in this case is not clear to me. Dr. Kaufman put forward some ideas. About 10 to 20 years ago, there was new work done that confirmed that niacin does indeed improve joint mobility. People can try this and see for themselves.

JM: Now, you had discussed previously the differences between the use of niacin and niacinamide for cholesterol and for psychiatric issues. In psychiatric issues, the niacinamide, outside of the nausea, seems to be providing useful benefits. Is there a differentiation with respect to the use of sleep, for the joint disorders, and for the joint pain also?

AS: As far as I know, using niacinamide or niacin will work for sleep and for arthritis. Dr. Kaufman used niacinamide; he preferred it. Dr. Hoffer used niacin. He preferred it. They both got good results. Dr. Kaufman reported in 5,000 patients' years of use, he didn't have a single reported side effect at all. Dr. Hoffer reported in 55 years of use, he probably had under a dozen serious side effects, out of I don't know how many thousands of patients.

JM: Well, that's certainly a powerful testimony. You know, I really want to thank you for bringing this form of treatment to everyone's attention by co-writing the book with Dr. Hoffer. I was wondering if there's any closing comment you wanted to make to kind of summarize it.

AS: Yes. Professor Harold Foster is the third author of *Niacin: The Real Story*. And I want to give credit to Harry for all the wonderful work that he did. He was a close friend of Abram's. They died in the same year. Abram was very advanced in age. Harry, unfortunately, died prematurely. It's for their memory that I went ahead, finished this book, and made it available to the public. I just couldn't think of a better tribute to these wonderful teachers, researchers, and doctors than to make sure that everybody had a chance to make up their own mind and see for themselves.

I owe a great deal of credit to a lot of different people who have taught me what I know today. That includes my children because it's in having a family that you really learn. I want to pass on your kind words to those that really deserve it.

Orthomolecular physicians have been curing disease with vitamins for 75 years. I tell my readers and your readers and listeners that if your doctor is not using vitamins, you have an old-fashioned doctor.

Clinical Experiences with a Vitamin B₃ Dependent Family[1]

JONATHAN E. PROUSKY, ND

Reprinted with permission from the Journal of Orthomolecular Medicine

A vitamin dependency occurs when there is a defect in the binding of the vitamin-related coenzyme to its apoenzyme. The only way to correct a vitamin dependency is to obtain daily amounts much greater than recommended dietary allowances. I believe that the most common vitamin dependency among patients with mental illnesses is vitamin B₃.

These three cases involve members of the same family. Each case improved clinically upon taking megadoses (500 to 1,500 milligrams per day) of the vitamin. A fourth member of this family has schizophrenia. This is significant since recent postmortem biopsies of brain tissues have shown defects in the ability of schizophrenic patients to generate adequate amounts of vitamin B₃ coenzymes from tryptophan. Families share similar genetics and environmental factors, and thus this family likely shares varying degrees of the ability to synthesize adequate amounts of vitamin B₃ coenzymes. If schizophrenic genes are common among the entire human population, then the majority of people will suffer from slight-to-severe defects in this biosynthetic pathway.

INTRODUCTION

The 16th edition of the *Merck Manual of Diagnosis and Therapy* defines a vitamin dependency as that which relates to "coenzyme function and results from an apoenzyme abnormality that can be overcome by administration of doses of the appropriate vitamin that are many times the recommended dietary allowance (RDA)."[2] In the 17th edition of this prestigious medical text, the definition of a vitamin dependency was slightly modified as resulting "from a genetic defect in the metabolism of the vitamin or in the binding of the vitamin-related coenzyme to its apoenzyme."[3] The authors note that to correct the altered metabolic pathway, vitamin doses of 1,000 times the RDA are sometimes necessary.

Thus, a vitamin dependency is only correctable by increasing the intake of a particular vitamin to levels greater than could be achieved from dietary sources alone. This is not unreasonable since many enzyme systems within the body require optimal doses of vitamins to remedy defects in the synthesis of vital metabolic products to sustain adequate health. In Pauling's famous 1968 publication, he reasoned that: "mental disease is for the most part caused by abnormal reaction rates, as determined by genetic constitution and diet, and by abnormal molecular concentrations of essential substances."[4] He described how megavitamin therapy would be necessary for the optimal treatment of mental disease since the saturating capacity would be much greater for defective enzymes that have diminished combining capacity for their respective substrates. In other words, an enzyme-catalyzed reaction could be corrected by increasing the concentration of its substrate through the use of optimal doses of vital micronutrients.

Other reports have since corroborated Pauling's original ideas that vitamin doses in excess of those obtained from diet are valuable therapeutic interventions for the treatment of mental illnesses. Some of these reports are cited. The illnesses include anxiety,[5-8] bipolar disorder,[9] depression,[10] and schizophrenia.[11] A 2002 report validated the concept of vitamin dependencies for the treatment of 50 common genetic diseases. In this report, the need for doses of vitamins far in excess of RDA amounts (i.e., optimal doses) were deemed necessary as a means of increasing coenzyme concentrations and correcting defective enzymatic activity.[12] The authors stated that the "examples discussed here are likely to represent only a small fraction of the total number of defective enzymes that would be responsive to therapeutic vitamins."

In light of the evidence, it is common for the "orthomolecularly-inclined" clinician to consider vitamin dependencies when proposing various differential diagnoses in the evaluation of patients. Hoffer and Osmond devised a simple classification to determine the potential causes of schizophrenia.[13] Their classification easily covers all the mental illnesses that plague us today. I have added "omega-3 essential fatty acid deficiency" to their classification based on the initial work of Rudin involving substrate pellagra,[14] and on more recent published works by Horrobin[15] and Stoll.[16] Thus, in the workup of the mentally ill it is best to consider the following potential causes:

Vitamin Dependencies

Vitamin B_3 (niacin or niacinamide)

Vitamin B_6 (pyridoxine)

Others such as vitamin C (ascorbic acid), vitamin B_{12} (cobalamin), and the rest of the B-complex vitamins

Mineral Disturbances

Deficiencies (e.g., chromium, manganese, selenium, zinc)

Excesses (e.g., copper, lead, mercury)

Cerebral Allergies

Food

Inhalant

Food Additives

Omega-3 Essential Fatty Acid Deficiency

Vitamin dependencies were listed first in Hoffer and Osmond's classification scheme. Even though vitamin B_3 was given priority consideration as the most common cause of the schizophrenic syndrome, I believe that the vast majority of all psychiatric patients suffer from a vitamin B_3 dependency. Here, I present three cases of non-schizophrenic individuals from the same family who all suffered varying degrees of mental disturbances, and who all responded well to optimal doses of vitamin B_3.

CASE #1

This 18-year-old Caucasian female presented to my office on July 6, 2005. She described a history of social anxiety disorder (social phobia) since primary school where she found it very difficult to talk with her peers and to attend school functions. She would often hide in the washrooms to avoid uncomfortable situations. At one time she was told that she might have learning problems. She completed high school and received grades in the high 90s. She was a talented opera singer and loved artistic endeavors such as reading poems and creating drawings. Although she felt that her social anxiety was much improved, she complained of stuttering when reading aloud.

After incorporating a whole-foods diet, her moods improved despite the occasional mood swings prior to menses. Physical examination was unremarkable. Although she was on a very good orthomolecular plan when I saw her, I had her change the 500 milligrams of inositol hexaniacinate that she was taking once daily to 500 milligrams of niacinamide twice daily. A follow-up on August 31, 2005, revealed significant improvements in her abilities to relate to peers and to enjoy the Arts Camp she attended. She had one "meltdown" at the camp which led to crying and the need to be alone. Despite this, she reported that she was doing really well most of the time. Prior to this visit, she had seen a psychiatrist who told the patient that her social phobia required prescription medication for the next two years. She declined the prescription, and instead agreed to have her niacinamide increased to 1,500 milligrams daily.

One of my final visits with her took place on October 29, 2005. She informed me that she was relatively stable considering the recent circumstances at home. Her schizophrenic brother had become verbally abusive and sometimes physically violent. He would not seek proper treatment. I still keep in touch with her and e-mail her mother on occasion to follow-up. She remained stable since commencing with the niacinamide treatment and she has not required the use of prescription medication.

CASE #2

The mother of case #1 came to my office on August 6, 2005. This 46-year-old female described a history of anxiety since age 7. She reported repeated bouts of anxiety and panic that became worse during the past 7 to 8 years. The recent difficulties at home due to her son's mental illness made her anxiety much worse. Daily meditation that used to be beneficial seemed to have lost its effectiveness. Physical examination revealed stage 1 hypertension, but was otherwise unremarkable. I had her complete the Beck Anxiety Inventory (BAI). Her score was 39, indicating that it was persistently high and in need of treatment. Like her daughter, she was already on a good orthomolecular plan.

I recommended that she start with 500 milligrams of niacinamide. On September 14, 2005, she returned for a follow-up. She had yet to start the niacinamide and was using diet to manage. She felt that even with the enormous amount of stress she was under, the anxiety was not preventing her from functioning adequately in her business as an interior designer. During her third visit on October 29, 2005, she reported a worsening of her anxiety since the situation with her son was not good. She began taking 500 milligrams of niacinamide during the last month. She came for another follow-up on May 24, 2006. Her stress level was still extremely high. Her son began medication sometime in December 2005, but has not shown any signs of progress. He was arrested several times and was verbally and physically abusive to her, as well as to her husband and daughter. She found that 1,500 milligrams of niacinamide at bedtime helped her relax and sleep better. She would only take 1,500 milligrams on "bad" days, and then reduce the dose to 500 milligrams on "good" days. A BAI was repeated on October 23, 2006. Her score had decreased from a 39 to a 26. She believed that the niacinamide was responsible for her improvements.

CASE #3

The husband of case #2 came to see me on February 27, 2006. He wanted me to review his orthomolecular plan and consider possible adjustments to it. His onset of stress occurred when his son was diagnosed with schizophrenia a couple of years ago. He described several bouts of heart palpitations and sleep problems following his son's diagnosis. He decided to put himself on niacinamide (1,000 milligrams at bedtime) and immediately he felt much better.

Niacinamide significantly improved his quality of life, his ability to sleep, and even helped with his creativity. He meditated regularly and felt that this helped his stress levels. Physical examination was unremarkable. I increased his niacinamide to 1,000 milligrams twice daily. I had a follow-up appointment with him on May 1, 2006. He reduced his dose of niacinamide to 1,000 milligrams at bedtime since he felt too sedated at work with the additional 1,000 milligrams. He felt much better since his stress reactions had resolved. We decided that there was no further need for follow-up visits unless he felt the need.

DISCUSSION

Hoffer has reported that a significant amount of modern mood disorders (i.e., anxiety and depression) and schizophrenia are the result of a vitamin B$_3$ dependency.[17] Both the daughter and mother suffered from chronic anxiety, and the father suffered from anxiety reactions that were precipitated by his son's mental illness.

Although each patient was taking other nutrients prior to consulting me, niacinamide added further benefit when daily dosages much greater than RDA amounts (500 to 1,500 milligrams) were prescribed. Their positive clinical responses to niacinamide supplementation confirmed my initial diagnosis of a vitamin B$_3$ dependency for each treated member of the family. Notwithstanding the clinical use of sophisticated laboratory tests (e.g., testing for individual coenzyme enzymopathies), all vitamin dependencies are confirmed in this manner.

When contrasting the clinical features of pellagra to that of a vitamin B$_3$ dependency, the main difference is that the former is characterized by more extreme manifestations. Pellagra is commonly referred to as a disease of the four Ds (diarrhea, dermatitis, dementia, and death), but more insidious symptoms develop long before the four Ds. Such symptoms include achlorhydria, anorexia, anxiety psychosis, cheilosis, constipation, delirium, dermatitis occurring on sun-exposed areas, diminished strength, glossitis, intermittent stupor, melancholia, nausea, paralysis of extremities, peripheral neuritis, stomatitis, weight loss, and vomiting.[18–22] Thus, pellagra is characterized by diverse clinical manifestations mainly involving the dermatological, gastrointestinal, and neuropsychiatric systems. This deficiency condition is prevented and cured by obtaining the minimal daily amounts (i.e., approximately 13 to 20 milligrams) of vitamin B$_3$. A vitamin B$_3$ dependency, on the other hand, would present as a subclinical (i.e., lesser) form of the deficiency or pellagrous condition. Treatment would require optimal dose quantities for its control and possible eradication. The differences between deficiency and dependency are quantitative since both conditions are manifestations of not obtaining adequate amounts of vitamin B_3. Hoffer eloquently pointed out that, "the borderline between vitamin-deficiency and vitamin-dependency conditions is merely a quantitative one when one considers prevention and cure."[23] At present, we are more apt to see patients suffering from the clinical manifestations of a vitamin B_3 dependency since profound malnutrition and starvation are rare occurrences. In this family, all the treated members had a vitamin B_3 dependency. Even though I did not formally evaluate and treat the son, he had schizophrenia—another vitamin B_3 dependent condition.[17] Hoffer hypothesized that vitamin B_3 dependency is inherited. He formulated this hypothesis from the clinical experiences he had with more than 100 families during a 10-year period.[24] If one parent is vitamin B_3 dependent, Hoffer noted that one-quarter of the children will be similarly affected. If two parents are vitamin B_3 dependent, then more three-quarters of the children will have the same dependency. Even with a good diet, Hoffer discovered that patients require 3 to 12 grams daily to effectively treat their vitamin B_3 dependency. In my report, the three family members were able to benefit from smaller daily dosages (500 to 1,500 milligrams) of vitamin B_3 than those advocated by Hoffer; they might have had more clinical benefits if they tolerated higher daily gram doses.

Why did the three members of the same family develop the same susceptibility? It is difficult to know, except that all these family members would share the same genes and environmental factors. They all experienced varying amounts of chronic severe psychosocial stress. When that combined with a history of not meeting their unique nutritional needs, a vitamin B_3 dependency developed. It appears that the "key" reason for this familial tendency resides with their schizophrenic son. It is known that patients with this disease do not manufacture adequate amounts of vitamin B_3 coenzymes (i.e., nicotinamide adenine dinucleotide; NAD) to meet their physiological requirements. In 1973, Hoffer hypothesized that schizophrenic patients likely have defects in their metabolism of tryptophan and that such defects or deficiencies in the ensuing reactions would cause a backup of indole metabolites in the precursor chain.[23] He further hypothesized that such defects would lead to an underproduction of NAD, possibly leading to an increased production of adrenochrome and its derivatives.

A recent postmortem report assessing the brain tissues of schizophrenic patients supports the notion that schizophrenic patients do not manufacture enough NAD.[25] In this report, an upregulation of the enzyme tryptophan[2,4] dioxygenase (TDO2) was found among schizophrenic patients but not among the controls. The brain tissues of the schizophrenic patients showed significant elevations of kynurenine (1.9 fold, p=0.02), TDO2 mRNA (1.7 fold, p=0.049), and the density of TDO2-positive white matter glial cells (p=0.01). In schizophrenia, the TDO2 enzyme was found to be upregulated, causing an overproduction of pathway intermediates (e.g., kynurenine). This upregulation might be responsible for the evolution of some schizophrenic symptoms. Instead of linking this upregulation to some defective factor in the TDO2 gene, the authors suggested that it might be due to a diminished niacin effect; possibly, the result of depressed production or reduced signal transduction via the niacin receptor. They recommended that niacin or its congeners are necessary regulators of this biochemical pathway and should be capable of restoring homeostasis. Since schizophrenia is a disease with a genetic basis,[26] I believe that all the family members described in this report have the same genetic fault, but with varying degrees of phenotypic expression: two had a history of chronic anxiety, one had episodes of anxiety, and one had a diagnosis of schizophrenia. All of them are vitamin B$_3$ dependent, and they all require optimal daily amounts of the vitamin to have a reasonable quality of life.

When looking beyond this genetically susceptible family, vitamin B$_3$ dependency might actually be a common problem among the entire human population. Horrobin hypothesized that schizophrenic genes have shaped humanity, provided us with important evolutionary advantages, and spread into the population.[27] Although schizophrenia affects one to two percent of the population, he feels that the genes for it are common among the entire population. The one to two percent would carry all four or more of the genes responsible for the full expression of the disease, while most other people would carry one, two, or three of these genes. Thus, the majority of the population could potentially have slight-to-severe defects in the capacity to synthesize adequate amounts of vitamin B$_3$ coenzymes from tryptophan.

This is similar to what Hoffer recently reported.[28] He believes that we now rely more on preformed vitamin B_3 from our foods since our genetic ability to synthesize niacin has declined as a conservation measure (i.e., to use more of our metabolic machinery for other purposes). Hoffer hypothesizes that this genetic loss/defect was exaggerated on or around 1800 when pure white flour was manufactured and introduced into the population. Thus, the syndrome of vitamin B_3 dependency arose—a prevalent syndrome of modern society provoked by a combination of genetic conservation, chronic psychosocial stress, and inadequate nutrition.

CONCLUSION

The family that I reported on all responded well to optimal doses of vitamin B_3. They likely suffer from a biochemical defect in the ability to synthesize vitamin B_3 coenzymes from tryptophan. When this defect occurs in the presence of chronic psychosocial stress and inadequate nutrition, a vitamin B_3 dependency will result. Schizophrenia, a vitamin B_3 dependent condition, has been identified as a disease where the production of NAD is reduced. All humans likely suffer from slight-to-severe defects in this biosynthetic pathway due to the permeation of schizophrenic genes into the population. In my humble opinion, vitamin B_3 dependency is likely to be the main cause of the majority of psychiatric problems that are encountered clinically.

ACKNOWLEDGMENTS

Written consent was obtained from these patients for publication of this report. The author would like to thank Mr. Robert Sealey for his editing suggestions.

Vitamin Deficiency, Megadoses, and Some Supplemental History

A LETTER BY WILLIAM KAUFMAN, MD, PHD, APRIL 7, 1992

Reprinted with the kind permission of Charlotte Schnee Kaufman

My attention has been called to the cover story on vitamins which appeared in the April 6, 1992, *TIME* magazine. Another major article on nutrition appeared in the March 10, 1992, *New York Times*.[1] Both articles were probably inspired by a New York Academy of Sciences meeting held in Arlington, Virginia, some weeks ago on the theme of vitamins, nutrition, and health.

I will comment on *TIME*'s feature article on vitamins a little later. Now, I'll list the vitamins that were first available commercially from 1934 through 1940 from Merck and Co. More than a half century ago, I started to use these vitamins in the successful treatment of my patients who had a variety of health problems.

1934 Ascorbic Acid (vitamin C)

1937 Thiamine Hydrochloride (vitamin B_1)

1938 Nicotinic acid (niacin)

1938 Nicotinic acid amide (niacinamide)

1938 Riboflavin (vitamin B_2)

1940 Pyridoxine Hydrochloride (vitamin B$_6$)

1940 Alpha-tocopherol (vitamin E)

1940 Vitamin K I

1940 Menadione (Has strong vitamin K activity)

1940 Calcium pantothenate (vitamin B$_5$)

Vitamins A and D were available before 1934, biotin in 1943, and beta-carotene, vitamin B$_{12}$, and folic acid soon thereafter.

Thus, none of these vitamins are "Johnny-come-lately's." In over a half century, a huge medical literature is available on the diagnosis of vitamin deficiencies and the safe therapeutic use of vitamins even when some were used in megadoses. Food as food and additional vitamins, macro- and micro-minerals supplements are often important factors in improving the health and well-being of many millions of people in this country.

DIET

First of all, food and water must serve as the basis for diets, nutrition, and the support of life provided the food can be eaten by the person, then be digested, metabolized properly and used to run the machinery of life, supply needed energy, and provide materials for cellular repair. However, it has never been proven scientifically with double-blind controls that food and water alone can provide all the nutrients in amounts that will ensure optimal long-term health to all individuals.

Humans display considerable biochemical individuality, and therefore there are also differences in nutritional needs for different people. A diet that is healthful for a non-allergic person may make another person allergic to some of the components of such a diet quite ill. Foods can greatly vary in their nutritional content at the time of purchase. Food tables will not dependably tell you the vitamin and mineral content of the food you are purchasing. Simply putting vinegar on a freshly cut coleslaw salad will cause a 53 percent loss of vitamin C content in an hour. Potatoes are a good source of vitamin C, but reconstituting dehydrated potato flakes to make mashed potatoes and keeping them on the steam table for an hour will eliminate nearly all the vitamin C. Oranges and potatoes held in storage for many months before being sold to grocery stores will have a decreased nutritional value. Cooking foods in a conventional manner can cause considerable loss of both heat labile and heat stable vitamins as well as of minerals. A nutritionally important oil has been genetically engineered out of soybeans to decrease spoilage which simultaneously decreased this type of soybean's nutritional value.

Now that preservation of some foods by exposure to heavy doses of radiation is being allowed, it would not be surprising if these foods have their nutritional value diminished plus the possibility that some of the molecular changes in the foods caused by the radiation may engender toxic substances which over time might cause ill-health. Milling wheat to make white flour causes a 70 to 80 percent loss of vitamins and minerals which, despite the so-called current "enrichment," leaves white bread inferior to whole wheat bread nutritionally because of the loss of vitamin B_6, vitamin E, chromium, manganese, and fiber, all of which have not been corrected by additional supplementation.

DOCTORS WHO BELIEVE FOOD ALONE SUPPLIES ALL NUTRITIONAL NEEDS

Doctors who believe that you can get all the nourishment including vitamins and minerals you need to sustain optimal health throughout life from food alone can be very smug. They have the equivalent of an orthodox religious belief: "food is everything." They don't have to concern themselves with the fact that the nutritional value of foods their patient eats may be greatly inferior to the listed nutritional values given in food tables. They don't have to concern themselves looking for evidence of malnutrition as long as the patient eats food that sustains his weight. The patient's diet may not include whole grains or organ meats, a diet that will cause the patient to have a chromium deficiency which deepens over time leading to important and potentially lethal forms of degenerative diseases which the "food is everything" doctor will mistakenly ascribe to aging alone. These "food is everything" doctors don't have to trouble themselves with thinking about how a patient's health can be improved over the long term by providing him with the additional beneficial vitamins, macro- and micro- mineral supplements tailored to his actual nutritional needs.

During the early part of World War II, American soldiers whose severe wound infections were treated with penicillin had to save all their urine so that the penicillin which had been excreted in their urine could be recovered and then used to treat other GI's with life-threatening wound infections. If one only considered the penicillin that was excreted in the urine and not the benefits that the soldier had in having his infection cured by penicillin, one could sneer that penicillin's only function was to give the soldier an expensive urine. If one considered only the function of penicillin in the soldier's body, one would have to marvel at the miracle of its curing a potentially lethal infection.

The two-liner attributed to Dr. Victor Herbert in *TIME*'s vitamin article—"We get all the vitamins we need in our diets. Taking supplements only gives you an expensive urine"—completely overlooks the benefits vitamin supplements can produce in our bodies before being excreted in our urine.

MOST DOCTORS ARE NUTRITIONALLY ILLITERATE

The subject of nutrition is not taught well in most medical schools. Thus, medical students, residents, doctors, and medical faculty may not even be able to recognize classic vitamin deficiencies. The University of Alabama's Dr. Butterworth referred to in the *TIME* magazine article on vitamins was a guest lecturer at Yale University School of Medicine some twenty years ago when I attended his lecture. During his talk on the nutrition of surgical patients, Dr. Butterworth showed a large number of color slides of a patient who had classic pellagra and of another patient who had classic scurvy. Not a single medical student, resident, dietician, or faculty member attending the lecture was able to make the correct diagnosis. If doctors fail to recognize classic vitamin deficiencies, these afflicted patients cannot receive prompt life-saving vitamin treatment. But even worse, medical students are not taught to recognize the enormously prevalent non-classic vitamin deficiency (and micro- and macro-mineral deficiency) disorders which impair the health and well-being of many millions of Americans. Unless such conditions are recognized, they cannot receive "curative" treatment. Furthermore, such undiagnosed non-classic vitamin (and mineral) deficiency patients instead of being given the "curative" vitamins (and minerals) they need, they often are given drugs which they do not need. Thus, in addition to unneeded pharmacologic effects, they are also exposed to the drugs' health-reducing side effects.

In 1992, what do United States medical schools teach medical students about nutrition? In her column entitled "Eating Well," which appeared in the April 1,1992, *New York Times*, Marian Burros gives a stunning answer to this question.

> Only about one-third of the 125 or so medical schools require students to take courses in nutrition. And, most of the courses are short. The one at Cornell is eight hours. . . . The University of Alabama at Birmingham is one of the exceptions, requiring 52 hours of nutrition education for its medical students. . . . The remaining two-thirds of this country's medical schools only offer elective courses.[2]

Is it any wonder that most doctors are nutritional illiterates? Is it any wonder why doctors who are nutritional illiterates often hide their lack of nutritional knowledge under the aegis "food provides all the nutrition a person will ever need"?

For the last half century, there have been recommendations that nutrition should be taught in medical schools as a required course. Currently, experts suggest that all medical schools should devote at least 40 hours to teaching medical students nutrition.

LINUS PAULING

I have had an "off and on" correspondence with Dr. Linus Pauling for several decades. He has referred to my use of niacinamide in the treatment of arthritis in some of his publications on nutrition. Some years ago, Pauling's foundation invited me to come to California to work with Dr. Pauling on cancer research. Unfortunately, at that time I could not make such a move.

I think the three reporters who made the denigrating statement in *TIME*'s vitamin article—"Certainly Linus Pauling lost much of his Nobel-Laureate luster when he began championing Vitamin C back in the 1970s as a panacea for everything from the common cold to cancer"—were very remiss in not first reading and then calling attention in their article to the important government-sponsored meeting which resulted in the following report:

Vitamin C

Biologic Functions and Relation to Cancer. Sponsored by National Cancer Institute and National Institute of Diabetes and Digestive and Kidney Diseases. September 10–12, 1990, Bethesda, Maryland

There has been considerable public interest in the possibility of a role of this vitamin (vitamin C) in cancer. In order that this debate might take place in a rigorous and informed manner, we attempted to bring together not only the latest research on basic actions, such as free-radical scavenging or enzyme functions, but also some of the basic laboratory and animal studies relating to cancer.

The well-known antioxidant and free-radical scavenging activities (of vitamin C) are discussed in the first series of papers. Because free-radical damage and formation of lipid peroxides are suspected in carcinogenesis as well as cardiovascular disease, this (vitamin C) may be important for disease prevention.

Approximately half of the symposium addressed the role of ascorbate in cancer prevention or as adjuvant in cancer therapy, primarily in animal models. In vitro studies included research on oncogenic transformations and effects on the HIV virus. Moreover, several researchers presented data that suggest a role for ascorbate in reducing the toxicity or improving the effectiveness of conventional (anti-cancer) therapies. Finally, a review is presented of all human epidemiologic studies between vitamin C and cancer prevention.

EPIDEMIOLOGIC DATA ON THE ROLE OF ASCORBIC ACID IN CANCER PREVENTION

Abstract by Gladys Block with Marilyn Menkes

The evidence for a protective effect of vitamin C or some component of fruits is strong and consistent for cancers of the esophagus, larynx, oral cavity and pancreas and there is strong evidence for cancers of the stomach and cervix. . . . While it is likely that ascorbic acid, carotenoids, folate, and other factors in fruits and vegetables act jointly, an increasingly important role for ascorbic acid (vitamin C) in cancer prevention would appear to be emerging.[3]

I cannot take the time to note all the titles of abstracts that indicate vitamin C inhibits the growth of cancer. However, to give you the flavor, I will cite just three:

1. Inhibiting effect of ascorbic acid on the growth of human mammary tumor xenografts in mice
2. Inhibition by vitamin C of incidence and severity of renal tumors induced by estradiol or diethylstilbesterol
3. Reduced incidence and tumor burden in spontaneous mouse mammary tumors and UV-induced tumors with increasing ascorbic acid

Thus, Linus Pauling's view that vitamin C has important anti-cancer properties is gaining substantial support in current laboratory and animal experiments. Where are the people who formerly ridiculed his ideas that vitamin C has anti-cancer actions?

A word about vitamin C for colds: In the early 1940s, the health service of one Midwest university prescribed vitamin C to relieve students' nasal congestion associated with colds. Although Charlotte and I go decades without having colds, we have used 250 milligram doses of vitamin C to decongest our nasal membranes when these get congested from a variety of allergies. However, this effect of vitamin C has a short half-life. Thus, it needs to be given at one-and-a-half to two-hour intervals during the day and upon awakening during the night. This keeps the nasal membranes decongested, reduces pain and discomfort, and prevents sinusitis. Usually, in 24 hours there is no further need to take vitamin C in this manner.

THE FDA

The *TIME* magazine article points out that the FDA are planning to destroy the RDA (Recommended Dietary Allowance) system as a practical guide to the amounts of various nutrients that would be required to provide decent nutrition to infants, children and adolescents, adult males of different ages, women of different ages, pregnant and lactating women. According to the article in *TIME*, the FDA plans replacing the RDA system with the so-called Reference Daily Intake (RDI).

The RDI system proposes to ignore the RDAs for different age groups and sexes.

> Instead of endorsing an allotment appropriate to ravenous fast-growing teenage males, it would simply average the RDAs for different age groups. The new figures are considerably lower, and are a better barometer of nutritional needs. Essentially they reflect the requirements of adult women.

This new system the FDA have created slashes the RDAs of vitamin A, Bs, C, E, and other nutrients from 10 to 80 percent. This will allow food manufacturers to put food products on the market legally that are much less nutritious than the ones that now have to conform to the RDA system.

There is already an enormous amount of malnutrition in this country because the large population of the poor cannot afford decent nutrition and much of their ill-health and lack of initiative is based on such malnutrition. The FDA will worsen this situation with its reduction of the RDAs.

One of the very important documents in the field of nutrition is the Bulletin of the National Research Council Number 109 November 1943 "Inadequate Diets and Nutritional Deficiencies in the United States, Their Prevalence and Significance," published by the National Research Council, National Academy of Sciences, Washington, D.C. This was the "Report of the Committee on Diagnosis and Pathology of Nutritional Deficiencies.

Food and Nutrition Board." Its conclusions and recommendations are just as applicable to today's widespread malnutrition as they were when this report was issued.

Items taken from the Summary and Conclusions of this Report

All the evidence from numerous surveys over the past ten years to the present among persons of all ages in many localities is without exception in complete agreement that inadequate diets are widespread in the nation. Although an appreciable percentage of diets failing to meet the Council's recommended dietary allowances were more than 50 percent deficient in amounts of several essential nutriments, most of the diets were less than 50 percent deficient. Accordingly, there is widespread prevalence of moderately deficient diets.

All the data from numerous surveys with new methods among persons of all ages in many regions are entirely in accord in showing that deficiency states are rife throughout the nation. Relatively few are the traditional severe acute types. Most are milder in intensity and gradual in their course. Predominantly they are subacute or chronic states: some marked, but very many mild or moderate. . . .

From this evidence it is clear that there is both a preventive and corrective problem. On the preventive side, it is evident that production of sufficient food should be maintained, and that effective distribution of proper food is needed. For the latter, it would seem advisable to give further consideration to the program of judicious enrichment of appropriate foods since this would add much to the guarantee of successful nutrition. It is also evident that diet education must be intensified and extended to the utmost and raised to new heights of effectiveness.

On the corrective side, there is need for detection and therapeutic treatment of deficiency states among the population. For this project it is necessary to disseminate the new diagnostic methods among the medical and public health professions. Foremost among the steps in this direction would be (1) preparation of a handbook on methods of detecting deficiency states (2) establishment of training centers for instruction in the medical aspects of nutrition, especially the diagnosis of deficiency states; and (3) introduction of adequate courses in nutrition, particularly its clinical aspects, into medical schools.

The conditions that existed nutritionally in the 1930s and early 1940s are just about the same as exist now in the working poor, in those on public assistance and even in those better off economically. The suggestions made about the need for prevention and curative measures are just as needed today as they were in the 1930s and 1940s. So is the need for adequate instruction in nutrition for every medical student in every medical school. So is proper nutritional enrichment of foods.

What the FDA is planning is to destroy the RDA system of nutritional standards and substituting an illogical system, RDI, that promotes a severe reduction of nutritional standards in a manner which if followed would ensure a great increase in nutritional deficiencies in the population of the United States.

What is astonishing in the *TIME* magazine article is that leaders in nutrition make such statements: "The long-term effects of high-dose supplements are still unknown, and doctors warn of dangers even in the short term," advises Dr. Walter Willett of the Harvard School of Public Health. "At this time, I don't take megadoses. I'm not ruling out that in two or three years we might change our mind."

What has been known for more than a half century is that vitamins even in properly chosen megadoses (and macro- and micro-mineral supplements) can greatly improve the long-term health and well-being of many persons eating their ordinary diets. Some of these older observations that vitamins can improve health are just being rediscovered as if they were brand-new scientific findings. The rediscoverers of old and proven observations can't believe their own findings. They call their conclusions tentative, and seem afraid of recommending vitamin megadoses that should be widely used in nutritional treatment.

If doctors want to know the long-term effects of various vitamin megadoses, they have to go back and study the literature. Since most articles and books on this subject cannot be found by electronic means, it requires that they make such a literature search manually.

The FDA's rejection of the three nutritional applications (which proposed to use vitamins to treat disease) as being premature also is part of the anti-nutritional bias. Just think: if a nutritional approach would delay myocardial infarctions by ten or fifteen years, would not this be a crippling blow to the profits of pharmaceutical companies that produce cardiac medications and cholesterol-reducing agents?

My wife, Charlotte, and I have taken megadoses of vitamins (and appropriate amounts of macro-and micro-minerals). The fact that we are alive today is attributable to the beneficial effects of this nutritional supplementation. Dr. Linus Pauling has taken megadoses of vitamin C for decades.

One fascinating thing is that from 2 to 5 percent of all hospital admissions result from severe adverse effects from prescription drugs. Yet, doctors have no compunction in prescribing these.

APPENDIX 7

Remembering
Dr. William Kaufman

BY ABRAM HOFFER, MD, PHD

I met Bill Kaufman by letter in 1958, when I received a letter in which he pointed out an error I had made in our first report on the treatment of schizophrenia with vitamin B$_3$. In our report we had written that as far as we knew, we were the first physicians to use these large gram dosages of nicotinic acid and nicotinamide. We should have known better. Bill wrote that he had been using these large gram doses since the mid-1940s. I promptly wrote to apologize and asked for his reprints. Very soon two books arrived, both dealing with his use of this vitamin for the treatment of the arthritides and diseases of aging. They were amazing, well written, very precise, very clinical, and totally surprising. I had prided myself on being honest about prior claims in medicine and decided I could make amends only by writing a review of his books. I sent my review to Bill to make sure of its accuracy and he returned it with many excellent suggestions for editorial changes. Bill was a much better writer than I was. I made these changes and then showed the article to Dr. Irwin Hilliard, the chair of the Department of Medicine at the College of Medicine, University of Saskatchewan, at Saskatoon. He read it and agreed that I should submit it for publication. It was accepted by the *Canadian Medical Association Journal*.[1] I also added a few patients of my own who, given this vitamin for other reasons, told me, to their surprise and to mine, that their joint pains and arthritis had also improved. A few years later when I was in New York I met him. We had lunch together. From that moment on we were friends and whenever I could, I visited him at his office in the big city. After he retired, we continued our relationship. I was really sorry when Charlotte, his loving wife, told me that at age 90, he had died.

This anecdote about my first connection with Bill will, I hope, make it easier for the reader to remember what Bill did, his major contribution, the proof that large doses of vitamin B_3 were safe and, even more importantly, therapeutic for the arthritides and other diseases of aging.

Bill was one of three most eminent pioneers in orthomolecular medicine, long before the word was coined by Linus Pauling in 1968. He used nicotinamide in gram doses, usually four doses each day because it is so water soluble, for a large series of cases of arthritis with great success and published his two books before 1949. His CV is described in 20 pages. He published 66 papers in medical journals, more than 100 reviews of medical books for the International Archives of Allergy and Applied Immunology, of which he was editor for many years, 25 magazine articles, as well as poetry, radio programs, and unproduced plays. He won many honors and awards, including the Tom Spies Memorial Award in Nutrition in 1978, an Award of Merit by the American College of Allergies in 1981, and was cited for his work in gerontology by the International Association of Gerontology in 1983.

Why was Bill Kaufman's important discovery rejected? Only in the past few years was his discovery examined by a controlled study and confirmed. But during the years many orthomolecular physicians observed that their patients became better, and I made his vitamin a permanent part of my arthritis regimen. I think there were several reasons his work was not recognized. First, by the time Bill began his work, the vitamin-as-prevention paradigm was fully established. This paradigm insisted that vitamins were to be used only for the classical deficiency diseases and only in small amounts, the recommended daily allowances. Bill's work contradicted both of these essential pillars of that old paradigm.

Arthritis is not a vitamin deficiency disease, or if it is, was never so recognized, and he used doses 1,000 times larger than those needed to prevent diseases such as scurvy and pellagra. The old paradigm forbade any serious examination of this work. Secondly, about the same time the corticosteroid hormones were developed, were taken on by Merck and Company and the Nobel Prize was awarded to a scientist working for the Mayo Clinic in

Rochester where the early studies of the effect of these steroids on arthritis was completed. The worldwide publicity was immense.

These steroids marked the introduction of the wonder drugs of that decade. The idea that steroids must be used became so well established that there was no time to even think about Bill's work. This is a pity, for in contrast to the steroids, which even today have a limited use in acute cases, there is nothing as efficacious for many of these patients as vitamin B3 as described by Bill 55 years ago. But the most important reason is vitamins cannot be patented. Think of the millions of arthritis sufferers who could have been helped if Bill's work had caught on, if the steroids had not been developed, and so on.

We must honor Bill because of the great pioneering research he completed, using large doses of vitamin B3, what I call optimum doses, so long ago and with such great success. He was one of four most eminent pioneers. The others were Wilfrid and Evan Shute in Ontario with vitamin E for heart disease, and Fred Klenner in North Carolina with vitamin C for viral and other killing diseases, including polio.

APPENDIX 8

Vitamin B$_3$: Niacin and Its Amide[1]

**A LETTER FOR DOCTORS AND PATIENTS BY
ABRAM HOFFER, MD, PHD, OCTOBER 1995**

The first water water-soluble were numbered in sequence according to priority of discovery. But after their chemical structure was determined they were given scientific names. The third one to be discovered was the anti-pellagra vitamin before it was shown to be niacin. But the use of the number B$_3$ did not stay in the literature very long. It was replaced by nicotinic acid and its amide (also known medically as niacin and its amide). The name was changed to remove the similarity to nicotine, a poison.

The term vitamin B$_3$ was reintroduced by my friend Bill Wilson, co-founder of Alcoholics Anonymous. We met in New York in 1960. Humphry Osmond and I introduced him to the concept of megavitamin therapy. We described the results we had seen with our schizophrenic patients, some of whom were also alcoholics. We also told him about its many other properties. It was therapeutic for arthritis, for some cases of senility, and it lowered cholesterol levels.

Bill was very curious about it and began to take niacin, 3 grams daily. Within a few weeks fatigue and depression which had plagued him for years were gone. He gave it to 30 of his close friends in AA and persuaded them to try it. Within six months he was convinced that it would be very helpful to alcoholics. Of the 30, 10 were free of anxiety, tension, and depression in one month. Another 10 were well in two months. He decided that the chemical or medical terms for this vitamin were not appropriate. He wanted to persuade members of AA, especially the doctors in AA, that this would be a useful addition to treatment, and he needed a term that could be more readily popularized. He asked me the names that had been used. I told him it was originally known as vitamin B_3. This was the term Bill wanted. In his first report to physicians in AA, he called it "The Vitamin B_3 Therapy." Thousands of copies of this extraordinary pamphlet were distributed. Eventually the name came back and today even the most conservative medical journals are using the term vitamin B_3.

Bill became unpopular with the members of the board of AA International. The medical members who had been appointed by Bill felt that he had no business messing about with treatment using vitamins. They also "knew" vitamin B_3 could not be therapeutic as Bill had found it to be. For this reason, Bill provided information to the medical members of AA outside of the National Board, distributing three of his amazing pamphlets. They are now not readily available.

Vitamin B_3 exists as the amide in nature, in nicotinamide adenine dinucleotide (NAD). Pure nicotinamide and niacin are synthetics. Niacin was known as a chemical for about 100 years before it was recognized to be vitamin B_3. It is made from nicotine, a poison produced in the tobacco plant to protect itself against its predators, but in the wonderful economy of nature which does not waste any structures, when the nicotine is simplified by cracking open one of the rings, it becomes the immensely valuable vitamin B_3.

Vitamin B_3 is made in the body from the amino acid tryptophan. On the average 1 milligram of vitamin B_3 is made from 60 milligrams of tryptophan, about 1.5 percent Since it is made in the body it does not meet the definition of a vitamin; these are defined as substances that cannot be made. It should have been classified with the amino acids, but long usage of the term vitamin has given it permanent status as a vitamin. The 1.5 percent conversion rate is a compromise based upon the conversion of tryptophan to N-methyl nicotinamide and its metabolites in human subjects. I suspect that one day in the far distant future none of the tryptophan will be converted into vitamin B_3 and it then will truly be a vitamin. According to Horwitt,[2] the amount converted is not inflexible but varies with patients and conditions. For example, women pregnant in their last three months convert tryptophan to niacin metabolites three times as efficiently as in non-pregnant females. There is also evidence that contraceptive steroids (estrogens) stimulate tryptophan oxygenase, the enzyme that converts the tryptophan into niacin.

This observation raises some interesting speculations. Women, on average, live longer than men. It has been shown for men that giving them niacin increases their longevity.[3] Is the increased longevity in women the result of greater conversion of tryptophan into niacin under the stimulus of their increase in estrogen production? Does the same phenomenon explain the decrease in the incidence of coronary disease in women?

The best-known vitamin deficiency disease is pellagra. More accurately it is a tryptophan deficiency disease since tryptophan alone can cure the early stages. Pellagra was endemic in the American South until the beginning of the last World War. It can be described by the four D's: dermatitis, diarrhea, dementia, and death. The dementia is a late-stage phenomenon. In the early stages it resembles much more the schizophrenias, and can only with difficulty be distinguished from it. The only certain method used by early pellagrologists was to give their patients small amounts of nicotinic acid. If they recovered, they diagnosed them pellagra; if they did not, they diagnosed them schizophrenia. This was good for some of their patients but was not good for psychiatry since it prevented any continuing interest in working with the vitamin for their patients who did not recover fast, but who might have done so had they given them a lot more for a much longer period of time, the way we started doing in Saskatchewan. I consider it one of the schizophrenic syndromes.

INDICATIONS

I have been involved in establishing two of the major uses for vitamin B3, apart from its role in preventing and treating pellagra. These are its action in lowering high cholesterol levels[4] and in elevating high-density lipoprotein cholesterol levels (HDL), and its therapeutic role in the schizophrenias and other psychiatric conditions. It has been found helpful for many other diseases or conditions. These are psychiatric disorders including children with learning and behavioral disorders, the addictions including alcoholism and drug addiction, the schizophrenias, some of the senile states. Its efficacy for a large number of both mental and physical conditions is an advantage to patients and to their doctors who use the vitamin, but is difficult to accept by the medical profession raised on the belief that there must be one drug for each disease, and that when any substance appears to be too effective for many conditions, it must be due entirely to its placebo effect, something like the old snake oils.

I have thought about this for a long time and have within the past year become convinced that this vitamin is so versatile because it moderates or relieves the body of the pernicious effect of chronic stress. It therefore frees the body to carry on its routine function of repairing itself more efficiently. The current excitement in medicine is the recognition that hyperoxidation, the formation of free radicals, is one of the basic damaging processes in the body. These hyperexcited molecules destroy molecules and damage tissues at the cellular level and at the tissue level.

All living tissue which depends on oxygen for respiration has to protect itself against these free radicals. Plants use one type of antioxidants and animals use another type. Fortunately, there is a wide overlap and the same antioxidants such as vitamin C are used by both plants and animals. There is growing recognition that adrenaline becoming adrenochrome plays a major role in the reactions to stress. I have elaborated on this in a further report for this journal.[5]

The catecholamines, of which adrenaline is the best-known example, and the aminochromes, of which adrenochrome is the best-known example, are intimately involved in stress reactions. Therefore, to moderate the influence of stress or to negate it, one must use compounds which prevent these substances from damaging the body. Vitamin B_3 is a specific antidote to adrenaline, and the antioxidants such as vitamin C, vitamin E, beta-carotene, selenium, and others protect the body against the effect of the free radicals by removing them more rapidly from the body. Any disease or condition which is stress related ought therefore to respond to the combined use of vitamin B_3 and these antioxidants provided they are all given in optimum doses, whether small or large as in orthomolecular therapy. I will therefore list briefly the many indications for the use of vitamin B_3.

For each condition I will describe one case to illustrate the therapeutic response. For each condition I can refer to hundreds and thousands of case histories and have already in the literature described many of them in detail.[6]

PSYCHIATRIC

Children with Learning and/or Behavioral Disorders

In 1960 seven-year-old Bruce came to see me with his father. Bruce had been diagnosed as intellectually disabled. He could not read, could not concentrate, and was developing serious behavioral problems such as cutting school without his parents' knowledge. He was being prepared for special classes for the disabled. He excreted large amounts of kryptopyrrole, the first child to be tested. I started him on nicotinamide, 1 gram three times a day. Within four months he was well. He graduated from high school, is now married, has been fully employed and has been paying income tax. He is one case out of approximately 1,500 patients I have seen since 1960.

Current treatment is more complicated as described in this journal.[7]

Organic Confusional States, Non-Alzheimer's Forms of Dementia, Electroconvulsive Therapy-Induced Memory Disturbances

In 1954 I observed how nicotinic acid relieved a severe case of post ECT amnesia in one month. Since then, I have routinely given it in conjunction with ECT to markedly decrease the memory disturbance that may occur during and after this treatment. I would never give any patient ECT without the concomitant use of nicotinic acid. It is very helpful, especially in cardio-vascular-induced forms of dementia as it reverses sludging of the red blood cell and permits proper oxygenation of the cells of the body. For further information see *Niacin Therapy in Psychiatry*.[8]

In September 1992, Mr. C., 76 years old, requested help with his memory. He was terribly absentminded. If he decided to do something, by the time he arrived where he wanted to do it he had forgotten what it was he wanted to do. His short-term memory was very poor and his long-term memory was beginning to be affected. I started him on a comprehensive vitamin program including niacinamide 1.5 grams daily. Within a month he began to improve. I added niacin to his program. By February 1993 he was normal. April 26, 1993, he told me he had been so well he had concluded he no longer needed any niacin and decreased the dose from 3.0 grams to 1.5 grams daily. He remained on the rest of the program. Soon he noted that his short-term memory was failing him again. I advised him to stay on the full dose the rest of his life.

An antidote against d-LSD,9,10 and against adrenochrome

See Abram Hoffer's *Orthomolecular Medicine for Physicians*.[6]

Alcoholism

Bill Wilson conducted the first clinical trial of the use of nicotinic acid for treating members of Alcoholics Anonymous.[9] He found that 20 out of 30 subjects were relieved of their anxiety, tension, and fatigue in two months of taking this vitamin, 1 gram three times a day. I found it very useful in treating patients who were both alcoholic and schizophrenic. The first large trial was conducted by David Hawkins, who reported a better than 90 percent recovery rate on about 90 patients. Since then, it has been used by many physicians who treat alcoholics. Dr. Russell Smith in Detroit has reported the largest series of patients.[10]

PHYSICAL

Cardiovascular

Of the two major findings made by my research group in Saskatchewan, the nicotinic acid-cholesterol connection is well known, and nicotinic acid is used worldwide as an economical, effective, and safe compound for lowering cholesterol and elevating high-density cholesterol. As a result of my interest in nicotinic acid, Altschul, Hoffer and Stephen[4] discovered that this vitamin, given in gram doses per day, lowered cholesterol levels. Since then, it was found it also elevates high-density lipoprotein cholesterol, thus bringing the ratio of total over HDL to below 5.

In the National Coronary Study, Canner[3] showed that nicotinic acid decreased mortality and prolonged life. Between 1966 and 1975, five drugs used to lower cholesterol levels were compared to placebo in 8,341 men, ages 30 to 64, who had suffered a myocardial infarction at least three months before entering the study. About 6,000 were alive at the end of the study. Nine years later, only niacin had decreased the death rate significantly from all causes. Mortality decreased 11 percent and longevity increased by two years. The death rate from cancer was also decreased.

This was a very fortunate finding because it led to the approval by the FDA of this vitamin in megadoses for cholesterol problems and opened up the use of this vitamin in large doses for other conditions as well. This occurred at a time when the FDA was doing its best not to recognize the value of megavitamin therapy. Its position has not altered over the past four decades.

Our finding opened up the second major wave of interest in vitamins. The first wave started around 1900 when it was shown that these compounds were very effective in small doses in curing vitamin deficiency diseases and in preventing their occurrence. This was the preventive phase of vitamin use. The second wave recognized that they have therapeutic properties not directly related to vitamin deficiency diseases but may have to be used in large doses. This was the second or present wave wherein vitamins are used in therapy for more than deficiency diseases. Our discovery that nicotinic acid was hypocholesterolemic compound is credited as the first paper to initiate the second wave and paved the way for orthomolecular medicine which came along several years later.

Arthritis

I first observed the beneficial effects of vitamin B₃ in 1953 and 1954. I was then exploring the potential benefits and side effects from this vitamin. Several of the patients who were given this vitamin would report after several months that their arthritis was better. At first this was a surprise since in the psychiatric history I had taken I had not asked about joint pain. This report of improvement happened so often I could not ignore it. A few years later I discovered that Prof. W. Kaufman had studied the use of this vitamin for the arthritides before 1950 and had published two books describing his remarkable results.[11] Since that time this vitamin has been a very important component of the orthomolecular regimen for treating arthritis.

The following case illustrates both the response which can occur and the complexity of the orthomolecular regimen. Patients who are early into their arthritis respond much more effectively and are not left with residual disability.

K.V. came to my office April 15, 1982. She was in a wheelchair pushed by her husband. He was exhausted, depressed, and she was one of the sickest patients I have ever seen. She weighed under 90 pounds. She sat in the chair on her ankles, which were crossed beneath her body because she was not able to straighten them out. Her arms were held in front of her, close to her body, and her fingers were permanently deformed and claw-like. She told me she had been deeply depressed for many years because of the severe pain and her major impairment. As she was being wheeled into my office, I saw how ill she was and immediately concluded there was nothing I could do for her, and had to decide how I could let her know without sending her even deeper into despair. However, I changed my mind when she suddenly said, "Dr. Hoffer, I know no one can ever cure me but if you could only help me with my pain. The pain in my back is unbearable. I just want to get rid of the pain in my back." I realized then she had a lot of determination and inner strength and that it was worthwhile to try and help her.

She began to suffer from severe pain in her joints in 1952. In 1957 it was diagnosed as arthritis. Until 1962 her condition fluctuated and then she had to go into a wheelchair some part of the day. She was still able to walk, although not for long, until 1967. In 1969 she depended on the wheelchair most of the time, and by 1973 she was there permanently. For a while she was able to propel herself with her feet. After that she was permanently dependent on help. For the three years before she saw me, she had gotten some home care but most of the care was provided by her husband. He had retired from his job when I first saw them. He provided the nursing care equivalent to four nurses on 8-hour shifts including holiday time. He had to carry her to the bathroom, bathe her, cook, and feed her. He was as exhausted as she was, but he was able to carry on.

She was severely deformed, especially her hands, suffered continuous pain, worse in her arms, and hips and her back. Her ankles were badly swollen, and she had to wear pressure bandages. Her muscles also were very painful most of the day. She was able to feed herself and to crochet with her few useful fingers, but it must have been extremely difficult. She was not able to write nor type, which she used to do with a pencil. A few months earlier she had been suicidal. On top of this severe pain and discomfort she had no appetite, and a full meal would nauseate her. Her skin was dry, she had patches of eczema, and she had white areas in her nails.

I advised her to eliminate sugar, potatoes, tomatoes, and peppers (about 10 percent of arthritics have allergic reactions to the solanine family of plants). She was to add niacinamide 500 milligrams four times daily (following the work of W. Kaufman), ascorbic acid 500 milligrams four times daily (as an anti-stress nutrient and for subclinical scurvy), pyridoxine 250 milligrams per day (found to have anti-arthritic properties by Dr. J. Ellis), zinc sulfate 220 milligrams per day (the white areas in her nails indicated she was deficient in zinc), flaxseed oil 2 tablespoons, and cod liver oil 1 table-spoon per day (her skin condition indicated she had a deficiency of omega 3 essential fatty acids). The detailed treatment of arthritis and the references are described in my book.[12]

One month later a new couple came into my room. Her husband was smiling, relaxed, and cheerful as he pushed his wife in in her chair. She was sitting with her legs dangling down, smiling as well. I immediately knew that she was a lot better. I began to ask her about her various symptoms she had had previously. After a few minutes she impatiently broke in to say, "Dr. Hoffer, the pain in my back is all gone." She no longer bled from her bowel, she no longer bruised all over her body, she was more comfortable, the pain in her back was easily controlled with aspirin and was gone from her hips (it had not helped before). She was cheerful and laughed in my office. Her heart was regular at last. I added inositol niacinate 500 milligrams four times daily to her program.

She came back June 17, 1982, and had improved even more. She was able to pull herself up from the prone position on her bed for the first time in 15 years, and she was free of depression. I increased her ascorbic acid to 1 gram four times daily and added vitamin E 800 IU. Because she had shown such dramatic improvement, I advised her she need no longer come to see me.

September 1, 1982, she called me on the telephone. I asked her how she was getting along. She said she was making even more progress. I then asked her how she had been able to get to the phone. She replied she was able to get around alone in her chair. Then she added she had not called for herself but for her husband. He had been suffering from a cold for a few days, she was nursing him, and she wanted some advice for him.

After another visit October 28, 1983, I wrote to her doctor:

Today Mrs. K.V. reported she had stayed on the whole vitamin program very rigorously for 18 months, but since that time had slacked off somewhat. She is regaining a lot of her muscle strength, can now sit in her wheelchair without difficulty, can also wheel herself around in her wheelchair but, of course, cannot do anything useful with her hands because her fingers are so awful. She would like to become more independent and perhaps could do so if something could be done about her fingers and also about her hip. I am delighted she has arranged to see a plastic surgeon to see if something can be done to get her hand mobilized once more. I have asked her to continue with the vitamins but because she had difficulty taking so many pills, she will instead take a multivitamin-multimineral supplement that can be dissolved in juice. She will also take inositol niacinate 3 grams daily.

I saw her again March 24, 1988. About four of her vertebrae had collapsed and she was suffering more pain, which was alleviated by Darvon. It had not been possible to treat her hands surgically. She had been able to eat by herself until six months before this last visit. She had been taking small amounts of vitamins. She was able to use a motorized chair. She had been depressed. I wrote to her doctor:

> She had gone off the total vitamin program about two or three years ago. It is very difficult for her to swallow, and I can understand her reluctance to carry on with this. I have therefore suggested that she take a minimal program which would include inositol niacinate 3 grams daily, ascorbic acid 1 gram three times, linseed oil 2 capsules and cod liver oil 2 capsules. Her spirits are good, and I think she is coming along considering the severe deterioration of her body as a result of the arthritis over the past few decades.

She was last seen by her doctor in the fall of 1989.

Her husband was referred. I saw him May 18, 1982. He complained of headaches and a sense of pressure about his head present for three years. This followed a series of light strokes. I advised him to take niacin 3 grams daily plus other vitamins including vitamin C. By September 1983 he was well and when seen last March 24, 1988, was still normal.

Juvenile Diabetes

Dr. Robert Elliot, Professor of Child Health Research at University of Auckland Medical School, is testing 40,000 five-year-old children for the presence of specific antibodies that indicate diabetes will develop. Those who have the antibodies will be given nicotinamide. This will prevent the development of diabetes in most of the children who are vulnerable. According to the *Rotarian* for March 1993 this project began eight years ago and has 3,200 relatives in the study. Of these, 182 had antibodies and 76 were given nicotinamide. Only 5 have become diabetic compared to 37 that would have been expected. Since 1988 over 20,100 schoolchildren have been tested. None have become diabetic compared to 47 from the untested comparable group. A similar study is underway in London, Ontario.

Cancer

Recent findings have shown that vitamin B_3 does have anti-cancer properties. This was discussed at a meeting in Texas in 1987.[13] The topic of this international conference was "Niacin, Nutrition, ADP-Ribosylation, and Cancer," and it was the 8th conference of this series.

Niacin, niacinamide, and nicotinamide adenine dinucleotide (NAD) are interconvertible via a pyridine nucleotide cycle. NAD, the coenzyme, is hydrolyzed or split into niacinamide and adenosine dinucleotide phosphate (ADP-ribose). Niacinamide is converted into niacin, which in turn is once more built into NAD. The enzyme which splits ADP is known as poly (ADP-ribose) polymerase, or poly (ADP) synthetase, or poly (ADP-ribose) transferase. Poly (ADP-ribose) polymerase is activated when strands of deoxyribonucleic acid (DNA) are broken. The enzyme transfers NAD to the ADP-ribose polymer, binding it onto a number of proteins. The poly (ADP-ribose) activated by DNA breaks helps repair the breaks by unwinding the nucleosomal structure of damaged chromatids. It also may increase the activity of DNA ligase. This enzyme cuts damaged ends off strands of DNA and increases the cell's capacity to repair itself. Damage caused by any carcinogenic factor, radiation, chemicals, is thus to a degree neutralized or counteracted.

Jacobson and Jacobson, conference organizers, hypothesized that niacin prevents cancer. They treated two groups of human cells with carcinogens. The group given adequate niacin developed tumors at a rate only 10 percent of the rate in the group deficient in niacin. Dr. M. Jacobson is quoted as saying, "We know that diet is a major risk factor, that diet has both beneficial and detrimental components. What we cannot assess at this point is the optimal amount of niacin in the diet. . . . The fact that we don't have pellagra does not mean we are getting enough niacin to confer resistance to cancer." About 20 milligrams per day of niacin will prevent pellagra in people who are not chronic pellagrins. The latter may require 25 times as much niacin to remain free of pellagra.

Vitamin B$_3$ may increase the therapeutic efficacy of anti-cancer treatment. In mice, niacinamide increased the toxicity of irradiation against tumors. The combination of normobaric carbogen with nicotinamide could be an effective method of enhancing tumor radiosensitivity in clinical radiotherapy where hypoxia limits the outcome of treatment. Chaplin, Horsman and Aoki[14] found that nicotinamide was the best drug for increasing radiosensitivity compared to a series of analogues. The vitamin worked because it enhanced blood flow to the tumor. Nicotinamide also enhanced the effect of chemotherapy. They suggested that niacin may offer some cardioprotection during long-term adriamycin chemotherapy.

Further evidence that vitamin B$_3$ is involved in cancer is the report by Nakagawa, Miyazaki, Okui, Kato, Moriyama, and Fujimura[15] that in animals there is a direct relationship between the activity of nicotinamide methyl transferase and the presence of cancer. Measuring the amount of N-methyl nicotinamide was used to measure the activity of the enzyme. In other words, in animals with cancer there is increased destruction of nicotinamide, thus making less available for the pyridine nucleotide cycle. This finding applied to all tumors except the solid tumors, Lewis lung carcinoma and melanoma B-16.

Gerson[16] treated a series of cancer patients with special diets and with some nutrients including niacin 50 milligrams 8 to 10 times per day, dicalcium phosphate with vitamin D, vitamins A and D, and liver injections. He found that all the cancer cases were benefited in that they became healthier and in many cases the tumors regressed. In a subsequent report Gerson elaborated on his diet. He now emphasized a high potassium over sodium diet, ascorbic acid, niacin, brewer's yeast, and Lugol's (aqueous) iodine. Right after the war, there was no ready supply of vitamins as there is today. I would consider the use of these nutrients in combination very original and enterprising. Dr. Gerson was the first physician to emphasize the use of multivitamins and some multiminerals. More details are in Hoffer.[17]

Additional evidence that vitamin B$_3$ is therapeutic for cancer arises from the National Coronary Study.[3]

Concentration Camp Survivors

In 1960 I planned to study the effect of nicotinic acid on a large number of aging people living in a sheltered home. A new one had been built. I approached the director of this home, Mr. George Porteous. I arranged to meet him and told him what I would like to do and why. I gave him an outline of its properties, its side effects, and why I thought it might be helpful. Mr. Porteous agreed, and we started this investigation. A short while after my first contact Mr. Porteous came to my office at University Hospital. He wanted to take nicotinic acid himself, he told me, so that he could discuss the reaction more intelligently with people living in his institution. He wanted to know if it would be safe to do so.

That fall he came again to talk to me and this time he said he wanted to tell me what had happened to him. Then I discovered he had been with the Canadian troops who had sailed to Hong Kong in 1940, had been promptly captured by the Japanese, and had survived 44 months in one of their notorious prisoner of war camps.

Twenty-five percent of the Canadian soldiers died in these camps. They suffered from severe malnutrition from starvation and nutrient deficiency. They suffered from beriberi, pellagra, scurvy, infectious diseases, and brutality from the guards.

Porteous, a physical education instructor, had been fit weighing about 190 pounds when he got there. When he returned home, he weighed only two-thirds of that. On the way home in a hospital ship the soldiers were fed and given extra vitamins in the form of rice polishings. There were few vitamins available then in tablets or capsules. He seemingly recovered but had remained very ill. He suffered from both psychological and physical symptoms. He was anxious, fearful, and slightly paranoid. Thus, he could never be comfortable sitting in a room unless he sat facing the door. This must have arisen from the fear of the guards. Physically he had severe arthritis. He could not raise his arms above his shoulders. He suffered from heat and cold sensitivity. In the morning he needed his wife's help in getting out of bed and to get started for the day. He had severe insomnia. For this he was given barbiturates in the evening and to help awaken him in the morning, he was given amphetamines.

Later I read the growing literature on the Hong Kong veterans and there is no doubt they were severely and permanently damaged. They suffered from a high death rate due to heart disease, crippling arthritis, blindness, and a host of other conditions.

Having outlined his background he then told me that two weeks after he started to take nicotinic acid, 1 gram after each meal, he was normal. He was able to raise his arms to their full extension, and he was free of all the symptoms which had plagued him for so long. When I began to prepare my report,[18] I obtained his Veterans Administration Chart. It came to me in two cardboard boxes and weighed over ten pounds, but over 95 percent of it was accumulated before he started on the vitamin. For the ten years after he started on the vitamin there was very little additional material. One could judge the efficacy of the vitamin by weighing the chart paper before and after he started on it. Porteous remained well as long as he stayed on the vitamin until his death when he was Lieutenant Governor of Saskatchewan. In 1962, after having been well for two years, he went on a holiday to the mountains with his son and he forgot to take his nicotinic acid with him. By the time he returned home almost the entire symptomatology had returned.

Porteous was enthusiastic about nicotinic acid and began to tell all his friends about it. He told his doctor. His doctor cautioned him that he might damage his liver. Porteous replied that if it meant he could stay as well as he was until he died from a liver ailment, he would still not go off it. His doctor became an enthusiast as well and within a few years had started over 300 of his patients on the vitamin. He never saw any examples of liver disease from nicotinic acid.

I have treated over 20 prisoners from Japanese camps and from European concentration camps since then with equally good results. I estimated that one year in these camps was equivalent to four years of aging, i.e., four years in camp would age a prisoner the equivalent of 16 years of normal living.

George Porteous wanted every prisoner of war from the eastern camps treated as he had been. He was not successful in persuading the Government of Canada that nicotinic acid would be very helpful, so he turned to fellow prisoners, both in Canada (Hong Kong Veterans) and to American Ex-Prisoners of War. These American veterans suffered just as much as had the Canadian soldiers since they were treated in exactly the same abysmal way. The ones who started on the vitamin showed the same response. Recently one of these soldiers, a retired officer, wrote to me after being on nicotinic acid 20 years that he felt great, owed it to the vitamin, and that when his arteries were examined during a simple operation, they were completely normal. He wrote, "About two years ago, I was hit, was bleeding down the neck. The MDs took the opportunity to repair me. They said the arteries under the ears look like they had never been used."

There is an important lesson from the experiences of these veterans and their response to megadoses of nicotinic acid. This is that every human exposed to severe stress and malnutrition for a long enough period of time will develop a permanent need for large amounts of this vitamin and perhaps for several others.

This is happening on a large scale in Africa, where the combination of starvation, malnutrition, and brutality is reproducing the conditions suffered by the veterans. Those who survive will be permanently damaged biochemically, and will remain a burden to themselves and to the community where they live. Will society have the good sense to help them recover by making this vitamin available to them in optimum doses?

DOSES

The optimum dose range is not as wide as it is for ascorbic acid, but it is wide enough to require different recommendations for different classes of diseases. As is always the case with nutrients, each individual must determine their own optimum level. With nicotinic acid this is done by increasing the dose until the flush (vasodilation) is gone, or is so slight it is not a problem.

One can start with as low a dose as 100 milligrams taken three times each day after meals and gradually increase it. I usually start with 500 milligrams each dose and often will start with 1 gram per dose especially for cases of arthritis, for schizophrenics, for alcoholics, and for a few elderly patients. However, with elderly patients it is better to start small and work it up slowly.

No person should be given nicotinic acid without explaining to them that they will have a flush which will vary in intensity from none to very severe. If this is explained carefully, and if they are told that in time the flush will not be a problem, they will not mind. The flush may remain too intense for a few patients and the nicotinic acid may have to be replaced by a slow-release preparation or by some of the esters, for example, inositol niacinate. The latter is a very good preparation with very little flush and most find it very acceptable even when they were not able to accept the nicotinic acid itself. It is rather expensive but with quantity production the price might come down.

The flush starts in the forehead with a warning tingle. Then it intensifies. The rate of the development of the flush depends upon so many factors it is impossible to predict what course it will follow.

The following factors decrease the intensity of the flush: a cold meal, taking it after a meal, taking aspirin before, using an antihistamine in advance.

The following factors make the flush more intense: a hot meal, a hot drink, an empty stomach, chewing the tablets and the rate at which the tablets break down in liquid.

From the forehead and face the flush travels down the rest of the body, usually stopping somewhere in the chest but may extend to the toes. With continued use the flush gradually recedes and eventually may be only a tingling sensation in the forehead. If the person stops taking the vitamin for a day or more the sequence of flushing will be re-experienced. Some people never do flush and a few only begin to flush after several years of taking the vitamin. With nicotinamide there should be no flushing, but I have found that about 2 percent will flush. This may be due to rapid conversion of the nicotinamide to nicotinic acid in the body.

When the dose is too high for both forms of the vitamin the patients will suffer from nausea at first, and then if the dose is not reduced it will lead to vomiting. These side effects may be used to determine what is the optimum dose. When they do occur, the dose is reduced until it is just below the nausea level. With children the first indication may be loss of appetite. If this does occur the vitamin must be stopped for a few days and then may be resumed at a lower level. Very few can take more than 6 grams per day of the nicotinamide. With nicotinic acid it is possible to go much higher. Many schizophrenics have taken up to 30 grams per day with no difficulty. The dose will alter over time and if on a dose where there were no problems, they may develop in time. Usually this indicates that the patient is getting better and does not need as much. I have divided all patients who might benefit from vitamin B$_3$ into the following categories.

Category 1. These are people who are well or nearly well, and have no obvious disease. They are interested in maintaining their good health or in improving it. They may be under increased stress. The optimum dose range varies between 0.5 to 3 grams daily. The same doses apply to nicotinamide.

Category 2. Everyone under physiological stress, such as pregnancy and lactation, suffering from acute illness such as the common cold or flu, or other diseases that do not threaten death. All the psychiatric syndromes are included in this group including the schizophrenias and the senile states. It also includes the very large group of people with high blood cholesterol levels or low HDL when it is desired to restore these blood values to normal. The dose range is 1 gram to 10 grams daily. For nicotinamide the range is 1 ½ grams to 6 grams.

Nicotinamide does not affect cholesterol levels.

SIDE EFFECTS

Here are Dr. John Marks' conclusions:[19]

A tingling or flushing sensation in the skin after relatively large doses (in excess of 75 milligrams) of nicotinic acid is a rather common phenomenon. It is the result of dilation of the blood vessels that is one of the natural actions of nicotinic acid and one for which it is used therapeutically. Whether this should therefore be regarded as a true adverse reaction is a moot point. The reaction clears regularly after about 20 minutes and is not harmful to the individual. It is very rare for this reaction to occur at less than three times the RDA, even in very sensitive individuals. In most people much larger quantities are required. The related substance nicotinamide only very rarely produces this reaction and in consequence this is the form generally used for vitamin supplementation.

Doses of 200 milligrams to 10 grams daily of the acid have been used therapeutically to lower blood cholesterol levels under medical control for periods of up to 10 years or more and though some reactions have occurred at these very high dosages, they have rapidly responded to cessation of therapy, and have often cleared even when therapy has been continued.

In isolated cases, transient liver disorders, rashes, dry skin, and excessive pigmentation have been seen. The tolerance to glucose has been reduced in diabetics and patients with peptic ulcers have experienced increased pain. No serious reactions have been reported however even in these high doses. The available evidence suggests that 10 times the RDA is safe (about 100 milligrams).

Dr. Marks is cautious about recommending that doses of 100 milligrams are safe. In my opinion, based upon 40 years of experience with this vitamin the dose ranges I have recommended above are safe. However, with the higher doses medical supervision is necessary.

Jaundice is very rare. Fewer than ten cases have been reported in the medical literature. I have seen none in ten years. When jaundice does occur, it is usually an obstructive type and clears when the vitamin is discontinued. I have been able to get schizophrenic patients back on nicotinic acid after the jaundice cleared and it did not recur.

Four serious cases have been reported, all involving a sustained-release preparation. Mullin, Greenson, and Mitchell[20] reported that a 44-year-old man was treated with crystalline nicotinic acid, 6 grams daily, and after 16 months was normal. He then began to take a sustained-release preparation, same dose. Within three days he developed nausea, vomiting, abdominal pain, dark urine. He had severe hepatic failure and required a liver transplant. Henkin, Johnson, and Segrest found three patients who developed hepatitis with sustained-release nicotinic acid. When this was replaced with crystalline nicotinic acid there was no recurrent liver damage.[21]

Since jaundice in people who have not been taking nicotinic acid is fairly common it is possible there is a random association. The liver function tests may indicate there is a problem when in fact there is not. Nicotinic acid should be stopped for five days before the liver function tests are given. One patient who had no problem with nicotinic acid for lowering cholesterol switched to the slow-release preparations and became ill. When he resumed the original nicotinic acid, he was well again with no further evidence of liver dysfunction. I have not seen any cases reported anywhere else. I have described much more fully the side effects of this vitamin elsewhere.[22]

Inositol hexaniacinate is an ester of inositol and nicotinic acid. Each inositol molecule contains six nicotinic acid molecules. This ester is broken down slowly in the body. It is as effective as nicotinic acid and is almost free of side effects. There is very little flushing, gastrointestinal distress, and other uncommon side effects. Inositol, considered one of the lesser important B vitamins, does have a function in the body as a messenger molecule and may add something to the therapeutic properties of the nicotinic acid.

CONCLUSION

Vitamin B_3 is a very effective nutrient in treating a large number of psychiatric and medical diseases but its beneficial effect is enhanced when the rest of the orthomolecular program is included. The combination of vitamin B_3 and the antioxidant nutrients is a great anti-stress program.

Contributor Biographies

Nick Fortino, PhD, has keen interest in niacin research. Andrew Saul was pleased to serve on Nick's PhD committee.

William Kaufman, MD, PhD, was so successful treating osteo- and rheumatoid-arthritis that he received mail simply addressed to "The Arthritis Doctor, Connecticut." Dr. Kaufman is a member of the Orthomolecular Medicine Hall of Fame.

Stephen McConnell is a lipidemiologist and researcher with an MSc in Cardiovascular and Renal Pathophysiology.

Jonathan Prousky, ND, is professor and Chief Naturopathic Medical Officer at the Canadian College of Naturopathic Medicine and author of many papers and books. Dr. Prousky is a member of the Orthomolecular Medicine Hall of Fame.

Joseph Mercola, DO, is a very well-known author, who has had the largest Internet presence, for the longest time, of any physician.

William B. Parsons, Jr., MD, was a prominent niacin researcher working at the Mayo Clinic. He is the author of *Cholesterol Control Without Diet: The Niacin Solution.*

Richard A. Passwater, PhD, is the author of *Supernutrition*, one of the first health books Andrew Saul ever read. Dr. Passwater is a member of the Orthomolecular Medicine Hall of Fame.

W. Todd Penberthy, PhD, is a biomedical researcher and continuing medical education writer who prepares courses for physicians to maintain their certification. https://https://www.cmescribe.com/resume/ He is a Contributing Editor for the *Orthomolecular Medicine News Service*.

Robert G. Smith, PhD, is Research Associate Professor of Neuroscience at the University of Pennsylvania Perelman School of Medicine and is Associate Editor of the *Orthomolecular Medicine News Service*. He is a specialist in retinal anatomy and physiology.

References

Foreword

1. Brown, B. (2006). "Niaspan® in the management of dyslipidaemia: The evidence." *European Heart Journal*, Supplement 8.

2. Villines, T.C., Stanek, E.J., Devine, P.J., Turco, M., Miller, M., Weissman, N.J., Griffen, L., and Taylor, A.J. (2010). "The ARBITER 6-HALTS Trial (Arterial Biology for the Investigation of the Treatment Effects of Reducing Cholesterol 6-HDL and LDL Treatment Strategies in Atherosclerosis): final results and the impact of medication adherence, dose, and treatment duration." *J Am Coll Cardiol* 55, 2721–2726.

3. Coleman, M. (2005). "Axon degeneration mechanisms: commonality amid diversity." *Nat Rev Neurosci 6*, 889–898.

4. Adalbert, R., Gillingwater, T.H., Haley, J.E., Bridge, K., Beirowski, B., Berek, L., Wagner, D., Grumme, D., Thomson, D., Celik, A., et al. (2005). "A rat model of slow Wallerian degeneration (WldS) with improved preservation of neuromuscular synapses." *Eur J Neurosci* 21, 271–277.

5. Araki, T., Sasaki, Y., and Milbrandt, J. (2004). "Increased nuclear NAD biosynthesis and SIRT1 activation prevent axonal degeneration." *Science* 305, 1010–1013.

6. Penberthy, W.T., and Tsunoda, I. (2009). "The importance of NAD in multiple sclerosis." *Curr. Pharm. Des.* 15, 64–99.

7. Lin, S.J., Defossez, P.A., and Guarente, L. (2000). "Requirement of NAD and SIR2 for life-span extension by calorie restriction in Saccharomyces cerevisiae." *Science* 289, 2126–2128.

8. Penberthy, W. Todd, and Kristian B. Axelsen (2022). "Table of NAD-Utilizing Enzymes."

9. Plascencia-Villa, G., and Perry, G. (2020). "Status and future directions of clinical trials in Alzheimer's disease." *Int Rev Neurobiol* 154, 3–50.

10. Moutinho, M., Puntambekar, S.S., Tsai, A.P., Coronel, I., Lin, P.B., Casali, B.T., Martinez, P., Oblak, A.L., Lasagna-Reeves, C.A., Lamb, B.T., et al. (2022). "The

niacin receptor HCAR2 modulates microglial response and limits disease progression in a mouse model of Alzheimer's disease." *Sci Transl Med* 14, eabl7634.

11. Manjarrez, Alejandra. "Could Vitamin Supplementation Help Alzheimer's Patients?" | *The Scientist Magazine*® https://www.the-scientist.com/news-opinion /could-vitamin-supplementation-help-alzheimer-s-patients-69897.

12. Sarkar, S., Yang, R., Mirzaei, R., Rawji, K., Poon, C., Mishra, M.K., Zemp, F.J., Bose, P., Kelly, J., Dunn, J.F., et al. (2020). "Control of brain tumor growth by reactivating myeloid cells with niacin." *Sci Transl Med* 12, eaay9924.

13. Rawji, K.S., Mishra, M.K., and Yong, V.W. (2016). "Regenerative Capacity of Macrophages for Remyelination." *Frontiers in Cell and Developmental Biology* 4, 47.

14. Guyton, J.R., and Bays, H.E. (2007). "Safety considerations with niacin therapy." *Am J Cardiol* 99, 22C-31C.

15. Pirinen, E., Auranen, M., Khan, N.A., Brilhante, V., Urho, N., Pessia, A., Hakkarainen, A., Kuula, J., Heinonen, U., Schmidt, M.S., et al. (2020). "Niacin Cures Systemic NAD+ Deficiency and Improves Muscle Performance in Adult-Onset Mitochondrial Myopathy." *Cell Metab* 31, 1078-1090.e5.

16. Kashyap, M.L., Ganji, S., Nakra, N.K., and Kamanna, V.S. (2019). "Niacin for treatment of nonalcoholic fatty liver disease (NAFLD): novel use for an old drug?" *J Clin Lipidol* 13, 873–879.

17. Shi, H., Enriquez, A., Rapadas, M., Martin, E.M.M.A., Wang, R., Moreau, J., Lim, C.K., Szot, J.O., Ip, E., Hughes, J.N., et al. (2017). "NAD Deficiency, Congenital Malformations, and Niacin Supplementation." *N Engl J Med* 377, 544–552.

Chapter 1: Why Should You Read This Book?

1. Kuhn, T. S. *The Structure of Scientific Revolutions*. Chicago, IL: Chicago University Press, 1962.

2. Moore, T. J. *Deadly Medicine: Why Tens of Thousands of Heart Patients Died in America's Worst Drug Disaster.* New York, NY: Simon and Schuster, 1995.

3. Abramson, J. *Overdo$ed America: The Broken Promise of American Medicine.* New York, NY: Harper Perennial, 2005.

4. Dean, C., T. Tuck. *Death by Modern Medicine.* Belleville, ON: Matrix Vérité Media, 2005.

5. Pauling, L. *How to Live Longer and Feel Better.* New York, NY: W.H. Freeman, 1986.

6. Pauling, L. "Orthomolecular Psychiatry." *Science* 160 (1968): 265–271.

7. Hoffer, A., A. W. Saul. *Orthomolecular Medicine for Everyone: Megavitamin Therapeutics for Families and Physicians.* Laguna Beach, CA: Basic Health Publications, 2008.

8. Ibid.

9. Ibid.

10. Williams, R. *Biochemical Individuality.* New York, NY: W. H. Freeman, 1956.

11. Foster, H. D. *Reducing Cancer Mortality: A Geographical Perspective.* Victoria, BC: Western Geographical Press, 1986.

12. Foster, H. D. *What Really Causes Alzheimer's Disease.* Victoria, BC: Trafford Publishing, 2004.

13. University of Maryland Medical Center, *Sulfur.*

14. Williams, S.R. *Nutrition and Diet Therapy,* 6th ed., St. Louis, MO: Times-Mirror/ Mosby, 1989: 239.

Chapter 2: What Is Niacin?

1. Gutierrez, D. "Niacin May Lower the Risk of Heart Disease." NaturalNews.com (Nov 7, 2008): http://www.naturalnews.com/024745_niacin_cholesterol _research.html

2. Penberthy, W T. "Nicotinic Acid-Mediated Activation of Both Membrane and Nuclear Receptors towards Therapeutic Glucocorticoid Mimetics for Treating Multiple Sclerosis." *PPAR Res* (2009): 853707.

3. Penberthy, W. T., I. Tsunoda. "The Importance of NAD in Multiple Sclerosis." *Curr Pharm Des* 15(1) (2009): 64–99. Review.

4. Penberthy, W. T. "Nicotinamide Adenine Dinucleotide Biology and Disease." *Curr Pharm Des* 15(1) (2009): 1–2.

5. Hoffer, A. "Patentable vs. Non-patentable Treatment," *J Orthomolecular Med* 14 (2nd Quarter 1999): Editorial.

6. Hoffer, A. "Megavitamin B₃ Therapy for Schizophrenia." *Can Psychiat Assoc J* 16 (1971): 499–504.

7. Dalton, T. A., R. S. Berry. "Hepatotoxicity Associated with Sustained-release Niacin." *Am J Med* 93(1) (Jul 1992): 102–4.

8. Henkin, Y., A. Oberman, D. C. Hurst, et al. "Niacin Revisited: Clinical Observations on an Important But Underutilized Drug." *Am J Med* 91 (1991): 239–246.

9. Henkin, Y., K. C. Johnson, J. P. Segrest. "Rechallenge With Crystalline Niacin After Drug-induced Hepatitis from Sustained-release Niacin." *J Am Med Assoc* 264 (1990): 241–243.

10. McKenney, J. M., J. D. Proctor, S. Harris, et al. "A Comparison of the Efficacy and Toxic Effects of Sustained- Vs. Immediate-release Niacin in Hypercholesterolemic Patients." *J Am Med Assoc* 271 (1994): 672–677.

11. Guyton, J. R., H. E. Bays. "Safety Considerations with Niacin Therapy." *Am J Cardiol* 19;99(6A) (Mar 2007): 22C–31C.

12. Loriaux, S. M., J. B. Deijen, J. F. Orlebeke, et al. "The Effects of Nicotinic Acid and Xanthinol Nicotinate on Human Memory in Different Categories of Age. A Double Blind Study." *Psychopharmacology (Berl)* 87(4) (1985): 390–5.

13. Perricone, N. V., D. Bagchi, B. Echard, et al. "Blood Pressure Lowering Effects of Niacin-bound Chromium (III) (NBC) in Sucrose-fed Rats: Renin-angiotensin System." *J Inorg Biochem* 102(7) (Jul 2008): 1541–8.

14. Preuss, H. G., D. Wallerstedt, N. Talpur, et al. "Effects of Niacin-bound Chromium and Grape Seed Proanthocyanidin Extract on the Lipid Profile of Hypercholesterolemic Subjects: A Pilot Study." *J Med* 31(5–6) (2000): 227–46.

15. Preuss, H. G., B. Echard, N. V. Perricone, et al. "Comparing Metabolic Effects of Six Different Commercial Trivalent Chromium Compounds." *J Inorg Biochem* 102(11) (Nov 2008): 1986–90.

16. Preuss, H. G., S. T. Jarrell, R. Scheckenbach, et al. "Comparative Effects of Chromium, Vanadium and Gymnema Sylvestre on Sugar-induced Blood Pressure Elevations in SHR." *J Am Coll Nutr* 17(2) (Apr 1998): 116–23.

Chapter 3. How Niacin Therapy Began

1. Elmore, J. G., A. R. Feinstein. "Joseph Goldberger: An Unsung Hero of American Clinical Epidemiology." *Ann Intern Med* 121(5) (Sep 1994): 372–5.

2. National Institutes of Health, Office of History. "Dr. Joseph Goldberger & the War on Pellagra." http://history.nih.gov/exhibits/goldberger/index.html

3. Wittenborn, J. R. "A Search for Responders to Niacin Supplementation." *Arch Gen Psychiat* 31 (1974): 547–552.

Chapter 4. How Niacin Works, and Why We Need More of It

1. Merialdi, M., L. E. Caulfield, N. Zavaleta, et al. "Randomized Controlled Trial of Prenatal Zinc Supplementation and the Development of Fetal Heart Rate." *Am J Obstet Gynecol* 190 (2004): 1106–1112.

2. Wu, G., F. W. Baze, T. A. Cudd, et al. "Maternal Nutrition and Fetal Development." *J Nut* 134 (2004): 2169–2172.

3. Ibid.

4. Hetzel, B. S. *The Story of Iodine Deficiency: An International Challenge in Nutrition.* Oxford, ENG: Oxford University Press, 1989.

5. Tan, J., R. Li, W. Zhu. "Medical Geography." In: M. Ren, C. Lin, eds. *Recent Development of Geographical Science in China.* Beijing: Science Press, 1990. 259–279.

6. Ibid.

7. Wu, Baze, Cudd, et al. "Maternal Nutrition." *J Nut* 134: 2169–2172.

8. Foster, H. D., A. Hoffer. "The Two Faces of L-Dopa: Benefits and Adverse Side-effects in the Treatment of Encephalitis Lethargica, Parkinson's Disease,

Multiple Sclerosis and Amyotrophic Lateral Sclerosis." *Med Hypotheses* 62(2) (2004): 177–181.

9. Foster, H. D. *What Really Causes Multiple Sclerosis.* Victoria, BC: Trafford Publishing, 2007.

10. Wu, Baze, Cudd, et al. "Maternal Nutrition." *J Nut* 134: 2169–2172.

11. Hartl, D. L., D. Freifelder, L. Synder. *Basic Genetics.* Boston, MA: Jones et Bartlett, 1988.

12. Ames, B. N., I. Elson-Schwab, E. A. Silver. "High-dose Vitamin Therapy Stimulates Variant Enzymes with Decreased Coenzyme Binding Affinity (Increased K_m): Relevance to Genetic Disease and Polymorphisms." *Am J Clin Nutr* 75 (2002): 616–658.

13. Ibid.

14. Ibid.

15. Barleer, G. W., G. L. Spaeth. "The Successful Treatment of Homocystinuria With Pyridoxine." *J Pediatr* 75 (1969): 463–478.

16. Neu, H. C. "The Crisis in Antibiotic Resistance." *Science* 257(5073) (1992): 1064–1073.

17. Foster, H. D. "Host-pathogen Evolution: Implications for the Prevention and Treatment of Malaria, Myocardial Infarction and AIDS." *Med Hypotheses.* 2008; 70: 21–25.

18. Mizuno, Y., S. I. Kawazu, S. Kano, et al. "In Vitro Uptake of Vitamin A by Plasmodium Falciparum." *Ann Trop Med Parasit* 97(3) (2003): 237–243.

19. Andrews, K. T., T. N. Tran, N. C. Wheatley, et al. "Targeting Histone Deacetylase Inhibitors for Anti-malarial Therapy." *Curr Top Med Chem* 9(3) (2009): 292–308.

20. Shankar, A. H., B. Genton, R. D. Semba, et al. "Effects of Vitamin A Supplementation on Morbidity Due to Plasmodium Falciparum in Young Children in Papua New Guinea: A Randomized Trial." *Lancet* 354(9174) (1999): 203–209.

21. Foster, H. D. "Coxsackie B Virus and Myocardial Infarction." *Lancet* 359(9308) (2002): 804.

22. Cermelli, C., M. Vincet, E. Scaltriti, et al. "Selenium Inhibition of Coxsackie B_5 Replication on the Etiology of Keshan Disease." *J Trace Elem Med Bio* 16(1) (2002): 41–46.

23. Kuklinski, B., E. Weissenbacher, A. Fähnrich. "Coenzyme Q_{10} and Antioxidants in Acute Myocardial Infarction." *Mol Aspects Med* 15(Suppl) (1994): 143–147.

24. Foster, H. D. *What Really Causes AIDS.* Victoria, BC: Trafford Publishing, 2002.

25. Namulema, E., J. Sparling, H. D. Foster. "Nutritional Supplements Can Delay the Progress of AIDS in HIV-infected Patients: Results from a Double-blinded, Clinical Trial at Mengo Hospital, Kampala, Uganda." *J Orthomolecular Med* 22(3) (2007): 129–136.

26. Xu, Q., C. G. Parks, L. A. Deroo, R. M. Cawthor, et al. "Multivitamin Use and Telomere Length in Women." *Am J Clin Nutr* 89(6) (2009): 1857–1863.

27. Bize, P., F. Criscuolo, N. B. Metcalfe, et al. "Telomere Dynamics Rather Than Age Predict Life Expectancy in the Wild." *P Biol Sci/R Soc.* 276(1662) (2009): 1679–1683.

28. Hoffer, A., H. D. Foster. *Feel Better, Live Longer with Vitamin B3: Nutrient Deficiency and Dependency.* Toronto, ON: CCNM Press, 2007.

29. Miller, C.L., J. R. Dulay. "The High-affinity Niacin Receptor HM74A is Decreased in the Anterior Cingulate Cortex of Individuals with Schizophrenia." *Brain Res Bull* 77(1) (Sep 5, 2008): 33–41.

30. Horrobin, D. *The Madness of Adam and Eve. How Schizophrenia Shaped Humanity.* London, ENG: Bantam Press, 2001.

31. Huxley, J., E. Mayr, H. Osmond, A. Hoffer. "Schizophrenia as a Genetic Morphism." *Nature* 204 (1964): 220–221.

32. Foster, Hoffer. "The Two Faces of L-Dopa." *Med Hypothesis* 62: 177–181.

33. Cleave, T.L. *Diabetes, Coronary Thrombosis, and the Saccharine Disease.* Bristol, ENG: John Wright & Sons, 1966.

34. Miller, Dulay. "The High-affinity Niacin Receptor HM74A." *Brain Res Bull* 77(1): 33–41.

35. Hoffer, A., H. D. Foster. *Feel Better, Live Longer With Niacin.* Toronto, ON: CCNM Press, 2007.

36. Hawthorn, T. Obituary. *Globe and Mail.* Toronto, ON: November 29, 2008.

37. Green, G. "Subclinical Pellagra." In: D. Hawkins, L. Pauling, eds. *Orthomolecular Psychiatry Treatment of Schizophrenia.* San Francisco, CA: WH Freeman, 1973. 411–433.

38. Kaufman, W. *The Common Form of Niacin Amide Deficiency Disease: Aniacinamidosis.* New Haven, CT: Yale University Press, 1943.

39. Kaufman, W. "Niacinamide: A Most Neglected Vitamin." *J Int Acad Prev Med* 8 (1983): 5–25.

40. Miller, Dulay. "The High-affinity Niacin Receptor HM74A." *Brain Res Bull* 77(1): 33–41.

41. Owen MJ, Sawa A, Mortensen PB. Schizophrenia. *Lancet.* 2016 Jul 2; 388:86-97. https://www.ncbi.nlm.nih.gov/pubmed/26777917.

42. Ledford, H. FDA advisers back gene therapy for rare form of blindness. Nature 550, 314 (2017). https://doi.org/10.1038/nature.2017.22819

43. Hoffer A, Osmond H, Smythies J. Schizophrenia; a new approach. II. Result of a year's research. J Ment Sci. 1954 Jan;100(418):29-45. doi: 10.1192/bjp.100.418.29. PMID: 13152519.

44. Hoffer A, Osmond H. Treatment of schizophrenia with nicotinic acid: a ten-year follow-up. *Acta Psychiat Scand* 1964, 40: 171–189. https://www.ncbi.nlm.nih.gov /pubmed/14235254.

45. Niacin and Schizophrenia: History and Opportunity. http://orthomolecular.org /resources/omns/v10n18.shtml.

46. To Give Credit Where Credit is Due. http://orthomolecular.org/resources /omns/v13n05.shtml.

47. Abram Hoffer Centenary. http://orthomolecular.org/resources/omns/v13n19 .shtml.

48. Pauling, L. Orthomolecular psychiatry. Varying the concentrations of substances normally present in the human body may control mental disease. *Science.* 1968 Apr 19;160:265-271. https://www.ncbi.nlm.nih.gov/pubmed/5641253 and https:// profiles.nlm.nih.gov/ps/access/MMBBJQ.pdf.

49. Xu XJ, Jiang GS. Niacin-respondent subset of schizophrenia—a therapeutic review. *Eur Rev Med Pharmacol Sci.* 2015;19:988-997. https://www.ncbi.nlm.nih. gov/pubmed/25855923.

50. Hoffer, A. *Adventures in Psychiatry: The Scientific Memoirs of Dr. Abram Hoffer.* KOS Publishing, 2005. ISBN-13: 978-0973194562.

51. Smesny S, Berger G, Rosburg T, et al. Potential use of the topical niacin skin test in early psychosis—a combined approach using optical reflection spectroscopy and a descriptive rating scale. *Psychiatr Res.* 2003 May-Jun;37:237-247. https://www .ncbi.nlm.nih.gov/pubmed/12650743.

52. Messamore, E. Niacin subsensitivity is associated with functional impairment in schizophrenia. *Schizophr Res.* 2012 May;137(1-3):180-4. https://www.ncbi.nlm. nih.gov/pubmed/22445461.

53. Lien YJ, Huang SS, Liu CM, et al. A genome-wide quantitative linkage scan of niacin skin flush response in families with schizophrenia. *Schizophr Bull.* 2013 Jan;39:68-76. https://www.ncbi.nlm.nih.gov/pubmed/21653277.

54. Nilsson BM, Holm G, Hultman CM, Ekselius L. Cognition and autonomic function in schizophrenia: inferior cognitive test performance in electrodermal and niacin skin flush non-responders. *Eur Psychiatry.* 2015 Jan;30:8-13. https://www. ncbi.nlm.nih.gov/pubmed/25169443.

55. Berger GE, Smesny S, Schäfer MR, et al. Niacin Skin Sensitivity Is Increased in Adolescents at Ultra-High Risk for Psychosis. *PLoS One.* 2016 Feb 19;11(2):e0148429. https://www.ncbi.nlm.nih.gov/pubmed/26894921.

56. Yao JK, Dougherty GG Jr, Gautier CH, Haas GL, Condray R, Kasckow JW, Kisslinger BL, Gurklis JA, Messamore E. Prevalence and Specificity of the Abnormal Niacin Response: A Potential Endophenotype Marker in Schizophrenia. *Schizophr Bull.* 2016 Mar;42(2):369-376. https://www.ncbi.nlm.nih.gov/ pubmed/26371338.

57. Sun L, Yang X, Jiang J, et al. Identification of the Niacin-Blunted Subgroup of Schizophrenia Patients from Mood Disorders and Healthy Individuals in Chinese Population. *Schizophr Bull.* 2017 Oct 25. https://www.ncbi.nlm.nih.gov /pubmed/29077970.

58. Langbein K, Schmidt U, Schack S, et al. State marker properties of niacin skin sensitivity in ultra-high-risk groups for psychosis—An optical reflection spectroscopy study. *Schizophr Res.* 2017 Jun 8. pii: S0920-9964(17)30335-3. https://www. ncbi.nlm.nih.gov/pubmed/28602647.

59. Ross, BM. Methylnicotinate stimulated prostaglandin synthesis in patients with schizophrenia: A preliminary investigation. *Prostaglandins Leukot Essent Fatty Acids.* 2017 May 19. pii: S0952-3278(16)30227-7. https://www.ncbi.nlm.nih.gov/ pubmed/28552466.

60. Messamore, E. The niacin response biomarker as a schizophrenia endophenotype: A status update. *Prostaglandins Leukot Essent Fatty Acids.* 2017 Jun 30. pii: S0952-3278(16)30249-6. https://www.ncbi.nlm.nih.gov/pubmed/28688777.

61. Lim SY, Kim EJ, Kim A, et al. Nutritional Factors Affecting Mental Health. *Clin Nutr Res.* 2016 Jul; 5:143-52. https://www.ncbi.nlm.nih.gov/pubmed/27482518.

62. Kim EJ, Lim SY, Lee HJ, et al. Low dietary intake of n-3 fatty acids, niacin, folate, and vitamin C in Korean patients with schizophrenia and the development of dietary guidelines for schizophrenia. *Nutr Res.* 2017 Sep;45:10-18. https://www. ncbi.nlm.nih.gov/pubmed/29037327.

63. Pawelczyk T, Piatkowska-Janko E, Bogorodzki P, et al. Omega-3 fatty acid supplementation may prevent loss of gray matter thickness in the left parieto-occipital cortex in first episode schizophrenia: A secondary outcome analysis of the OFFER randomized controlled study. *Schizophr Res.* 2017 Oct 24. pii: S0920-9964(17)30621-7. https://www.ncbi.nlm.nih.gov/pubmed/29079060.

64. Marx W, Moseley G, Berk M, Jacka F. Nutritional psychiatry: the present state of the evidence. *Proc Nutr Soc.* 2017 Nov;76:427-436. https://www.ncbi.nlm.nih. gov/pubmed/28942748.

65. Cieslak K, Feingold J, Antonius D, et al. Low vitamin D levels predict clinical features of schizophrenia. *Schizophr Res.* 2014 Nov;159:543-545. https://www. ncbi.nlm.nih.gov/pubmed/25311777.

66. Chiang M, Natarajan R, Fan X. Vitamin D in schizophrenia: a clinical review. *Evid Based Ment Health.* 2016 Feb;19:6-9. https://www.ncbi.nlm.nih.gov /pubmed/26767392.

67. Akinlade KS, Olaniyan OA, Lasebikan VO, Rahamon SK. Vitamin D Levels in Different Severity Groups of Schizophrenia. *Front Psychiatry.* 2017 Jun 13;8:105. https://www.ncbi.nlm.nih.gov/pubmed/28659835.

68. Berridge, MJ. Vitamin D deficiency: infertility and neurodevelopmental diseases (attention deficit hyperactivity disorder, autism and schizophrenia). *Am J Physiol Cell Physiol.* 2017 Oct 25:ajpcell.00188.2017. https://www.ncbi.nlm.nih.gov /pubmed/29070492.

69. Goel H, Dunbar RL. Niacin Alternatives for Dyslipidemia: Fool's Gold or Gold Mine? Part II: Novel Niacin Mimetics. *Curr Atheroscler Rep.* 2016 Apr;18:17. https://www.ncbi.nlm.nih.gov/pubmed/26932224.

70. Dunbar RL, Goel H, Tuteja S, et al. Measuring niacin-associated skin toxicity (NASTy) stigmata along with symptoms to aid development of niacin mimetics. J Lipid Res. 2017 Apr;58:783-797. https://www.ncbi.nlm.nih.gov /pubmed/28119443.

Chapter 5. How to Take Niacin

1. "Doctors Say, Raise the RDAs Now." *Orthomolecular Medicine News Service*, Oct 30, 2007. http://orthomolecular.org/resources/omns/v03n10.shtml

2. Passwater, R. A. *Supernutrition,* New York, NY: Pocket Books, 1991.

3. Merck Manual, Online Medical Library, Home Ed. "Disorders of Nutrition and Metabolism: Vitamins."

4. Troppmann, L., K. Gray-Donald, T. Johns. "Supplement Use: Is There Any Nutritional Benefit?" *J Am Diet Assoc* 102(6) (June 1, 2002): 818–825.

5. Ibid

6. Rohte, O., D. Thormählen, P. Ochlich. ["Elucidation of the Mechanism of Nicotinic Acid Flush in Animal Experimentation."] [Article in German] *Arzneimittelforschung* 7(12) (1977): 2347–52.

7. Kunin, R. A. "Manganese and Niacin in the Treatment of Drug-induced Dyskinesias." *J Orthomol Psych,* 5(1) (1976): 4–27.

8. Kaijser, L., B. Eklund, A. G. Olsson, et al. "Dissociation of the Effects of Nicotinic Acid on Vasodilatation and Lipolysis by a Prostaglandin Synthesis Inhibitor, Indomethacin, in Man." *Med Biol* 57(2) (Apr 1979): 114–7.

9. Estep, D. L., G. R. Gay, R. T. Rappolt, Sr. "Preliminary Report of the Effects of Propranolol HCl on the Discomfiture Caused by Niacin." *Clin Toxicol* 11(3) (1977): 325–8.

10. Boyle, E. "Niacin and the Heart." Paper delivered at Int. Conf. Alcoholics Anonymous Physicians, New York, 1967 (excerpted in *A Second Communication to A.A.'s Physicians,* Bedford Hills, NY: 1968).

11. Cheng, K., T. J. Wu, K. K. Wu, et al. "Antagonism of the Prostaglandin D2 Receptor 1 Suppresses Nicotinic Acid-induced Vasodilation in Mice and Humans." *P Natl Acad Sci USA.* 103(17) (Apr 25, 2006): 6682–7.

12. Bicknell, F., F. Prescott. *The Vitamins in Medicine,* 3rd ed., p 379. London, ENG: William Heinemann Medical Books Ltd, 1953. Reprint: Milwaukee, WI: Lee Foundation for Nutritional Research.

13. Dajani HM, Lauer AK. Optical coherence tomography findings in niacin maculopathy. *Can J Ophthalmol* 2006; 41:197–200.

14. Freisberg L, Rolle, TJ, Ip MS. Diffuse Macular Edema in Niacin-Induced Macu-lopathy May Resolve with Dosage Decrease. *Retinal Cases & Brief Reports* 5:227–228 doi: 10.1097/ICB.0b013e3181e180c0.

15. Millay RH, Klein ML, Illingworth DR. Niacin maculopathy. *Ophthalmology* 1998; 95:930–936.

16. See Fraunfelder FW, Fraunfelder FT, and Illingworth DR. Adverse ocular effects associated with niacin therapy. *Br J Ophthalmol* 1995; 79:54–56. See also Fraunfelder FW. Ocular side effects from herbal medicines and nutritional sup-plements. *Amer J Ophthalmol* 2004; 138:639–647.

Chapter 6. Safety of Niacin

1. Gummin DD, Mowry JB, Beuhler MC et al. 2020 Annual Report of the American Association of Poison Control Centers' National Poison Data System (NPDS): 38th Annual Report. *Clinical Toxicology* 2021, 59:12. https://doi.org/10.1080/15563650.2021.1989785 or https://www.tandfonline.com/doi/abs/10.1080/15563650.2021.1989785.

2. https://osteopathic.org/2019/01/16/poll-finds-86-of-americans-take-vitamins-or-supplements-yet-only-21-have-a-confirmed-nutritional-deficiency/

3. Vague, P. H., B. Vialtettes, V. Lassmanvague, et al. "Nicotinamide May Extend Remission Phase in Insulin Dependent Diabetes." *Lancet* 1 (1987): 619–620.

4. Canner, P. L., C. D. Furberg, M. E. McGovern. "Benefits of Niacin in Patients With Versus Without the Metabolic Syndrome and Healed Myocardial Infarc-tion (from the Coronary Dug Project)." *Am J Cardiol* 97(4) (Feb 2006): 477–479.

5. Dube, M. P., et al. "Safety and Efficacy of Extended-release Niacin for the Treat-ment of Dyslipidaemia in Patients with HIV Infection: AIDS Clinical Trials Group Study A5148." *Antivir Ther* 11(8) (2006): 1081–1089.

6. Kirkey, A. "Diabetics Should Take Cholesterol-lowering Drugs, Study Finds." *Edmonton Journal* Jan 11, 2008.

7. Zhou, S. S., D. Li, W. P. Sun, et al. "Nicotinamide Overload May Play a Role in the Development of Type 2 Diabetes." *World J Gastroenterol* 15(45) (Dec 7, 2009): 5674–84.

8. Li, D., W. P. Sun, Y. M. Zhou al. "Chronic Niacin Overload May Be Involved in the Increased Prevalence of Obesity in US Children." *World J Gastroenterol* 16(19) (May 21, 2010): 2378–2387.

9. Mularski, R. A., R. E. Grazer, L. Santoni, et al. "Treatment Advice on the Inter-net Leads to a Life-threatening Adverse Reaction: Hypotension Associated with Niacin Overdose." *Clin Toxicol (Phila)* 44(1) (2006): 81–4.

10. Bays, H. E., D. Maccubbin, A. G. Meehan, et al. "Blood Pressure-lowering Effects of Extended-release Niacin Alone and Extended-release Niacin/Laropiprant Combination: A Post Hoc Analysis of a 24-Week, Placebo-controlled Trial in Dyslipidemic Patients." *Clin Ther* (1) (Jan 2009): 115–22.

11. Bays, H. E., D. J. Rader. "Does Nicotinic acid (Niacin) Lower Blood Pressure?" *Int J Clin Pract* 63(1) (Jan 2009): 151–9.

12. Parsons, W. B. Jr. *Cholesterol Control without Diet! The Niacin Solution.* 2nd ed., Scottsdale, AZ: Lilac Press, 2003.

13. A review can be found in *Journal of Orthomolecular Medicine,* Volume 14, 1999, 3rd quarter.

14. Parsons, W.B. (2000) *Cholesterol Control Without Diet!* 2nd ed, Lilac Press; ISBN-13: 978-0966256871

15. Gass, JD. (1973) Nicotinic acid maculopathy. *Am J Ophthalmol.* 76:500-510. https://www.ncbi.nlm.nih.gov/pubmed/4743805

16. Millay RH, Klein ML, Illingworth DR. (1988) Niacin Maculopathy. *Ophthalmology* 95:930-936. https://www.ncbi.nlm.nih.gov/pubmed/3174043

17. Dajani HM, Lauer AK. (2006) Optical coherence tomography findings in niacin maculopathy. *Can J Ophthalmol.* 41:197-200. https://www.ncbi.nlm.nih.gov/pubmed/16767207

18. Lee JG, Patel A, Bertolucci A, Rosen RB (2019) Optical Coherence Tomography, Fluorescein Angiography, and Electroretinography Features of Niacin Maculopathy: New Insight Into Pathogenesis. *Journal of VitreoRetinal Diseases,* 3:474-479.

19. Freisberg L, Rolle TJ, Ip MS. (2011) Diffuse macular edema in niacin-induced maculopathy may resolve with dosage decrease. *Retin Cases Brief Rep.* 5:227-228. https://www.ncbi.nlm.nih.gov/pubmed/25390170

20. Smith, RG (2012) *The Vitamin Cure for Eye Disease.* Basic Health Pubs, Inc. SBN-13: 978-1591202929

21. Bronstein AC, Spyker DA, Cantilena LR Jr, Green JL, Rumack BH, Giffin SL. 2009 Annual Report of the American Association of Poison Control Centers' National Poison Data System (NPDS): 27th Annual Report. *Clinical Toxicology* (2010). 48, 979–1178. The vitamin data mentioned in the inset are found in Table 22B.

22. http://www.doctoryourself.com/omns/v07n05.shtml.

23. http://www.doctoryourself.com/omns/v17n31.shtml.

24. http://www.doctoryourself.com/omns/v17n06.shtml.

25. http://www.doctoryourself.com/omns/v15n20.shtml.

26. http://www.doctoryourself.com/omns/v15n01.shtml.

27. http://www.doctoryourself.com/omns/v13n01.shtml.

28. http://www.doctoryourself.com/omns/v12n01.shtml.

29. http://www.doctoryourself.com/omns/v11n01.shtml.

30. http://www.doctoryourself.com/omns/v10n01.shtml.

31. http://www.doctoryourself.com/omns/v09n03.shtml.

32. http://www.doctoryourself.com/omns/v07n16.shtml.

33. http://www.doctoryourself.com/omns/v07n01.shtml.

34. Full text articles since 2012 are available for free download at https://aapcc.org/annual-reports. The "Vitamin" category is usually near the very end of the report. Special thanks to Jagan N. Vaman, MD, for assisting in researching this topic. All OMNS releases are archived for free access at http://www.doctoryourself.com/omns/index.shtml and also at http://www.orthomolecular.org/resources/omns/index.shtml.

35. Gonzalez-Heydrich, J., R. D. Wilens, A. Leichtner, et al. "Retrospective Study of Hepatic Enzyme Elevations in Children Treated with Olanzapine, Divalproic Acid and Their Combination." *J Am Acad Child Adolescent Psych* 42 (2003): 1227–33.

36. "Niacin for detoxification: A little-known therapeutic use." *J Orthomolecular Med* 2011, 26: 2, 85–92.

37. Kemper, K. J., K. L. Hood. "Does Pharmaceutical Advertising Affect Journal Publication About Dietary Supplements?" *BMC Complement Altern Med* 8(11) (Apr 9, 2008). Full text at https://bmccomplementmedtherapies.biomedcentral.com/articles/10.1186/1472-6882-8-11.

38. Ibid.

39. Vedantam, S. "Drug Studies Skewed Toward Study Sponsors: Industry-funded Research Often Favors Patent-holders, Study Finds." *The Washington Post,* April 11, 2006. https://www.nbcnews.com/id/wbna12275329.

40. Heres, S., J. Davis, K. Maino, et al. "Why Olanzapine Beats Risperidone, Risperidone Beats Quetiapine, and Quetiapine Beats Olanzapine: An Exploratory Analysis of Head-to-Head Comparison Studies of Second-Generation Antipsychotics." *Am J Psychiat* 163 (Feb 2006): 185–194. http://ajp.psychiatryonline.org/cgi/content/full/163/2/185

41. Angell, M. *The Truth about the Drug Companies.* New York, NY: Random House, 2004.

42. Ibid.

43. Stroup, T. S., Lieberman, J. A., J. P. McEvoy, et al. "Effectiveness of Olanzapine, Quetiapine, Risperidone, and Ziprasidone in Patients with Chronic Schizophrenia Following Discontinuation of a Previous Atypical Antipsychotic." *Am J Psychiat* 163(4) (Apr 2006): 611–22.

Chapter 7. Pandeficiency Disease

1. Marini, N. J., J. Gin, J. Ziegle, et al. "The Prevalence of Folate-remedial MTHFR Enzyme Variants in Humans." *P Natl Acad Sci USA* 105(23) (Jun 10, 2008): 8055–60.

2. Cleave, T. L. *The Saccharine Disease.* New Canaan, CT: Keats Publishing, 1975.

3. Cleave, T. L. *Diabetes, Coronary Thrombosis, and the Saccharine Disease.* Bristol, ENG: John Wright & Sons, 1966.

4. Hoffer, A., M. Walker. *Orthomolecular Nutrition.* New Canaan, CT: Keats Publishing, 1978.

5. Yudkin, J. *Sweet and Dangerous.* New York, NY: Peter H Wyden, 1972.

6. Challem, J., B. Berkson, M. D. Smith. *Syndrome X: The Complete Nutritional Program to Prevent and Reverse Insulin Resistance.* New York, NY: Wiley, 2000.

7. Marini, Gin, Ziegle, et al. "The Prevalence of Folate-remedial MTHFR." *P Natl Acad Sci USA* 105(23): 8055–60.

8. Ames, B. N., I. Elson-Schwab, E. A. Silver. "High-dose Vitamin Therapy Stimulates Variant Enzymes With Decreased Coenzyme Binding Affinity (Increased K(m)): Relevance to Genetic Disease and Polymorphisms." *Am J Clin Nutr* 75(4) (Apr 2002): 616–58.

9. Hoffer, Walker. *Orthomolecular Nutrition.*

10. USDA Economic Research Service. "U.S. Sugar Consumption Continues to Grow." *USDA Agr Outlook* (March 1997).

11. Hoffer, A., A. W. Saul. *Orthomolecular Medicine for Everyone: Megavitamin Therapeutics for Families and Physicians.* Laguna Beach, CA: Basic Health Publications, 2008.

12. *Diagnostic and Statistical Manual of Mental Disorders,* published by the American Psychiatric Association.

13. Baker, S. M. "What's 'Biomedical'?" *Autism Res Rev Int* 21 (2007): 3. Guest editorial.

Chapter 8. Reversing Arthritis with Niacinamide: The Pioneering Work of William Kaufman, MD, PhD

1. Kaufman, W. *The Common Form of Joint Dysfunction: Its Incidence and Treatment.* Brattleboro, VT: E. L. Hildreth & Company, 1949. After being out of print for several decades, Dr. Kaufman's detailed clinical experience treating arthritis with megadoses of niacinamide has been posted in its entirety at http://www.doctoryourself.com and is freely available for online reading.

2. Kaufman, W. "The Use of Vitamins to Reverse Certain Concomitants of Aging." *J Am Geriatr Soc* 3 (1955): 927–936.

3. Because this privately-printed book was published in 1949 and is long out of print, we are grateful to Charlotte Kaufman for enabling the full text of Dr. Kaufman's *The Common Form of Joint Dysfunction* to be published at www.doctoryourself.com. The book's 248 references are posted at http://www.doctoryourself.com/kaufman11.html.

4. A concise summary of his niacinamide therapy (pages 20 to 29 of his book) is posted at doctoryourself.com/kaufman5.html.

5. Jonas, W. B., C. P. Rapoza, W. F. Blair. "The Effect of Niacinamide in Osteoar-thritis: A Pilot Study." *Inflamm Res* 45 (July 1996): 330–334.

6. A complete listing of all Dr. Kaufman's work will be found at http://www. doctoryourself.com/biblio_kaufman.html. His letter, "What Took the FDA So Long to Come Out in Favor of Folic Acid?" is posted at http://www. doctoryourself.com/kaufman4.html. Also of interest:

   Kaufman, W. Niacinamide therapy for joint mobility. *Conn. State Med. J.* 17:584-589, 1953.

   Kaufman, W. Niacinamide, a most neglected vitamin. 1978 Tom Spies Memorial Lecture. *J. Int. Acad. of Preventive Med.* 8:5-25,1983.

   Kaufman, W. Niacinamide improves mobility in degenerative joint disease. Abstract published in Program of the American Association for the Advance-ment of Science for its meeting in Philadelphia, May 24-30, 1986.

   In 2002, Dr. Kaufman's papers were acquired by the University of Michigan, Special Collections Library, 7th Floor, Harlan Hatcher Graduate Library, Ann Arbor, Ml 48109. Email: special.collections@umich.edu. Phone: (734) 764-9377.

7. See page 21.

8. The pattern of recovery from joint dysfunction in response to niacinamide therapy, and the numerical limits of increments in the value of the Joint Range Index which are considered to be satisfactory for the first month of therapy and for succeeding months, are described on page 24.

9. See page 153.

10. See pages 187 and 188.

11. See page 79.

12. See page 115.

13. See page 76.

14. See page 21.

15. Lukaczer, D., *Nutr Sci* (Nov 1999).

16. Hoffer, A. "Treatment of Arthritis by Nicotinic Acid and Nicotinamide." *Can Med Assoc J* 81 (1959): 235–238.

17. Gardiner, H., A. Berenson. "10 Voters on Panel Backing Pain Pills Had Industry Ties." *New York Times,* February 25, 2005.

18. Hoffer, A., H. D. Foster. *Feel Better, Live Longer with Vitamin B3: Nutrient Deficiency and Dependency.* Toronto, ON: CCNM Press, 2007.

19. Psaty, B. M., Kronmal, R. A. "Reporting Mortality Findings in Trials of Rofecoxib for Alzheimer Disease or Cognitive Impairment: A Case Study Based on Doc-uments from Rofecoxib Litigation." *J Am Med Assoc*; 299(15) (Apr 16, 2008): 1813-7.

20. Ross, J. S., K. P. Hill, D. S. Egilman, et al. "Guest Authorship and Ghostwriting in Publications Related to Rofecoxib: A Case Study of Industry Documents from Rofecoxib Litigation." *J Am Med Assoc* 299(15) (Apr 16, 2008): 1800–12. For more on this topic, see Hill, et al., "The ADVANTAGE Seeding Trial" in the For Further Reading section of this book.

21. DeAngelis, C. D., P. B. Fontanarosa. "Impugning the Integrity of Medical Science: The Adverse Effects of Industry Influence." *J Am Med Assoc* 299(15) (Apr 16, 2008): 1833–5.

22. Taylor, P. "Health Care, Under the Influence." *Globe and Mail*, Toronto, ON: Apr 26, 2008.

23. The golden age of vitamin discovery occurred between 1930 and 1940 with several Nobel prizes awarded for these discoveries. Dr. W. Kaufman was caught up in the excitement of those heady days in nutrition. The vitamins-as-prevention paradigm had finally become established and had made it possible to identify, isolate, and synthesize these vitamins. And none of these nutrients were captured by companies because they were not patentable. According to this paradigm vitamins were only useful to prevent the occurrence of the vitamin deficiency diseases such as beri beri, pellagra, scurvy, etc. and were to be used only in very small doses for these conditions after they had been diagnosed. This paradigm still reigns over most of the world but is being rapidly eroded in North America. Dr. Kaufman was not aware that his work was one of the major blows against this early paradigm since he used very large doses of a vitamin for conditions not considered to be deficiency diseases.

24. This was amazing. Compare it with any medical school today. Canadian medical schools may provide their students as much as 1 or 2 hours of academic nutrition but never any instruction in clinical nutrition and how it is used to fight disease. In 1949 to 1950, in my fourth-year medicine, in the course on therapeutics, the professor spent at least one third of the time discussing nutrition for each disease he was covering.

25. Dr. Kaufman's reaction must have been intense indeed. This does occur with a very small proportion of patients, and they all have to be told in advance all about the flush. However, it is not life-threatening and no one has ever died from the niacin flush. With very sensitive patients it is a good idea to start with small doses and gradually increase them. Niacin is safe and today is used to decrease cholesterol levels, to increase high-density lipoprotein cholesterol and to decrease triglycerides. It is the gold standard for cholesterol lowering agents. It also decreases mortality and increases longevity. Doctors skilled in the use of niacin have no difficulty with their patients and there are many ways of dealing with this. It is in most cases a nuisance or irritant, not a major side effect or complication.

26. This is an excellent description of most modern diets.

Chapter 9. Children's Learning and Behavioral Disorders

1. "NTP Toxicology and Carcinogenesis Studies of Methylphenidate Hydrochloride" (CAS No. 298–59–9) in "F344/N Rats and B6C3F1 Mice (Feed Studies)." *Natl Toxicol Prog Tech Rep Ser* 439 (Jul 1995): 1–299.

2. Kaufman, W. *The Common Form of Joint Dysfunction: Its Incidence and Treatment.* Brattleboro, VT: E. L. Hildreth & Company, 1949.

3. Much of this article originally appeared in the *Journal of Orthomolecular Medicine* 2003, Vol 18, p 29-32. Free full text at http://orthomolecular.org/library/jom/2003/pdf/2003-v18n01-p029.pdf.

4. Hoffer, A. *Healing Children's Attention and Behavior Disorders: Complementary Nutritional and Psychological Treatments.* Toronto, ON: CCNM Press, 2004.

5. Ibid.

6. Hoffer, A., A. W. Saul. *Orthomolecular Medicine for Everyone: Megavitamin Therapeutics for Families and Physicians.* Laguna Beach, CA: Basic Health Publications, 2008.

7. Riordan, H. D. *Medical Mavericks: Volume Three.* Wichita, KS: Bio-Communications Press, 2005. Also: Saul, A. W. "The Pioneering Work of Ruth Flinn Harrell: Champion of Children." *J Orthomolecular Med* 19(1) (2004): 21–26.

8. Harrell, R. F., R. H. Capp, D. R. Davis, et al. "Can Nutritional Supplements Help Mentally Retarded Children? An Exploratory Study." *P Natl Acad Sci USA* 78 (1981): 574–578.

9. Saul. "The Pioneering Work of Ruth Flinn Harrell." *J Orthomolecular Med* 19(1): 21–26.

10. Anyone wishing to learn more about Dr. Harrell's research is advised to read Dr. Saul's 2004 article in the *Journal of Orthomolecular Medicine*, "The Pioneering Work of Ruth Flinn Harrell: Champion of Children" and also the description of her research in Dr. Hugh Desaix Riordan's book *Medical Mavericks, Volume 3.* The article by Dr. Harrell and colleagues, published in the *Proceedings of the National Academy of Science USA* in 1981, is also well worth reading

11. Hoffer, A., H. D. Foster. *Feel Better, Live Longer with Niacin.* Toronto, ON: CCNM Press, 2007.

12. Ieraci, A., D. G. Herrera. "Nicotinamide Protects Against Ethanol-induced Apoptolic Neurodegeneration in the Developing Mouse Brain." *PloS Med* 3(4) (Apr 2006): e101.

13. Gesch, C. B. "Food for Court: Diet and Crime." *Magistrate* 61(5) (2005): 137–139.

14. Ibid.

15. Gesch, C. B., S. M. Hammond, S. E. Hampson, et al. "Influence of Supplementary Vitamins, Minerals and Essential Fatty Acids on the Antisocial Behavior of Young Adult Prisoners. Randomized, Placebo-controlled Trial." *Brit J Psychiat* 181 (2002): 22–28.

16. Challem, J. "Mean Streets or Mean Minerals?" *The Nutrition Report 2001.*

Chapter 10. Mental Illness

1. National Park Service, USA. "Aviation: From Sand Dunes to Sonic Booms: Wright Brothers," https://archives.iupui.edu/handle/2450/680

2. Hoffer, A. *Healing Schizophrenia: Complementary Vitamin and Drug Treatments.* Toronto, ON: CCNM Press, 2004.

3. Miller, C. L., J. R. Dulay. "The High-affinity Niacin Receptor HM74A Is Decreased in the Anterior Cingulate Cortex of Individuals with Schizophrenia." *Brain Res Bull* 77(1) (Sep 5, 2008): 33–41.

4. Hawkins, R., L. Pauling. *Orthomolecular Psychiatry.* San Francisco, CA: WH Freeman, 1973.

5. Miller, Dulay. "The High-affinity Niacin Receptor HM74A." *Brain Res Bull* 77(1): 33–41.

6. Hoffer, A., H. D. Foster. *Feel Better, Live Longer with Vitamin B3: Nutrient Deficiency and Dependency.* Toronto, ON: CCNM Press, 2007.

7. Miller, C. L., P. Murakami, I. Ruczinski, et al. "Two Complex Genotypes Relevant to the Kynurenine Pathway and Melanotropin Function Show Association with Schizophrenia and Bipolar Disorder." *Schizophr Res* 113(2–3) (Sep 2009): 259–67.

8. Miller, Dulay. "The High-affinity Niacin Receptor HM74A." *Brain Res Bull* 77(1): 33–41.

9. Lorenzen, A., C. Stannek, H. Lang, et al. "Characterization of a G protein-coupled Receptor for Nicotinic Acid." *Mol Pharmacol* 2001 Feb;59(2):349–57.

10. Pike, N. B., A. Wise. "Identification of a Nicotinic Acid Receptor: Is This the Molecular Target for the Oldest Lipid-lowering Drug?" *Curr Opin Investig Drugs* 5(3) (Mar 2004): 271–5.

11. el-Zoghby, S. M., A. K. el-Shafei, G. A. Abdel-Tawab, et al. "Studies on the Effect of Reserpine Therapy on the Functional Capacity of the Tryptophan-niacin Pathway in Smoker and Non-smoker Males." *Biochem Pharmacol* 19(5) (May 1970): 1661–7.

12. Liu, C. M., S. S. Chang, S. C. Liao, et al. "Absent Response to Niacin Skin Patch Is Specific to Schizophrenia and Independent of Smoking." *Psychiat Res* 152(2–3) (Aug 30, 2007): 181–7.

13. Hoffer, A., H. D. Foster. "Why Schizophrenics Smoke but Have a Lower Incidence of Lung Cancer: Implications for the Treatment of Both Disorders." *J Orthomolecular Med* 15 3rd Q 2000. Full text at: http://orthomolecular.org/library /jom/2000/pdf/2000-v15n03-p141.pdf

14. Prousky, J. E. "Vitamin B3 for Nicotine Addiction." *J Orthomolecular Med* 19 1st Q 2004. 56. Full text at: http://www.orthomolecular.org/library/jom/2004 /pdf/2004-v19n01-p056.pdf

15. Agnew, N., A. Hoffer: "Nicotinic Acid Modified Lysergic Acid Diethylamide Psychosis." *J Ment Sci* 101 (1955): 12–27.

16. Lewis, N. D., Z. A. Piotrowski. "Clinical Diagnosis of Manic-depressive Psychosis." *P Am Psychopathol Assoc* (1952–1954): 25–8.

17. Weiser, M., A. Reichenberg, J. Rabinowitz, et al. "Association Between Nonpsychotic Psychiatric Diagnoses in Adolescent Males and Subsequent Onset of Schizophrenia." *Arch Gen Psychiat* 58(10) (Oct 2001): 959–64.

18. Redelmeier, D. A., D. Thiruchelvam, N. Daneman. "Delirium After Elective Surgery Among Elderly Patients Taking Statins." *Can Med Assoc J* 179(7) (Sep 23, 2008): 645–52.

19. Marcantonio, E. R. "Statins and Postoperative Delirium." *Can Med Assoc J* 179(7) (Sep 23, 2008): 627–8.

Chapter 11. Cardiovascular Disease

1. Wachter, K. "National Heart, Lung, and Blood Institute Halts Niacin Study Early; No Added Reduction in CV Events." *Internal Medicine News Digital Network* May 26, 2011. https://www.mdedge.com/cardiology/article/35092/cardiology/nhlbi-halts-niacin-study-early-no-added-reduction-cv-events

2. http://pediatrics.aappublications.org/content/128/Supplement_5/S213.full.

3. http://www.aap.org/en-us/about-the-aap/corporate-relationships/Pages/Friends-of-Children-Fund-President%27s-Circle.aspx.

4. To learn more, visit:

   How niacin (Vitamin B₃) lowers high cholesterol safely http://orthomolecular.org/resources/omns/v01n10.shtml.

   Cholesterol-lowering drugs for eight-year-old kids? http://orthomolecular.org/resources/omns/v04n08.shtml.

   How the American Medical Association sells 100% of all physicians' names to advertisers: http://www.mmslists.com/news-articles/article.asp?ID=98.

5. Carlson, LA. Nicotinic acid: the broad-spectrum lipid drug. A 50th anniversary review. *J Intern Med.* Aug 2005;258(2):94-114.

6. Kowalski, RA. *The New 8-Week Cholesterol Cure: The Ultimate Program for Preventing Heart Disease.* Harper Collins; 2001.

7. Creider JC, Hegele RA, Joy TR. Niacin: another look at an underutilized lipid-lowering medication. Nature reviews. *Endocrinology.* Sep 2012;8(9):517-528.

8. Hoffer A, Osmond H. Treatment of Schizophrenia with Nicotinic Acid. A Ten Year Follow-Up. *Acta Psychiatr Scand.* 1964;40:171-189. Also, Osmond H, Hoffer A. Massive niacin treatment in schizophrenia. Review of a nine-year study. *Lancet.* Feb 10 1962;1:316-319.

9. Guyton JR, Bays HE. Safety considerations with niacin therapy. *Am J Cardiol.* Mar 19 2007;99(6A):22C-31C.

10. Horrobin, DF. Schizophrenia: a biochemical disorder? *Biomedicine.* May 1980;32(2):54-55. Messamore E, Hoffman WF, Janowsky A. The niacin skin

flush abnormality in schizophrenia: a quantitative dose-response study. *Schizophr Res.* Aug 1 2003;62(3):251-258. Liu CM, Chang SS, Liao SC, Hwang TJ, Shieh MH, Liu SK, ... Hwu HG. Absent response to niacin skin patch is specific to schizophrenia and independent of smoking. *Psychiatry Res.* Aug 30 2007;152(2-3):181-187.

11. UniproKB database of the Swiss Institute of Bioinformatics. Penberthy WT. Niacin, Riboflavin, and Thiamine. In: Stipanuk MH, Caudill MA, eds. Biochemical, physiological, and molecular aspects of human nutrition. 3rd ed. St. Louis, Mo.: Elsevier/Saunders; 2013:p.540-564.

12. Ames BN, Elson-Schwab I, Silver EA. High-dose vitamin therapy stimulates variant enzymes with decreased coenzyme binding affinity (increased K(m)): relevance to genetic disease and polymorphisms. *Am J Clin Nutr.* Apr 2002;75(4):616-658.

13. Avila MD, Escolar E, Lamas GA. Chelation therapy after the Trial to Assess Chelation Therapy (TACT): results of a unique trial. *Curr Opin Cardiol.* Jul 11 2014.

14. Husten, L (2012) HPS2-THRIVE: No Benefit, Signal of Harm for Niacin Therapy. *Forbes.* http://www.forbes.com/sites/larryhusten/2012/12/20/hps2-thrive -no-benefit-signal-of-harm-for-niacin-therapy.

15. Roberts H, Hickey S. (2011) *The Vitamin Cure for Heart Disease: How to Prevent and Treat Heart Disease Using Nutrition and Vitamin Supplementation.* Basic Health Publications. ISBN-13: 978-1591202646.

16. HPS2-THRIVE Collaborative Group. (2013) HPS2-THRIVE randomized placebo-controlled trial in 25 673 high-risk patients of ER niacin/laropiprant: trial design, pre-specified muscle and liver outcomes, and reasons for stopping study treatment. *Eur Heart J.* 2013 Feb 26. doi: 10.1093/eurheartj/eht055.

17. Parsons, WB. (1998) *Cholesterol Control Without Diet! The Niacin Solution.* Scottsdale, Ariz: Lilac Press, ISBN-13: 978-0966256871.

18. Canner, P.L., Berge, K.G., Wenger, N.K., Stamler, J., Friedman, L., Prineas, R.J., and Friedewald, W. (1986) Fifteen year mortality in Coronary Drug Project patients: long-term benefit with niacin. *J Am Coll Cardiol,* 8(6): 1245-1255.

19. Carlson, L.A. (2005) Nicotinic acid: the broad-spectrum lipid drug. A 50th anniversary review. *J Intern Med,* 258(2): 94-114.

20. Guyton, J.R., and Bays, H.E. (2007) Safety considerations with niacin therapy. *Am J Cardiol,* 99(6A): 22C-31C.

21. Sood A, Arora R. (2009) Mechanisms of flushing due to niacin and abolition of these effects. *J Clin Hypertens* (Greenwich). 11(11):685-689. doi: 10.1111/j.1559-4572.2008.00050.x.

22. Vosper, H. (2011) Extended release niacin-laropiprant in patients with hypercholesterolemia or mixed dyslipidemias improves clinical parameters. *Clin Med Insights Cardiol.* 5:85-101. doi: 10.4137/CMC.S7601.

23. Tuohimaa P, Järvilehto M. (2010) Niacin in the prevention of atherosclerosis: significance of vasodilatation. *Med Hypotheses* 75(4):397-400.

24. 1956

25. 1961, 1961a, 1962

26. 1981

27. 1968

28. 1981

29. 1982

30. Altschul, R., I. H. Herman. "Influence of Oxygen Inhalation on Cholesterol Metabolism." *Arch Biochem Biophys* 1954 51(1) (Jul): 308–9.

31. Altschul, R., A. Hoffer, J. D. Stephen. "Influence of Nicotinic Acid on Serum Cholesterol in Man." *Arch Biochem Biophys* 54 (1955): 558–559.

32. Simonson, E., A. Keys. "Research in Russia on Vitamins and Atherosclerosis." *Circulation* (Nov 24, 1961): 1239–48.

33. Grundy, Grundy, Mok, et al. "Influence of Nicotinic Acid." *J Lipid Res* 1: 24–36.

34. National Institutes of Health. NIH Consensus Development Conference Statement. "Lowering Blood Cholesterol to Prevent Heart Disease." 5(7) December 10–12, 1984. Final Panel Statement.

35. National Institutes of Health. NIH Consensus Development Program. http://consensus.nih.gov/1984/1984Cholesterol047html.htm

36. Saul, A. W. "Orthomolecular Medicine on the Internet." *J Orthomolecular Med,* 20(2) (2005): 70–74.

37. https://medlineplus.gov/.

38. May 2022.

39. Illingworth, D. R., B. E. Phillipson, J. H. Rapp, et al. "Colestipol Plus Nicotinic Acid in Treatment of Heterozygous Familial Hypercholesterolaemia." *Lancet.* 1(8215) (Feb 7, 1981): 296–8.

40. Kane, J. P., M. J. Malloy, P. Tun, et al. "Normalization of Low-density-lipoprotein Levels in Heterozygous Familial Hypercholesterolemia with a Combined Drug Regimen." *New Engl J Med* 304(5) (Jan 29, 1981): 251–8.

41. Cheraskin, E., W. M. Ringsdorf, Jr. "The Biologic Parabola: A Look at Serum Cholesterol." *J Amer Med Assoc* 247(3) (Jan 15, 1982): 302.

42. Ueshima, H., M. Iida, Y. Komachi. "Is It Desirable to Reduce Total Serum Cholesterol Level as Low as Possible?" *Prev Med* 8(1) (Jan 1979): 104–5.

43. Hoffer, A., M. J. Callbeck. "The Hypocholesterolemic Effect of Nicotinic Acid and Its Relationship to the Autonomic Nervous System." *J Ment Sci* 103 (1957): 810–820.

44. Hoffer, A., P. O. O'Reilly, M. J. Callbeck. "Specificity of the Hypocholesterolemic Activity of Nicotinic Acid." *Dis Nerv Syst* 20 (1959): 286–288.

45. O'Reilly, P. O., M. J. Callbeck, A. Hoffer. "Sustained-Release Nicotinic Acid (Nicospan). Effect on (1) Cholesterol Levels and (2) Leukocytes." *Can Med Assoc J* 80: 359–362, 1959.

46. El-Enein, A. M. A., Y. S. Hafez, H. Salem, et al. "The Role of Nicotinic Acid and Inositol Hexanicotinate as Anti-cholesterolemic and Antilipemic Agents." *Nutrition Rep Int* 28 (1983): 899–911.

47. Mahadoo, J., L. B. Jaques, C. J. Wright. "Lipid metabolism: the histamine-glycosaminoglycan-histaminase connection." *Med Hypotheses* 7(8) (Aug 1981): 1029–38.

48. Szatmari, A., A. Hoffer, R. Schneider. "The Effect of Adrenochrome and Niacin on the Electroencephalogram of Epileptics." *Am J Psychiatry* 111(8) (Feb 1955): 603–16.

49. Hoffer, A., H. Osmond. "A Perceptual Hypothesis of Schizophrenia." *Psychiatry Dig* 28(3) (Mar 1967): 47–53.

50. Goldsborough, C. E. "Nicotinic Acid in the Treatment of Ischaemic Heart Disease." *Lancet* 2 (1960): 675–677.

51. Inkeles, S., D. Eisenberg. "Hyperlipidemia and Coronary Atherosclerosis: A Review." *Medicine* (*Baltimore*) (60(2) (Mar 1981): 110–23.

52. Maynard, K. I. "Natural Neuroprotectants After Stroke." *Sci Med* 8(5) (Jun 28, 2008): 258–267.

53. Mason, M. "An Old Cholesterol Remedy Is New Again." *New York Times* January 23, 2007. http://www.nytimes.com/2007/01/23/health/23consume.html?_r=1&oref=slogin.

54. Adams, M. "Vitamin B₃ Beats Big Pharma's Zetia Cholesterol Drug." NaturalNews.com, March 30, 2010, http://www.naturalnews.com/028473_Zetia_Vitamin_B3.html.

Chapter 12. Other Clinical Conditions That Respond to Niacin

1. Canner, P. L., K. G. Berge, N. K. Wenger, et al. "Fifteen Year Mortality in Coronary Drug Project Patients: Long-term Benefit with Niacin." *J Am Coll Cardiol* 8(6) (Dec 1986): 1245–55.

2. Ames, B. N., J. Elson-Schwab, E. A. Silver. "High-dose Vitamin Therapy Stimulates Variant Enzymes with Decreased Coenzyme-binding Affinity (Increased K(m)): Relevence to Genetic Disease and Polymorphism." *Am J Clin Nutr* 75 (2002): 616–658.

3. Ames, B. N. "Increasing Longevity by Tuning Up Metabolism." *Eur Mol Org* 6 (2005): S20-S24.

4. Gutierrez, H. "Micronutrient Deficiency Responsible for Cancer and other Diseases, Proclaims Scientist." NaturaNews.com November 4, 2008 http://www.naturalnews.com/024703_cancer_deficiency_health.html

5. Pauling, L. *How to Live Longer and Feel Better.* Corvallis, OR: Oregon State University Press, 2006.

6. Wysong, P. "High HDL Cholesterol May Protect Against Dementia." *Medical Post* Toronto, ON: August 10, 2004.

7. Westphal, C. H., M. A. Dipp, L. Guarente. "A Therapeutic Role for Sirtuins in Diseases of Aging?" *Trends Biochem Sci* 32(12) (December 1, 2007): 555–560.

8. Kaneko, S., J. Wang, M. Kaneko, et al. "Protecting Axonal Degeneration by Increasing Nicotinamide Adenine Dinucleotide Levels in Experimental Autoimmune Encephalomyelitis Models." *J Neurosci* 26(38) (Sep 20, 2006): 9794–804.

9. Sasaki, Y., A. Toshiyuki, J. Milbrandt. "Stimulation of Nicotinamide Adenine Dinucleotide Biosynthetic Pathways Delays Axonal Degeneration after Axotomy." *J Neurosci* 26(33) (August 16, 2006): 8484–8491.

10. Yang, H., T. Yang, J. A. Baur, et al. "Nutrient-sensitive Mitochondrial NAD+ Levels Dictate Cell Survival." *Cell* 130(6) (Sep 21, 2007): 1095–107.

11. Silverman, D. H. S., C. J. Dy, S. A. Castellon, et al. "Altered Frontocortical, Cerebellar, and Basal Ganglia Activity in Adjuvant-treated Breast Cancer Survivors 5–10 Years After Chemotherapy." *Breast Cancer Res Tr* 103(3) (Jul 2007): 303–11. Epub 2006 Sep 29.

12. Silverman, D. H. S., S. A. Castellon, P. A. Ganz. "Cognitive Dysfunction Associated with Chemotherapy for Breast Cancer." *Future Neurol* 2(3) (May 2007): 271–277.

13. Hoffer, A., A. W. Saul. *Orthomolecular Medicine for Everyone: Megavitamin Therapeutics for Families and Physicians.* Laguna Beach, CA: Basic Health Publications, 2008.

14. Hoffer, A., A. W. Saul. *The Vitamin Cure for Alcoholism.* Laguna Beach, CA: Basic Health Publications, 2008. See also Hoffer's *Adventures in Psychiatry.*

15. Junqueira-Franco, M. V. M., L. E. Troncon, P. G. Chiarello, et al. "Intestinal Permeability and Oxidative Stress in Patients with Alcoholic Pellagra." *Clin Nutr* 25 (2006): 977–983.

16. CBC News. "Lower-status Monkeys More Likely to Opt for Cocaine Over Food: Study." http://www.cbc.ca/news/technology/story/2008/04/07/monkeys-cocaine.html

17. ScienceDaily. "Subordinate Monkeys More Likely to Choose Cocaine Over Food." *ScienceDaily* (Apr 7, 2008). http://www.sciencedaily.com/releases/2008/04/080406153354.htm

18. Williams, R. J., M. K. Roach. "Impaired and Inadequate Glucose Metabolism in the Brain as an Underlying Cause of Alcoholism—An Hypothesis." *P Natl Acad Sci USA* 56(2) (Aug 1966): 566–571. https://www.pnas.org/doi/epdf/10.1073/pnas.56.2.566

19. For more information about William Griffith Wilson:

Hoffer, A. *Vitamin B3: Niacin and Its Amide.* http://www.doctoryourself.com /hoffer_niacin.html.

Hoffer, A., A. W. Saul. *The Vitamin Cure for Alcoholism.* Laguna Beach, CA: Basic Health Publications, 2008.

Wilson, B. *The vitamin B3 therapy: The first communication to AA's physicians.* Bedford Hills, NY:/Private publication. 1967.

Wilson, B. *A second communication to AA's physicians.* Bedford Hills, NY:/Private publication. 1968.

20. Foster, H. D. *What Really Causes Alzheimer's Disease.* Victoria, BC: Trafford Publishing, 2004.

21. Morris, M. C., D. A. Evans, P. A. Bienias, et al. "Dietary Niacin and the Risk of Incident Alzheimer's Disease and of Cognitive Decline." *J Neurol Psychiatry* 75 (2004): 1093–1099.

22. Green, K. N., J. S. Steffan, H. Martinez-Coria, et al. "Nicotinamide Restores Cognition in Alzheimer's' Disease Transgenic Mice via a Mechanism Involving Soirtuin Inhibition and Selective Reduction of Thr231-Phosphotau." *J Neurosci* 45 (2008): 11500 to11510.

23. Foster. *What Really Causes Alzheimer's Disease.*

24. Evans, D. A., J. L. Bienias, et al. "Dietary Niacin and the Risk of Incident Alzheimer's Disease and of Cognitive Decline." *Neurol Neurosurg Psychiat* 75 (2004):1093–1099.

25. Zandi, P. P., J. C. Anthony, A. S. Khachaturian, et al. "Reduced Risk of Alzheimer Disease in Users of Antioxidant Vitamin Supplements: The Cache County Study." *Arch Neurol* 61 (2004): 82–88.

26. For more information about Henry Turkel:

Turkel, H. "Medical amelioration of Down syndrome incorporating the orthomolecular approach." *J Orthomolecular Psych* 4 (1975):102–115.

Turkel, H. "Medical amelioration of Down syndrome incorporating the orthomolecular approach," in: *Diet Related to Killer Diseases V. Nutrition and Mental Health.* Hearing before the Select Committee on Nutrition and Human Needs of the United States Senate, Washington, DC: U.S. Government Printing Office, 1977: 291–304.

Turkel, H. *Medical treatment of Down syndrome and genetic diseases,* Southfield, MI: Ubiotica, 4th rev. ed., 1985.

Turkel, H. *New hope for the mentally retarded: Stymied by the FDA.* New York, NY: Vantage Press, 1972.

27. Pauling, L. *How to Live Longer and Feel Better.* Corvallis, OR: Oregon State University Press, 2006. Used with permission of the Linus Pauling Institute, Oregon State University.

28. Thiel, R. J. "Orthomolecular Therapy and Down Syndrome: Rationale and Clinical Results." Presentation at the 8th Annual Scientific Program of the Orthomolecular Health-Medicine Society, San Francisco, CA: March 1, 2002. http://www. health research.com/orthods.htm.

29. MacLeod, K. *Down Syndrome and Vitamin Therapy.* Ottowa, ON: Kemanso Publishing, 2003.

30. Li, J., M. Zhu, A. B. Manning-Bog, et al. "Dopamine and L-dopa Disaggregate Amyloid Fibrils: Implications for Parkinson's and Alzheimer's Disease." *FASEB J* 18(9) (Jun 2004): 962–4.

31. Religa, D., H. Laudon, M. Styczynska, et al. "Amyloid ß Pathology in Alzheimer's Disease and Schizophrenia." *Am J Psychiat* 160 (May 2003): 867–872.

32. Purohit, D. P., D. P. Perl, V. Haroutunian, et al. "Alzheimer Disease and Related Neurodegenerative Diseases in Elderly Patients with Schizophrenia: A Postmortem Neuropathologic Study of 100 Cases." *Arch Gen Psychiat* 55 (1998): 205–211.

33. Arana, G. W. (2000). An overview of side effects caused by typical antipsychotics. *Journal of Clinical Psychiatry,* 61(8), 5-11. http://www.ncbi.nlm.nih.gov/pubmed/10811237.

34. Ciranni, M. A., Kearney, T. E., & Olson, K. R. (2009). Comparing acute toxicity of first- and second-generation antipsychotic drugs: A 10-year, retrospective cohort study. *The Journal of Clinical Psychiatry,* 70(1), 122-129. http://www.ncbi.nlm.nih.gov/pubmed/19192473

35. Ho, B. C., Andreasen, N. C., Ziebell, S., Pierson, R., & Magnotta, V. (2011). Long-term antipsychotic treatment and brain volumes: A longitudinal study of first-episode schizophrenia. *Archives of General Psychiatry,* 68(2), 128. http://www. ncbi.nlm.nih.gov/pubmed/21300943.

36. Pope, H. G., Keck, P. E., & McElroy, S. L. (1986). Frequency and presentation of neuroleptic malignant syndrome in a large psychiatric hospital. *The American Journal of Psychiatry,* 143(10), 1227-1233. http://www.ncbi.nlm.nih.gov/pubmed /2876647.

37. Saddichha, S., Manjunatha, N., Ameen, S., & Akhtar, S. (2008). Diabetes and schizophrenia-effect of disease or drug? Results from a randomized, double blind, controlled prospective study in first-episode schizophrenia. *Acta Psychiatrica Scandinavica,* 117, 342-347. http://www.ncbi.nlm.nih.gov/pubmed/18307585.

38. Woods, S. W., Morgenstern, H., Saksa, J. R., Walsh, B. C., Sullivan, M. C., Money, R., Hawkins, K. A., Gueorguieva, R. V., & Glazer, W. M. (2010). Incidence of tardive dyskinesia with atypical and conventional antipsychotic medications: Prospective cohort study. *The Journal of Clinical Psychiatry,* 71(4), 463-475. http:// www.ncbi.nlm.nih.gov/pmc/articles/PMC3109728/.

39. Angell, M. (2004). *The truth about the drug companies: How they deceive us and what to do about it.* New York, N.Y.: Random House LLC.

40. Berenson, A. (2007, January 05). Lilly settles with 18,000 over zyprexa. *The New York Times*, pp. 1-2. Retrieved from http://www.nytimes.com/2007/01/05/business/05drug.html?_r=0.

41. Kendall, T. (2011). The rise and fall of atypical antipsychotics. *The British Journal of Psychiatry*, 199(4), 266-268. doi:10.1192/bjp.bp.110.083766.

42. Moynihan, R., & Alan, C. (2005). *Selling sickness: How the world's biggest pharmaceutical companies are turning us all into patients.* New York, N.Y.: Nation Books.

43. Moynihan, R., Heath, I., & Henry, D. (2002). Selling sickness: the pharmaceutical industry and disease mongering. *British Medical Journal*, 324(7342), 886. http://www.ncbi.nlm.nih.gov/pubmed/11950740.

44. Scherer, F. M. (1993). Pricing, profits, and technological progress in the pharmaceutical industry. *The Journal of Economic Perspectives*, 7(3), 97-115. https://www.aeaweb.org/articles.php?doi=10.1257/jep.7.3.97.

45. Spielmans, G. I., & Parry, P. I. (2009). From evidence-based medicine to marketing-based medicine: Evidence from internal industry documents. *Journal of Bioethical Inquiry*, 7(1), 13-29. doi:10.1007/s11673-010-9208-8.

46. Lieberman, J. A., Stroup, T. S., McEvoy, J. P., Swartz, M. S., Rosenback, R. A., Perkins, D. O., Keefe, R. S. E., Davis, S. M., Davis, C. E., Lebowitz, B. D., Severe, J., Hsiao, J. K. (2005). Effectiveness of antipsychotic drugs in patients with chronic schizophrenia. *The New England Journal of Medicine*, 353(12), 1209-1223. http://www.ncbi.nlm.nih.gov/pubmed/17335312.

47. Whitaker, R. (2010). *Anatomy of an epidemic: Magic bullets, psychiatric drugs, and the astonishing rise of mental illness in America.* New York, N.Y.: Crown Publishers.

48. Kuehn, B. M. (2010). Questionable antipsychotic prescribing remains common, despite serious risks. *Journal of the American Medical Association*, 303(16), 1582-1584. http://www.ncbi.nlm.nih.gov/pubmed/20424239.

49. Moran, M. (2011). Misuse of antipsychotics widespread in nursing homes. *Psychiatric News*, 46(11), 2. http://psychnews.psychiatryonline.org/newsarticle.aspx?articleid=108671.

50. 18. Ray, W. A., Federspiel, C. F., & Schaffner, W. (1980). A study of antipsychotic drug use in nursing homes: Epidemiologic evidence suggesting misuse. *American Journal of Public Health*, 70(5), 485-491. http://www.ncbi.nlm.nih.gov/pubmed/6103676.

51. Stevenson, D. G., Decker, S. L., Dwyer, L. L., Huskamp, H. A., Grabowski, D. C., Metzger, E. D., & Mitchell, S. L. (2010). Antipsychotic and benzodiazepine use among nursing home residents: Findings from the 2004 National Nursing Home Survey. *The American Journal of Geriatric Psychiatry: Official Journal of the American Association for Geriatric Psychiatry*, 18(12), 1078-1092. http://www.ncbi.nlm.nih.gov/pubmed/20808119.

52. Szaz, T. (1974). *The myth of mental illness: Foundations of a theory of personal conduct.* New York, N.Y.: Harper Perennial.

53. Pauling, L. (1968). Orthomolecular psychiatry. Varying the concentrations of substances normally present in the human body may control mental disease. *Science*, 160, 265-271. http://www.ncbi.nlm.nih.gov/pubmed/5641253.

54. Cleckley, H. M., Sydenstricker, V. P., & Geeslin, L. E. (1939). Nicotinic acid in the treatment of atypical psychotic states. *The Journal of the American Medical Association*, 112(21), 2107-2110. http://jama.jamanetwork.com/article.aspx?articleid=288714.

55. Hoffer, A. (1962). *Niacin Therapy in Psychiatry*. Springfield, Il: C. C. Thomas.

56. Hoffer, A. (1963). Nicotinic acid: An adjunct in the treatment of schizophrenia. *American Journal of Psychiatry*, 120, 171-173. http://www.ncbi.nlm.nih.gov/pubmed/13963912.

57. Hoffer, A. (1966). The effect of nicotinic acid on the frequency and duration of re-hospitalization of schizophrenic patients: A controlled comparison study. *International Journal of Neuropsychiatry*, 2(3), 234-240. http://www.ncbi.nlm.nih.gov/pubmed/4225426.

58. Hoffer, A. (1970a). Childhood schizophrenia: A case treated with nicotinic acid and nicotinamide. *Schizophrenia*, 2, 43-53. http://orthomolecular.org/library/jom/1970/pdf/1970-v02n01-p043.pdf.

59. Hoffer, A. (1973). A neurological form of schizophrenia. *Canadian Medical Association Journal*, 108, 186-194. http://www.ncbi.nlm.nih.gov/pmc/articles/PMC1941147/.

60. Hoffer, A. (1994). Chronic schizophrenic patients treated ten years or more. *Journal of Orthomolecular Medicine*, 9(1), 7-37. http://orthomolecular.org/library/jom/1994/pdf/1994-v09n01-p007.pdf.

61. Hoffer, A. (1996). Inside schizophrenia: Before and after treatment. *Journal of Orthomolecular Medicine*, 11(1), 45-48. http://orthomolecular.org/library/jom/1996/pdf/1996-v11n01-p045.pdf.

62. Hoffer, A. & Fuller, F. (2009). Orthomolecular treatment of schizophrenia. *Journal of Orthomolecular Medicine*, 24(3,4), 151-159. http://orthomolecular.org/library/jom/2009/pdf/2009-v24n01-p009.pdf.

63. Hoffer, A., & Osmond, H. (1964). Treatment of schizophrenia with nicotinic acid: A ten year follow up. *Acta Psychiatrica Scandinavica*, 40, 171-189. doi:10.1111/j.1600-0447.1964.tb05744.x.

64. Hoffer, A., & Osmond, H. (1980). Schizophrenia: Another long term follow-up in Canada. *Orthomolecular Psychiatry*, 9(2), 107-113. http://psycnet.apa.org/psycinfo/1981-13316-001.

65. Hoffer, A., Osmond, H., Callbeck, M. J., & Kahan, I. (1957). Treatment of schizophrenia with nicotinic acid and nicotinamide. *Journal of Clinical and Experimental Psychopathology*, 18(2), 131-157. http://www.ncbi.nlm.nih.gov/pubmed/13439009.

66. Tung-Yep, T. (1981). The use of orthomolecular therapy in the control of schizophrenia-a study preview. *The Australian Journal of Clinical Hypnotherapy*, 2(2), 111-116. http://schizophreniabulletin.oxfordjournals.org/content/12/1/141.full. pdf.

67. Verzosa, P. L. (1976). A report on a twelve-month period of treating metabolic diseases using mainly vitamins and minerals on the schizophrenias. *Orthomolecular Psychiatry*, 5(4), 253-260. http://www.orthomolecular.org/library/jom/1976/pdf /1976-v05n04-p253.pdf.

68. Gilmer, T. P., Dolder, C. R., Lacro, J. P., Folsom, D. P., Lindamer, L., Garcia, P., & Jeste, D. V. (2004). Adherence to treatment with antipsychotic medication and health care costs among Medicaid beneficiaries with schizophrenia. *American Journal of Psychiatry*, 161(4), 692-699. http://www.ncbi.nlm.nih.gov/pubmed /15056516.

69. McGrath, J., Saha, S., Chant, D., & Welham, J. (2008). Schizophrenia: A concise overview of incidence, prevalence, and mortality. *Epidemiologic Reviews*, 30, 67-76. http://www.ncbi.nlm.nih.gov/pubmed/18480098.

70. Prousky, J., A. Hoffer. *Anxiety: Orthomolecular Diagnosis and Treatment*. Toronto, ON: CCNM Press, 2006.

71. http://nationalpaincentre.mcmaster.ca/opioid/cgop_b_app_b06.html.

72. https://www.orpdl.org/durm/ROAD/Modules/Benzodiazepines/ BenzodiazepinesSlideSet.pdf

73. Lapin IP. (1981) Nicotinamide, inosine and hypoxanthine, putative endogenous ligands of the benzodiazepine receptor, opposite to diazepam are much more effective against kynurenine-induced seizures than against pentylenetetrazol-induced seizures. *Pharmacology Biochemistry and Behavior*, 14(5): 589-593.

74. Möhler H, Polc P, Cumin R, Pieri L, Kettler R. (1979) Nicotinamide is a brain constituent with benzodiazepine-like actions. *Nature*, 278(5704):563-5.

75. Tallman JF, Paul SM, Skolnick P, and Gallager DW. (1980) Receptors for the age of anxiety: pharmacology of the benzodiazepines. *Science*, 207(4428): 274-281.

76. Riond J, Mattei, Kaghad M, et al. (1991) Molecular cloning and chromosomal localization of a human peripheral-type benzodiazepine receptor. *Eur J Biochem*. 195(2):305-311.

77. Belelli D and Lambert JJ. (2005) Neurosteroids: endogenous regulators of the GABA(A) receptor. *Nat Rev Neurosci*, 6(7): 565-575.

78. Prousky, JE. (2004) Niacinamide's potent role in alleviating anxiety with its benzodiazepine-like properties: a case report. *J Orthomol Med*, 19(2): 104-110.

79. Prousky J and Seely D. (2005) The treatment of migraines and tension-type headaches with intravenous and oral niacin (nicotinic acid): systematic review of the literature. *Nutr J*, 4:3.

80. Bronson, PJ. (2011) A Biochemist's Experience with GABA. *J Orthomolecular Med*, 26:11-14.

81. Levy, TE (2009) *Curing the Incurable: Vitamin C, Infectious Diseases, and Toxins*, 3rd Edition, Livon Books, ISBN: 978-0977952021.

82. Cathcart, Robert F. III. (1981) The method of determining proper doses of vitamin C for the treatment of disease by titrating to bowel tolerance. *Journal of Orthomolecular Psychiatry*. 10:125-132.

83. Eighth International Symposium on ADP-Ribosylation. "Niacin Nutrition, ADP-Ribosylation and Cancer." Fort Worth, Texas, June 1987.

84. Hostetler, D. "Jacobsons Put Broad Strokes in the Niacin/Cancer Picture." *The D.O.*, 28 (Aug 1987): 103–104.

85. Hoffer, A. "The Psychophysiology of Cancer." *J Asthma Res* 8 (1970): 61–76.

86. Other forms of niacin include: nicotinamide riboside and nicotinamide mononucleotide. This article focuses on niacin/niacinamide.

87. Penberthy WT, Kirkland JB. Niacin [Internet]. In: *Present Knowledge in Nutrition*. John Wiley & Sons, Ltd, [cited 2021 Jan 1]; 293-306. https://onlinelibrary.wiley.com/doi/abs/10.1002/9781119946045.ch19.

88. Penberthy, WT. (2021) Vitamin B_1, B_2 & B_3 Functions [cited 2021 Jan 1]

89. Kirkland, JB. (2012) Niacin requirements for genomic stability. Mutation Research, 733: 14-20. https://pubmed.ncbi.nlm.nih.gov/22138132.

90. Spronck JC, Nickerson JL, Kirkland JB. (2007) Niacin deficiency alters p53 expression and impairs etoposide-induced cell cycle arrest and apoptosis in rat bone marrow cells. Nutrition and Cancer, 57: 88-99. https://pubmed.ncbi.nlm.nih.gov/17516866.

91. Koshland, DE. (1993) Molecule of the year. *Science*, 262: 1953. https://pubmed.ncbi.nlm.nih.gov/8266084/.

92. Boyonoski AC, Gallacher LM, ApSimon MM, et al. (1999) Niacin deficiency increases the sensitivity of rats to the short and long term effects of ethylnitrosourea treatment. *Molecular and Cellular Biochemistry*, 193: 83-87. https://pubmed.ncbi.nlm.nih.gov/10331642.

93. Galli U, Colombo G, Travelli C, Tron GC, Genazzani AA, Grolla AA. (2020) Recent Advances in NAMPT Inhibitors: A Novel Immunotherapic Strategy. *Frontiers in Pharmacology*, 11:656. https://pubmed.ncbi.nlm.nih.gov/32477131.

94. Heske, CM. (2019) Beyond Energy Metabolism: Exploiting the Additional Roles of NAMPT for Cancer Therapy. *Frontiers in Oncology*, 9:1514. https://pubmed.ncbi.nlm.nih.gov/32010616.

95. Mukherjee P, Augur ZM, Li M, et al. (2019) Therapeutic benefit of combining calorie-restricted ketogenic diet and glutamine targeting in late-stage experimental glioblastoma. *Communications Biology*, 2:200. https://pubmed.ncbi.nlm.nih.gov/31149644.

96. Seyfried TN, Mukherjee P, Iyikesici MS, et al. (2020) Consideration of Ketogenic Metabolic Therapy as a Complementary or Alternative Approach for Managing

Breast Cancer. *Frontiers in Nutrition*, 7:21. https://pubmed.ncbi.nlm.nih.gov/32219096.

97. McGinnis, W. R., T. Audhya, W. J. Walsh, et al. "Discerning the Mauve Factor, Alternative Therapies in Health and Disease, Part 1." *Alt Ther* 14(2) (Mar/Apr 2008):40–51. "Part 2" 14(3) (Jun 2008): 56–63.

98. Hoffer, A., H. D. Foster, "Schizophrenia and Cancer: The Adrenochrome Balanced Morphism." *Med Hypotheses* 62 (2004): 415–419.

99. Bartleman, A., R. Jacobs, J. B. Kirkland. "Niacin Supplementation Decreases the Incidence of Alklation-induced Nonlymphocytic Leukemia in Long-Evans Rats." *Nutr Cancer* 60 (2008): 251–258.

100. Jacobsen, E. L. "Niacin Deficiency and Cancer in Women." *J Am Coll Nutr* 12 (1993): 412–416.

101. Moalem, S. *Survival of the Sickest. A Medical Maverick Discovers Why We Need Disease.* New York, NY: HarperCollins Publishers, 2007.

102. Bartleman, Jacobs, Kirkland. "Niacin Supplementation ..." *Nutr Cancer* 60: 251–258.

103. Boyonoski, A. C., J. C. Spronck, R. M. Jacobs, et al. "Pharmacological Intakes of Niacin Increase Bone Marrow Poly(ADP-ribose) and the Latency of Ethylnitrosourea-induced Carcinogenesis in Rats." *J Nutr* 132(1) (Jan 2002): 115–20.

104. Boyonoski, A. C., J. C. Spronck, L. M. Gallacher, et al. "Niacin Deficiency Decreases Bone Marrow Poly(ADP-ribose) and the Latency of Ethylnitrosourea-induced Carcinogenesis in Rats." *J Nutr* 132(1) (Jan 2002): 108–14.

105. Boyonoski, A. C., L. M. Gallacher, M. M. ApSimon, et al. "Niacin Deficiency in Rats Increases the Severity of Ethylnitrosourea-induced Anemia and Leukopenia." *J Nutr* 130(5) (May 2000): 1102–7.

106. Sivapirabu, G., E. Yiasemides, G. M. Halliday, et al. "Topical Nicotinamide Modulates Cellular Energy Metabolism and Provides Broad-spectrum Protection Against Ultraviolet Radiation-induced Immunosuppression in Humans." *Br J Dermatol* 161(6) (Dec 2009): 1357–64.

107. Canadian Cancer Society. "More Canadian Children Surviving Cancer—Many Experience Future Health Issues; More Research Needed: Canadian Cancer Statistics. April 9, 2008.

108. Eighth International Symposium on ADP-Ribosylation. "Niacin Nutrition ...", June 1987.

109. For more information about niacin and cancer, see the report from the Linus Pauling Institute available at http://lpi.oregonstate.edu/infocenter/vitamins/niacin.

110. Kuzniarz, M., P. Mitchell, R. G. Cumming, et al. "Use of Vitamin Supplements and Cataract: the Blue Mountains Eye Study." *Am J Ophthalmol* 132(1) (2001): 19–26.

111. Chiu, C. J. "Nutritional Antioxidants and Age-related Cataract and Maculopathy." *Exp Eye Res* 84(2) (Feb 2007): 229–45.

112. Rabbani, G. H., T. Butler, P. K. Bardhan, et al. "Reduction of Fluid-loss in Cholera by Nicotinic Acid: A Randomised Controlled Trial." *Lancet* 2(8365–66) (Dec 24–31, 1983): 1439–1442.

113. Briend, A., S. K. Nath, M. Heyman, et al. "Comparative Effects of Nicotinic Acid and Nicotinamide on Cholera Toxin-induced Secretion in Rabbit Ileum." *J Diarrhoeal Dis Res* 11(2) (Jun 1993): 97–100.

114. Petersdorf, R. G., Adams, Braunwald, et al. *Harrison's Principles of Internal Medicine,* 10th ed., New York, NY: McGraw Hill, 1983.

115. Ng C-F, Lee C-P, Ho AL, et al. (2011) Effect of niacin on erectile function in men suffering erectile dysfunction and dyslipidemia. J Sex Med. 8:2883-2893. https://pubmed.ncbi.nlm.nih.gov/21810191.

116. Parsons, W (2000) *Cholesterol Control Without Diet.* Lilac Press. ISBN-13: 978-0966256871.

117. Nehra A, Jackson G, Miner M, et al. (2012) The Princeton III Consensus Recommendations for the Management of Erectile Dysfunction and Cardiovascular Disease. *Mayo Clin Proc* 87:766-778. https://pubmed.ncbi.nlm.nih.gov/22862865

118. Miner M, Seftel AD, Nehra A, et al. (2012) Prognostic utility of erectile dysfunction for cardiovascular disease in younger men and those with diabetes. *Am Heart J.* 164:21-28. https://pubmed.ncbi.nlm.nih.gov/22795278.

119. Carlson, LA (2005) Nicotinic acid: the broad-spectrum lipid drug. A 50th anniversary review. *J Intern Med.* 258:94-114. https://pubmed.ncbi.nlm.nih.gov/16018787.

120. Creider JC, Hegele RA, Joy TR (2012) Niacin: another look at an underutilized lipid-lowering medication. *Nat Rev Endocrinol.* 8:517-528. https://pubmed.ncbi.nlm.nih.gov/22349076.

121. Guyton JR, Bays HE (2007) Safety considerations with niacin therapy. *Am J Cardiol.* 99:22C-31C. https://pubmed.ncbi.nlm.nih.gov/17368274.

122. Pieper, JA (2002) Understanding niacin formulations. Am J Manag Care 8:S308-S314. https://pubmed.ncbi.nlm.nih.gov/12240702.

123. Preckshot, J (1999) Male impotency and the compounding pharmacist. Int J Pharm Compd. 3:80-83. https://pubmed.ncbi.nlm.nih.gov/23985547.

124. Canner PL, Berge KG, Wenger NK, et al. (1986) Fifteen-year mortality in Coronary Drug Project patients: long-term benefit with niacin. J Am Coll Cardiol. 8:1245-1255. https://pubmed.ncbi.nlm.nih.gov/3782631.

125. Kelly LE, Ohlsson A, Shah PS. (2017) Sildenafil for pulmonary hypertension in neonates. Cochrane Database Syst Rev. 8:CD005494. https://pubmed.ncbi.nlm.nih.gov/28777888.

126. Wang R, Jiang F, Zheng Q, et al. (2014) Efficacy and safety of sildenafil treatment in pulmonary arterial hypertension: a systematic review. Respir Med. 108:531-537. https://pubmed.ncbi.nlm.nih.gov/24462476.

127. Gentile V, Antonini G, Antonella Bertozzi M, et al. (2009) Effect of propionyl-L-carnitine, L-arginine and nicotinic acid on the efficacy of vardenafil in the treatment of erectile dysfunction in diabetes. Curr Med Res Opin. 25:2223-2228. https://pubmed.ncbi.nlm.nih.gov/19624286.

128. Tunstall-Pedoe H, Woodward M, Tavendale R, et al. (1997) Comparison of the prediction by 27 different factors of coronary heart disease and death in men and women of the Scottish Heart Health Study: cohort study. BMJ 315:722-729. https://pubmed.ncbi.nlm.nih.gov/9314758

129. Jacobson, TA (2013) Lipoprotein(a), cardiovascular disease, and contemporary management. Mayo Clin Proc. 88:1294-1311. https://pubmed.ncbi.nlm.nih.gov /24182706.

130. J Am Col Cardiol 39:7, p 1199-1203, 2002.

131. Int J Impot Res 6: p 33-36, 1994. For more on the effect of niacin on erectile function in men suffering erectile dysfunction and dyslipidemia:

   Ng CF, Lee CP, Ho AL, Lee VW. J Sex Med. 2011 Oct;8(10):2883-93. doi: 10.1111/j.1743-6109.2011.02414.x. Epub 2011 Aug 2. PMID: 21810191.

   Propionyl-L-carnitine, L-arginine, and niacin in sexual medicine: a nutraceutical approach to erectile dysfunction. Gianfrilli D, Lauretta R, Di Dato C, Graziadio C, Pozza C, De Larichaudy J, Giannetta E, Isidori AM, Lenzi A. Andrologia. 2012 May;44 Suppl 1:600-4. doi: 10.1111/j.1439-0272.2011.01234.x. Epub 2011 Oct 4. PMID: 21966881.

   Effect of propionyl-L-carnitine, L-arginine and nicotinic acid on the efficacy of vardenafil in the treatment of erectile dysfunction in diabetes. Gentile V, Antonini G, Antonella Bertozzi M, Dinelli N, Rizzo C, Ashraf Virmani M, Koverech A.

   Curr Med Res Opin. 2009 Sep;25(9):2223-8. doi: 10.1185/03007990903138416. PMID: 19624286.

   Effect of vitamins on sexual function: A systematic review. Ghanbari-Homaie S, Ataei-Almanghadim K, Mirghafourvand M. Int J Vitam Nutr Res. 2021 Mar 29:1-10. doi: 10.1024/0300-9831/a000703. Online ahead of print. PMID: 33779240.

132. Maupin, C. "Dr. Les Simpson—Rethinking the Pathogenesis of CFIDS." *The CFS Report.*

133. Simpson, L. O. "Altered Blood Rheology in the Pathogenesis of Diabetic and Other Neuropathies." *Muscle Nerve* 11(7) (Jul 1988): 725–44.

134. Simpson, L. O." Blood Pressure and Blood Viscosity." *NZ Med J* 101(853) (Sep 14, 1988): 581.

135. Oakley, A., J. Wallace. "Hartnup Disease Presenting in an Adult." *Clin Exp Dermatol* 19(5) (Sep 1994): 407–8.

136. Cachin, M., J. L. Beaumont. [Treatment of Migraine by Nicotinic Acid]. *Sem Hop* 27(24) Mar 30, 1951): 977–9.

137. Velling, D. A., D. W. Dodick, J. J. Muir. "Sustained-release Niacin for Prevention of Migraine Headache." *Mayo Clin Proc* 78(6) (Jun 2003): 770–1.

138. Prousky, J., D. Seely. "The Treatment of Migraines and Tension-type Headaches with Intravenous and Oral Niacin (Nicotinic Acid): Systematic Review of the Literature." *Nutr J* 4:3 (2005).

139. Kaneko, S., J. Wang, M. Kaneko, et al. "Protecting Axonal Degeneration by Increasing Nicotinamide Adenine Dinucleotide Levels in Experimental Auto-immune Encephalomyelitis Models." *J Neurosci.* 26(38) (Sep 20, 2006): 9794–804. https://www.ncbi.nlm.nih.gov/pmc/articles/PMC6674451/

140. Rauscher, M. "Vitamin B3 May Be Useful Against MS: Animal Study." Reuters Health.

141. Mount, H. T. "Multiple Sclerosis and other Demyelinating Diseases." *Can Med Assoc J* 108(11) (Jun 2, 1973): 1356–1358.

142. Klenner, F. R. "Response of Peripheral and Central Nerve Pathology to Mega-Doses of the Vitamin B-Complex and Other Metabolites." *J Appl Nutr* 1973, https://www.ncbi.nlm.nih.gov/pmc/articles/PMC6674451/

143. Klenner, F. R. "Clinical Guide to the Use of Vitamin C." http://www.seanet.com/~alexs/ascorbate/198x/smith-lh-clinical_guide_1988.htm.

144. Klenner, F. R. "Treating Multiple Sclerosis Nutritionally." *Cancer Control J* 2(3): 16–20. Frederick Klenner's detailed megavitamin protocol is posted at http://www.tldp.com/issue/ 11_00/klenner.htm.

145. "Peter's Promise" http://www.orthomolecular.com (accessed Jan 2011).

146. For more on Wee Yong, visit https://cumming.ucalgary.ca/departments/dcns/about/faculty/yong

147. Wahlberg, G., L. A. Carlson, J. Wasserman, et al. "Protective Effect of Nicotin-amide Against Nephropathy in Diabetic Rats." *Diabetes Res* 2 (1985): 307–312.

148. Condorelli, L. "Nicotinic Acid in the Therapy of the Cardiovascular Apparatus." In: R. Altschul, ed. *Niacin in Vascular Disorders and Hyperlipemia* Springfield, IL: CC Thomas, 1964.

149. Kidney Disease Statistics for the United States. NIDDK. National Institute of Diabetes and Digestive and Kidney Diseases. https://www.niddk.nih.gov/health-information/health-statistics/kidney-disease.

150. National Center for Health Statistics (2021) Deaths and Mortality. FastStats. https://www.cdc.gov/nchs/fastats/deaths.htm.

151. US Renal Data System. (2018) Chapter 1: Incidence, Prevalence, Patient Characteristics, and Treatment Modalities. 2:291-331. https://www.usrds.org/media/1736/v2_c01_incprev_18_usrds.pdf.

152. Ketteler M, Block GA, Evenepoel P, et al. (2018) Diagnosis, Evaluation, Prevention, and Treatment of Chronic Kidney Disease—Mineral and Bone Disorder: Synopsis of the Kidney Disease: Improving Global Outcomes 2017 Clinical Practice Guideline Update. Ann Intern Med 168:422-430. https://pubmed.ncbi.nlm.nih.gov/29459980.

153. Eto N, Miyata Y, Ohno H, Yamashita T. (2005) Nicotinamide prevents the development of hyperphosphataemia by suppressing intestinal sodium-dependent phosphate transporter in rats with adenine-induced renal failure. Nephrology Dialysis Transplantation 20:1378-1384. https://pubmed.ncbi.nlm.nih.gov/15870221.

154. Katai K, Tanaka H, Tatsumi S, et al. (1999) Nicotinamide inhibits sodium-dependent phosphate cotransport activity in rat small intestine. Nephrology Dialysis Transplantation 14: 1195-1201 (1999). https://pubmed.ncbi.nlm.nih.gov/10344361.

155. Fouque D, Vervloet M, Ketteler M. (2018) Targeting Gastrointestinal Transport Proteins to Control Hyperphosphatemia in Chronic Kidney Disease. Drugs 78:1171-1186. https://pubmed.ncbi.nlm.nih.gov/30022383.

156. Berns, JS. (2008) Niacin and Related Compounds for Treating Hyperphosphatemia in Dialysis Patients. Semin Dial 21:203-205. https://pubmed.ncbi.nlm.nih.gov/18363600.

157. Park, CW. (2013) Niacin in patients with chronic kidney disease: Is it effective and safe? Kidney Research and Clinical Practice 32:1-2. https://pubmed.ncbi.nlm.nih.gov/26889431.

158. Kang HJ, Kim DK, Lee SM, et al. (2013) Effects of low-dose niacin on dyslipidemia and serum phosphorus in patients with chronic kidney disease. Kidney Research and Clinical Practice 32:21-26. https://pubmed.ncbi.nlm.nih.gov/26889433.

159. Taketani Y, Masuda M, Yamanaka-Okumura H, et al. (2015) Niacin and Chronic Kidney Disease. J Nutr Sci Vitaminol 61:S173-S175. https://pubmed.ncbi.nlm.nih.gov/26598845.

160. Cheng SC, Young DO, Huang Y, Delmez JA, Coyne DW. (2008) A Randomized, Double-Blind, Placebo-Controlled Trial of Niacinamide for Reduction of Phosphorus in Hemodialysis Patients. Clin J Am Soc Nephrol. 3:1131-1138. https://pubmed.ncbi.nlm.nih.gov/18385391.

161. Charnow JA (2014) Niacin May Slow Chronic Kidney Disease (CKD) Progression. Renal and Urology News. https://www.renalandurologynews.com/home/conference-highlights/kidney-week-annual-meeting/kidney-week-2014/kidney-week-2014-general-news/niacin-may-slow-chronic-kidney-disease-ckd-progression.

162. Rao M, Steffes M, Bostom A, Ix JH. (2014) Effect of niacin on FGF23 concentration in chronic kidney disease. Am J Nephrol 39, 484-490. https://pubmed.ncbi.nlm.nih.gov/24854458.

163. Ginsberg C, Ix JH. (2016) Nicotinamide and phosphate homeostasis in chronic kidney disease: Curr Opin Nephrol Hyperten. 25:285-291. https://pubmed.ncbi.nlm.nih.gov/27219041.

164. Streja E, Kovesdy CP, Streja DA, et al. (2015) Niacin and Progression of CKD. Am J Kidney Dis. 65:785-798. https://pubmed.ncbi.nlm.nih.gov/25708553.

165. Rennick A, Kalakeche R, Seel L, Shepler B. (2013) Nicotinic Acid and Nicotinamide: A Review of Their Use for Hyperphosphatemia in Dialysis Patients. Pharmacotherapy. 33:683-690. https://pubmed.ncbi.nlm.nih.gov/23526664.

166. Khalid SA, Inayat F, Tahir MK, et al. (2019) Nicotinic Acid as a Phosphate-lowering Agent in Patients with End-stage Renal Disease on Maintenance Hemodialysis: A Single-center Prospective Study. Cureus 11:e4566. https://pubmed.ncbi.nlm.nih.gov/31281749.

167. Shimoda K, Akiba T, Matsushima T, et al. (1998) [Niceritrol decreases serum phosphate levels in chronic hemodialysis patients]. Nihon Jinzo Gakkai Shi 40:1-7. https://pubmed.ncbi.nlm.nih.gov/9513376.

168. Zeman M, Vecka M, Perlík F, et al. (2016) Pleiotropic effects of niacin: Current possibilities for its clinical use. Acta Pharm, 66:449-469. https://pubmed.ncbi.nlm.nih.gov/27749252.

169. Zhang Y, Ma T, Zhang, P. (2018) Efficacy and safety of nicotinamide on phosphorus metabolism in hemodialysis patients: A systematic review and meta-analysis. Medicine, 97: e12731. https://pubmed.ncbi.nlm.nih.gov/30313075.

170. Vasantha J, Soundararajan P, Vanitharani N, et al. (2011) Safety and efficacy of nicotinamide in the management of hyperphosphatemia in patients on hemodialysis. Indian J Nephrol. 21:245-249. https://pubmed.ncbi.nlm.nih.gov/22022084.

171. Lenglet A, Liabeuf S, El Esper N, et al. (2017) Efficacy and safety of nicotinamide in haemodialysis patients: the NICOREN study. Nephrol Dial Transplant. 32:870-879. https://pubmed.ncbi.nlm.nih.gov/27190329.

172. Liu X-Y, Yao J-R, Xu R, et al. (2020) Investigation of nicotinamide as more than an anti-phosphorus drug in chronic hemodialysis patients: a single-center, double-blind, randomized, placebo-controlled trial. Ann Transl Med. 8:530. https://pubmed.ncbi.nlm.nih.gov/32411753.

173. El Borolossy R, El Wakeel LM, El Hakim I, Sabri, N. (2016) Efficacy and safety of nicotinamide in the management of hyperphosphatemia in pediatric patients on regular hemodialysis. Pediatr Nephrol. 31:289-296. https://pubmed.ncbi.nlm.nih.gov/26420678.

174. Ketteler M, Wiecek A, Rosenkranz AR, et al. (2021) Efficacy and Safety of a Novel Nicotinamide Modified-Release Formulation in the Treatment of Refractory Hyperphosphatemia in Patients Receiving Hemodialysis—A Randomized

Clinical Trial. Kidney Int Rep. 6:594-604. https://pubmed.ncbi.nlm.nih.gov /33732974.

175. Raines NH, Ganatra S, Nissaisorakarn P, et al. (2021) Niacinamide May Be Associated with Improved Outcomes in COVID-19-Related Acute Kidney Injury: An Observational Study. Am Soc of Nephrol. Kidney360. https://kidney360.asnjournals.org /content/2/1/33.

176. Takahashi Y, Tanaka A, Nakamura T, et al. (2004) Nicotinamide suppresses hyperphosphatemia in hemodialysis patients. Kidney International. 65:1099-1104. https://www.kidney-international.org/article/S0085-2538(15)49804-7/fulltext.

177. Sampathkumar, K (2016) Niacin for phosphate control: A case of David versus Goliath. Indian J Nephrol. 26:237-238. https://pubmed.ncbi.nlm.nih.gov /27510758.

178. Sampathkumar K, Selvam M, Sooraj YS, et al. (2006) Extended release nicotinic acid—a novel oral agent for phosphate control. Int Urol Nephrol 38:171-174. https://pubmed.ncbi.nlm.nih.gov/16502077.

179. Edalat-Nejad M, Zameni F, Talaiei A. (2012) The effect of niacin on serum phosphorus levels in dialysis patients. Indian J Nephrol 22:174-178. https://pubmed. ncbi.nlm.nih.gov/23087550.

180. Shin S, Lee S. (2014) Niacin as a drug repositioning candidate for hyperphosphatemia management in dialysis patients. Ther Clin Risk Manag. 10:875-883. https://pubmed.ncbi.nlm.nih.gov/25342908.

181. Zahed NS, Zamanifar N, Nikbakht H. (2016) Effect of low dose nicotinic acid on hyperphosphatemia in patients with end stage renal disease. Indian J Nephrol 26:239-243. https://pubmed.ncbi.nlm.nih.gov/27512294.

182. Ralto KM, Rhee EP, Parikh SM. (2020) NAD+ homeostasis in renal health and disease. Nat Rev Nephrol. 16:99-111. https://pubmed.ncbi.nlm.nih.gov /31673160.

183. Palmer BF, Alpern RJ. (2003) Treating dyslipidemia to slow the progression of chronic renal failure. Am J Med. 114:411-412 (2003). https://pubmed.ncbi.nlm.nih.gov /12714133.

184. Cho K, Kim H, Rodriguez-Iturbe B, Vaziri ND. (2009) Niacin ameliorates oxidative stress, inflammation, proteinuria, and hypertension in rats with chronic renal failure. American Journal of Physiology-Renal Physiology 297. F106-F113. https://pubmed.ncbi.nlm.nih.gov/19420110.

185. Owada A, Suda S, Hata T. (2003) Antiproteinuric effect of niceritrol, a nicotinic acid derivative, in chronic renal disease with hyperlipidemia: a randomized trial. Am J Med 114:347-353. https://pubmed.ncbi.nlm.nih.gov/12714122.

186. Burge, NJ. (2017) Association of Niacin on Phosphate Control in Advanced-Stage Chronic Kidney Disease Patients within a VA Population. https:// www.semanticscholar.org/paper/Association-of-Niacin-on-Phosphate -Control-in-a-VA-Burge/988840c5343630c2e2319a85b4c05b61ecf75362.

187. Zhen X, Zhang S, Xie F, et al. (2021) Nicotinamide Supplementation Attenu-ates Renal Interstitial Fibrosis via Boosting the Activity of Sirtuins. Kidney Dis (Basel) 7:186-199. https://pubmed.ncbi.nlm.nih.gov/34179114.

188. Müller D, Mehling H, Otto B, et al. (2007) Niacin lowers serum phosphate and increases HDL cholesterol in dialysis patients. Clin J Am Soc Nephrol 2:1249-1254. https://pubmed.ncbi.nlm.nih.gov/17913971.

189. Liu D, Wang X, Kong L, Chen Z. (2014) Nicotinic Acid Regulates Glucose and Lipid Metabolism Through Lipid Independent Pathways. Curr Pharm Biotechno. 16:3-10. https://pubmed.ncbi.nlm.nih.gov/25429652.

190. Small C, Kramer HJ, Griffin KA, et al. (2017) Non-dialysis dependent chronic kidney disease is associated with high total and out-of-pocket healthcare expen-ditures. BMC Nephrol 18:3. https://pubmed.ncbi.nlm.nih.gov/28056852.

191. Golestaneh L, Alvarez PJ, Reaven NL, et al. (2017) All-cause costs increase exponentially with increased chronic kidney disease stage. Am J Manag Care 23:S163-S172. https://pubmed.ncbi.nlm.nih.gov/28978205.

192. Dharnidharka, V. R., Kwon, C. & Stevens, G. (2002) Serum cystatin C is superior to serum creatinine as a marker of kidney function: a meta-analysis. Am J Kidney Dis. 40:221-226. https://pubmed.ncbi.nlm.nih.gov/12148093.

193. Grubb, A. (2017) Cystatin C is Indispensable for Evaluation of Kidney Disease. EJIFCC 28:268-276 . https://pubmed.ncbi.nlm.nih.gov/29333146.

194. Finn, WF (1961-2011) PubMed, see: https://pubmed.ncbi.nlm.nih.gov/?term =finn+wf.

195. Shang D, Xie Q, Ge X, et al. (2015) Hyperphosphatemia as an independent risk factor for coronary artery calcification progression in peritoneal dialysis patients. BMC Nephrol 16:107. https://pubmed.ncbi.nlm.nih.gov/26187601.

196. Felsenfeld AJ, Levine BS, Rodriguez M. (2015) Pathophysiology of Calcium, Phosphorus, and Magnesium Dysregulation in Chronic Kidney Disease. Semin Dial 28:564-577. https://pubmed.ncbi.nlm.nih.gov/26303319.

197. Monckeberg's arteriosclerosis. Wikipedia (2020). https://en.wikipedia.org/wiki /Monckeberg%27s_arteriosclerosis.

198. de Brito-Ashurst, I, Varagunam M, Raftery MJ, Yaqoob MM. (2009) Bicarbonate supplementation slows progression of CKD and improves nutritional status. J Am Soc Nephrol 20:2075-2084. https://pubmed.ncbi.nlm.nih.gov/19608703.

199. Brauser, D (2010) Baking Soda May Slow Progression of Chronic Kidney Dis-ease. Medscape. http://www.medscape.com/viewarticle/706043.

200. Kumakura S, Sato E, Sekimoto A, et al. (2021) Nicotinamide Attenuates the Pro-gression of Renal Failure in a Mouse Model of Adenine-Induced Chronic Kidney Disease. Toxins (Basel) 13:50. https://pubmed.ncbi.nlm.nih.gov/33440677.

201. Hussain S., Singh A, Alshammari TM, et al. (2020) Nicotinamide Therapy in Dialysis Patients: A Systematic Review of Randomized Controlled Trials. Saudi J Kidney Dis Transpl 31:883-897. https://pubmed.ncbi.nlm.nih.gov/33229753.

202. He YM, Feng L, Huo D-M, Yang Z-H, Liao Y-H. (2014) Benefits and harm of niacin and its analog for renal dialysis patients: a systematic review and meta-analysis. Int Urol Nephrol 46:433-442. https://pubmed.ncbi.nlm.nih.gov/24114284.

203. Faivre A, Katsyuba E, Verissimo T, et al. (2021) Differential role of nicotinamide adenine dinucleotide deficiency in acute and chronic kidney disease. Nephrol Dial Transplant 36, 60-68 . https://pubmed.ncbi.nlm.nih.gov/33099633.

204. Hasegawa, K. (2019) Novel tubular—glomerular interplay in diabetic kidney disease mediated by sirtuin 1, nicotinamide mononucleotide, and nicotinamide adenine dinucleotide Oshima Award Address 2017. Clin Exper Nephrol 23:987-994. https://pubmed.ncbi.nlm.nih.gov/30859351.

205. Hasegawa, K. Wakino S, Sakamaki Y, et al. (2016) Communication from Tubular Epithelial Cells to Podocytes through Sirt1 and Nicotinic Acid Metabolism. Curr Hypertens Rev 12:95-104. https://pubmed.ncbi.nlm.nih.gov/26931474.

206. Ilkhani F, Hosseini B, Saedisomeolia A (2016) Niacin and Oxidative Stress: A Mini-Review. J Nutri Med Diet Care. 2:014. https://clinmedjournals.org/articles /jnmdc/journal-of-nutritional-medicine-and-diet-care-jnmdc-2-014.php.

207. Lenglet A, Liabeuf S, Guffroy P, et al. (2013) Use of Nicotinamide to Treat Hyperphosphatemia in Dialysis Patients. Drugs R D 13:165-173. https://pubmed.ncbi. nlm.nih.gov/24000048.

208. Matthews DR, Hosker JP, Rudenski AS, et al. (1985) Homeostasis model assessment: insulin resistance and beta-cell function from fasting plasma glucose and insulin concentrations in man. Diabetologia, 28:412-419. https://pubmed.ncbi. nlm.nih.gov/3899825.

209. Wallace TM, Levy JC, Matthews DR (2004) Use and abuse of HOMA modeling Diabetes Care 27:1487-1495. https://pubmed.ncbi.nlm.nih.gov/15161807.

210. Editorial (2018) Making more of multimorbidity: an emerging priority. The Lancet. 391:1637 https://www.thelancet.com/journals/lancet/article/PIIS0140-6736 (18)30941-3/fulltext.

211. Arias E, Heron M, Tejada-Vera B. (2013) United States life tables eliminating certain causes of death, 1999-2001. Natl Vital Stat Rep 61:1-128. https://pubmed. ncbi.nlm.nih.gov/24968617.

212. Canner PL, Berge KG, Wenger NK, et al. (1986) Fifteen year mortality in Coronary Drug Project patients: long-term benefit with niacin. J Am Coll Cardiol 8:1245-1255. https://pubmed.ncbi.nlm.nih.gov/3782631.

213. Wald, G., B. Jackson. "Activity and Nutritional Deprivation." *P Nat Acad Sci USA,* 30(9) (Sep 15, 1944): 255–263.

214. Kaufman, W. *The Common Form of Joint Dysfunction: Its Incidence and Treatment.* Brattleboro, VT: E. L. Hildreth & Company, 1949.

215. Hoffer, A., H. D. Foster. *Feel Better, Live Longer with Vitamin B3: Nutrient Deficiency and Dependency.* Toronto, ON: CCNM Press, 2007.

216. Foster, H. D. and A. Hoffer. "The Two Faces of L-DOPA: Benefits and Adverse Side Effects in the Treatment of Encephalitis Lethargica, Parkinson's Disease, Multiple Sclerosis and Amyotrophic Lateral Sclerosis." *Med Hypotheses* 62(2) (February 2004): 177–181.

217. Hoffer, Foster. *Feel Better, Live Longer with Vitamin B3.*

218. Foster, H. D., A. Hoffer. "Hyperoxidation of the Two Catecholamines, Dopamine and Adrenaline: Implications for the Etiologies and Treatment of Encephalitis Lethargica, Parkinson's Disease, Multiple Sclerosis, Amyotrophic Lateral Sclerosis, and Schizophrenia." In: *Oxidative Stress and Neurodegenerative Disorders,* Amsterdam: Elsevier, 2007, Ch 16, 369–382.

219. Evans, E. L., P. J. Matts. Skin Care Composition Containing Glycerin and a Vitamin B3 Compound That Increase and Repair Skin Barrier Function. Eur. Pat. Appl. (2004), EP 1459736; A1 20040922. Patent written in English.

220. Jacobson, E. L. et al. "A Topical Lipophilic Niacin Derivative Increases NAD, Epidermal Differentiation and Barrier Function in Photodamaged Skin." *Exp Dermatol* 16(6) (2007): 490–499.

221. Moro, O. Antiaging Topical Formulations Containing Niacin and Ubiquinones. Jpn. Kokai Tokkyo Koho (2005) JP 2005298370; A 20051027. Patent written in Japanese.

222. Sore, G., I. Hansenne. Peeling Composition Containing Vitamin B3 and Vitamin C. Fr. Demande (2005), FR 2861595; A1 20050506. Patent written in French.

223. Tanno, O. "The New Efficacy of Niacinamide in the Skin and the Application to the Skin Care Products of Cosmetics." *Fragrance J* 32(2) (2004): 35–39.

224. Yates, P. R., R. L. Charles-Newsham. Skin Lightening Compositions Comprising Vitamins and Flavonoids. PCT Int. Appl. (2005), WO 2005094770; A1 20051013.

225. Hoffer, Saul. *Orthomolecular Medicine for Everyone.*

226. Tang, H., J. Y. Lu, X. Zheng, et al. "The Psoriasis Drug Monomethylfumarate Is a Potent Nicotinic Acid Receptor Agonist." *Biochem Biophys Res Commun* 375(4) (Oct 31, 2008): 562–5.

227. Hoffer A, M. Walker. *Putting It All Together: The New Orthomolecular Nutrition.* New Canaan, CT: Keats Publishing Inc., 1996. Also: McGraw-Hill; 1998.

Chapter 13. Niacin for COVID: How Niacin, Niacinamide, and NAD Can Help with Long COVID-19

1. Raines NH, Ganatra S, Nissaisorakarn P, et al. (2021) Niacinamide May Be Associated with Improved Outcomes in COVID-19-Related Acute Kidney Injury: An Observational Study. Kidney360 2:33-41. https://pubmed.ncbi.nlm.nih.gov/35368823.

2. Pieper JA (2002) Understanding niacin formulations. Am J Manag Care 8:S308-S314. https://pubmed.ncbi.nlm.nih.gov/12240702

3. Kashyap ML, Ganji S, Nakra NK, et al. (2019) Niacin for treatment of nonalcoholic fatty liver disease (NAFLD): novel use for an old drug? J Clin Lipidol. 13:873-879. https://pubmed.ncbi.nlm.nih.gov/31706905

4. Ganji S, Hoa N, Kamanna J, et al. (2022) Niacin regresses collagen content in human hepatic stellate cells from liver transplant donors with fibrotic non-alcoholic steatohepatitis (NASH). Am J Transl Res. 14:4006-4014. https://pubmed.ncbi.nlm.nih.gov/35836902

5. Guyton JR. (2007) Niacin in cardiovascular prevention: mechanisms, efficacy, and safety. Curr Opin Lipidol. 18:415-420. https://pubmed.ncbi.nlm.nih.gov/17620858

6. McConnell S, Penberthy WT (2021) Reversing Chronic Kidney Disease with Niacin and Sodium Bicarbonate. Orthomolecular Medical News Service. http://orthomolecular.org/resources/omns/v17n22.shtml

7. Park YK, Sempos CT, Barton CN, et al. (2000) Effectiveness of food fortification in the United States: the case of pellagra. Am J Public Health 90:727-738. https://pubmed.ncbi.nlm.nih.gov/10800421

8. Li R, Li Y, Liang X, et al. (2021) Network Pharmacology and bioinformatics analyses identify intersection genes of niacin and COVID-19 as potential therapeutic targets. Brief Bioinform. 22:1279-1290. https://pubmed.ncbi.nlm.nih.gov/33169132

9. Zheng M, Schultz MB, Sinclair DA. (2022) NAD+ in COVID-19 and viral infections. Trends Immunol. 43:283-295. https://pubmed.ncbi.nlm.nih.gov/35221228

10. Heer CD, Sanderson DJ, Voth LS, et al. (2020) Coronavirus infection and PARP expression dysregulate the NAD metabolome: An actionable component of innate immunity. J Biological Chem. 295:17986-17996. https://pubmed.ncbi.nlm.nih.gov/33051211

11. Penberthy WT, Axelsen KB. (2022) Table of NAD-Utilizing Enzymes. https://www.cmescribe.com/vitamin-dependent-gene-databases

12. Ames BN, Elson-Schwab I, Silver EA. (2002) High-dose vitamin therapy stimulates variant enzymes with decreased coenzyme binding affinity (increased K(m)): relevance to genetic disease and polymorphisms. Am J Clin Nutr. 75:616-658. https://pubmed.ncbi.nlm.nih.gov/11916749

13. Suchard MS, Savulescu DM. (2022) Nicotinamide pathways as the root cause of sepsis - an evolutionary perspective on macrophage energetic shifts. FEBS J. 289:955-964. https://pubmed.ncbi.nlm.nih.gov/33686748

14. de Assis Barros D'Elia Zanella LGF, de Lima Galvão L (2021) The COVID-19 Burden or Tryptophan Syndrome: Autoimmunity, Immunoparalysis and Tolerance in a Tumorigenic Environment. J Infect Dis Epidemiol. 7:195. https://doi.org/10.23937/2474-3658/1510195

15. Penberthy, WT. (2007) Pharmacological targeting of IDO-mediated tolerance for treating autoimmune disease. Curr Drug Metab. 8:245-66. https://pubmed.ncbi.nlm.nih.gov/17430113

16. Hoffer A, Prousky J. (2008) Successful treatment of schizophrenia requires optimal daily doses of vitamin B3. Altern Med Rev. 13:287-291. https://www.researchgate.net/publication/24036385_The_proper_treatment_of_schizophrenia_requires_optimal_daily_doses_of_vitamin_B3

17. Nemani K, Li C, Olfson M, et al. (2021) Association of Psychiatric Disorders with Mortality Among Patients With COVID-19. JAMA Psychiatry 78:380-386. https://pubmed.ncbi.nlm.nih.gov/33502436

18. Dembosky, A. (2022) Having schizophrenia is the second biggest risk factor for dying from COVID-19. NPR. https://www.npr.org/2022/03/20/1087766160/having-schizophrenia-is-the-second-biggest-risk-factor-for-dying-from-covid-19

19. NIH COVID-19 Treatment Guidelines. (2022) Interleukin-6 Inhibitors. https://www.covid19treatmentguidelines.nih.gov/therapies/immunomodulators/interleukin-6-inhibitors

20. Murray, MF. (2003) Nicotinamide: an oral antimicrobial agent with activity against both Mycobacterium tuberculosis and human immunodeficiency virus. Clin Infect Dis. 36:453-460. https://pubmed.ncbi.nlm.nih.gov/12567303

21. Thomas T, Stefanoni D, Reisz JA, et al. (2020) COVID-19 infection alters kynurenine and fatty acid metabolism, correlating with IL-6 levels and renal status. JCI Insight 5:e140327. https://pubmed.ncbi.nlm.nih.gov/32559180

22. Kashi AA, Davis RW, Phair RD. (2019) The IDO Metabolic Trap Hypothesis for the Etiology of ME/CFS. Diagnostics (Basel) 9:82. https://pubmed.ncbi.nlm.nih.gov/31357483

23. Kats, D. (2021) Sufficient Niacin Supply: The Missing Puzzle Piece to COVID-19, and beyond? Preprint. https://doi.org/10.31219/osf.io/uec3r

24. Kwon WY, Suh GJ, Kim KS, et al. (2011) Niacin attenuates lung inflammation and improves survival during sepsis by downregulating the nuclear factor-κB pathway. Crit Care Med. 39:328-334. https://pubmed.ncbi.nlm.nih.gov/20975550

25. Gharote, M. (2021) potential role of nicotinamide supplementation in prevention of covid-19 transmission-a perspective. https://www.researchgate.net/publication/350800103_potential_role_of_nicotinamide_supplementation_in__prevention_of_covid-19_transmission-a_perspective

26. Jiang Y, Deng Y, Pang H, et al. (2022) Treatment of SARS-CoV-2-induced pneumonia with NAD+ and NMN in two mouse models. Cell Discov. 8:38. https://pubmed.ncbi.nlm.nih.gov/35487885

27. Pirinen E, Auranen M, Khan NA, et al. (2020) Niacin Cures Systemic NAD+ Deficiency and Improves Muscle Performance in Adult-Onset Mitochondrial

Myopathy. Cell Metab. 31:1078-1090.e5. https://pubmed.ncbi.nlm.nih.gov/32386566.

28. Wallace, A.E., W. B. Weeks. "Thiamine Treatment of Chronic Hepatitis B Infection." *Am J Gastroenterol* 96(3) (2001): 864–868.

29. Shoji, S. et al. "Thiamine Disulfide as a Potent Inhibitor of Human Immunodeficiency Virus (Type-1) Production. Biochemical and Biophysical Research Communications." 205(1) (1994): 967–75.

30. Murray, M. F. "Niacin as a Potential AIDS Preventive Factor." *Med Hypotheses* 53(5) (1999): 375–379.

31. Tang, A. M., N. M. Graham, A. J. Kirby, et al. "Dietary Micronutrient Intake and Risk of Progression to Acquired Immunodeficiency Syndrome (AIDS) in Human Immunodeficiency Virus Type 1 (HIV-1)-Infected Homosexual Men." *Am J Epidemiol* 138(11) (Dec 1, 1993): 937–51.

32. Fawzi, W. W., G. I. Msamanga, D. Spiegelman, et al. "A Randomized Trial of Multivitamin Supplements and HIV Disease Progression and Mortality." *New Engl J Med* 351(1) (Jul 1, 2004): 23–32.

33. Foster, H. D. *What Really Causes AIDS.* Victoria: Trafford Publishing, 2002

34. Foster, H. D. "Treating AIDS with Nutrition." Doctor Yourself Newsletter, 4(12) (May 20, 2004). http://www.doctoryourself.com/news/v4n12.txt

35. Bradfield, M., H. D. Foster." The Successful Orthomolecular Treatment of AIDS: Accumulating Evidence from Africa." *J Orthomolecular Med* 21(4) (2006). http://www.orthomolecular.org/library/jom/2006/pdf/2006-v21n04-p193.pdf.

Chapter 14. Niacin: Why the Original Megavitamin Is More Important Than Ever

1. Saul, A. *Doctor Yourself: Natural Healing That Works.* Basic Health Publications, Inc. Laguna Beach, CA; 2nd revised edition (August 13, 2012).

2. Mason, M. *New York Times*, January 23, 2007. An old cholesterol remedy is new again.

3. "The Effects of Vitamin and Mineral Supplementation on Symptoms of Schizophrenia: A Systematic Review and Meta-analysis." J. Firth (a1), B. Stubbs (a2) (a3), J. Sarris (a4) (a5), S. Rosenbaum (a6). DOI: 10.1017/S0033291717000022.

4. https://doi.org/10.1017/S0033291717000022 Published online: February, 16, 2017 Orthomolecular Psychiatry 10:2; 98-118 (1981).

5. www.orthomolecular.org/resources/omns/v09n30.shtml.

6. www.jneurosci.org/content/26/38/9794.long.

7. His detailed megavitamin protocol is posted for all interested persons to read at www.townsendletter.com/Klenner/KlennerProtocol_forMS.pdf.

8. You can read the entire archive at either http://www.doctoryourself.com/omns /index.shtml or http://orthomolecular.org/resources/omns/index.shtml. All articles are posted in Spanish and Portuguese, as well as in English.

9. Jonas WB, Rapoza CP, Blair WF. The effect of niacinamide in osteoarthritis: a pilot study. *Inflammatory Research* 45:330–334.

10. A summation of his niacinamide therapy (pages 20-29 of his book) is posted at www.doctoryourself.com/kaufman5.html.

11. www.doctoryourself.com/biblio_kaufman.html.

12. www.orthomolecular.org/resources/omns/v10n09.shtml. Readers may also enjoy the comments made by Dr. Kaufman in 1998 at www.doctoryourself.com /kaufman3.html.

13. Passwater, R.A. "From Pellagra to Trans Fats and Beyond, — How a Legendary Nutritional Scientist is Still Saving Countless Thousands from Premature Death." *WholeFoods Magazine*. 37 (9). 2014.

14. Ganji SH, Kamanna VS, Kashyap ML. J Nutr Biochem. 2003 Jun;14(6):298-305. See also: Kamanna VS and Kashyap ML. Am J Cardiol. 2008 Apr 17;101(8A):20B-26B.

15. Ritter, M. "Study Says Vitamin C Could Cut Liver Damage." Associated Press, October 11, 1986.

16. Photodermatology, Photoimmunology & Photomedicine (Melanoma and non-melanoma skin cancer chemoprevention: A role for nicotinamide? Minocha R., Damian D.L., & Halliday, G. Aug 8, 2017 DOI: 10.1111/phpp.12328.

17. Shi H., et al., NAD Deficiency, Congenital Malformations, and Niacin Supplementation. N Engl J Med 2017; 377:544-552August 10, 2017DOI: 10.1056/ NEJMoa1616361.

18. The entire 300-plus issue archive is available for free access at http://www. doctoryourself.com/omns/index.shtml and also at http://www.orthomolecular. org/resources/omns/index.shtml.

Appendix 1. The Introduction of Niacin as the First Successful Treatment for Cholesterol Control

1. Abridged and reprinted with permission of the *Journal of Orthomolecular Medicine*, 2000. 15:3. Footnotes renumbered.

2. Parsons, W. B. Jr, R. W. P. Achor, K. G. Berge, et al. "Changes in Concentration of Blood Lipids Following Prolonged Administration of Large Doses of Nicotinic Acid to Persons with Hypercholesterolemia: Preliminary Observations." *P Staff Meet Mayo Clinic*, 31 (1956): 377–390.

3. Altschul, R., A. Hoffer, J. D. Stephen. "Influence of Nicotinic Acid on Serum Cholesterol in Man." *Arch Biochem Biophys* 54 (1955): 558–559.

4. Altschul, R. *Niacin in Vascular Disorders and Hyperlipidemia.* Springfield, IL: Charles C. Thomas, 1964.

5. Altschul, Hoffer, Stephen. "Influence of Nicotinic acid . . ." *Arch Biochem Biophys* 1955: 558–559.

6. Parsons, W. B. Jr. *Cholesterol Control Without Diet! The Niacin Solution.* Scottsdale, AZ: Lilac Press, 1998.

7. The Coronary Drug Project Research Group. "Clofibrate and Niacin in Coronary Heart Disease." *J Am Med Assoc* 231 (1975): 360–381.

8. Canner, P. L., K. G. Berge, N. K. Wenger, et al., for the Coronary Drug Project Research Group. "Fifteen Year Mortality in Coronary Drug Project Patients: Long-term Benefit with Niacin." *J Am Coll Cardiol* 8 (1986): 1245–1255.

Appendix 2. The Historical Significance of 1940s Mandatory Niacin Enrichment: Niacin Rescues Cannibalistic Hamsters

1. Tissier ML, Handrich Y, Dallongeville O, Robin JP, Habold C. (2017) Diets derived from maize monoculture cause maternal infanticides in the endangered European hamster due to a vitamin B_3 deficiency. *Proc Biol Sci.* 2017 Jan 25;284(1847). pii: 20162168. doi: 10.1098/rspb.2016.2168. http://rspb.royalsocietypublishing.org/content/284/1847/20162168 PMID:28100816 https://www.ncbi.nlm.nih.gov/pubmed/28100816

2. Park, Y. K., Sempos, C. T., Barton, C. N., Vanderveen, J. E., & Yetley, E. A. (2000). Effectiveness of food fortification in the United States: the case of pellagra. *Am J Public Health*, 90(5), 727-738.

3. Hoffer, A. (2005). *Adventures in Psychiatry: The Scientific Memoirs of Dr. Abram Hoffer.* KOS Publishing.

4. Mawson, A., & Jacobs, K. (1978). Corn Consumption, Tryptophan, and Cross-National Homicide Rates. *Orthomolecular Psychiatry*, 7(4), 227-230.

5. Hoffer, A. (2009). *Psychiatry Yesterday (1950) and Today (2007): From Despair to Hope with Orthomolecular Psychiatry.* Trafford Publishing.

6. Etheridge, E. W. (1972). *The Butterfly Caste: A Social History of Pellagra in the South.* Westport, Conn: Greenwood Pub Co.

7. Roe, D.A. (1973). *A Plague of Corn: The Social History of Pellagra* (Ithaca NY: Cornell University Press).

8. Ames, B. N., Elson-Schwab, I., & Silver, E. A. (2002). High-dose vitamin therapy stimulates variant enzymes with decreased coenzyme binding affinity (increased $K(m)$): relevance to genetic disease and polymorphisms. *Am J Clin Nutr*, 75(4), 616-658.

9. Guyton, J. R., & Bays, H. E. (2007). Safety considerations with niacin therapy. *Am J Cardiol, 99(6A)*, 22C-31C.

10. Williams PA, Harder JM, Foxworth NE, Cochran KE, Philip VM, Porciatti V, Smithies O, John SW. (2017) Vitamin B3 modulates mitochondrial vulnerability and prevents glaucoma in aged mice. *Science.* Feb 17;355(6326):756-760. doi:10.1126/science.aal0092

11. Smith RG. (2012) *The Vitamin Cure for Eye Disease: How to Prevent and Treat Eye Disease Using Nutrition and Vitamin Supplementation.* Basic Health Pub. ISBN-13: 978-1591202929.

12. http://orthomolecular.org/resources/omns/v13n01.shtml.

Appendix 3. An Interview with Abram Hoffer, MD, PhD

1. *Cholesterol Control Without Diet*, Lilac Press, 2000.

2. Hoffer, Abram and Linus Pauling. *Healing Cancer: Complementary Vitamin and Drug Treatments.* CCNM Press, 2004.

3. *Townsend Letter for Doctors and Patients*, June 1996.

4. *Statistical Theory: The Relationship of Probability, Credibility, and Error*, Norton, 1957.

Appendix 4. A Special Interview with Andrew W. Saul

1. The *Journal of Orthomolecular Medicine*'s archives are online and they're free access at https://isom.ca/jom/ or at http://orthomolecular.org/library/jom/index.shtml.

Appendix 5. Clinical Experiences with a Vitamin B3 Dependent Family

1. Reprinted with permission from the *Journal of Orthomolecular Medicine.*

2. The Merck Manual of Diagnosis and Therapy: 16th edition. Rathway, NJ. Merck Research Laboratories. 1992; 959.

3. The Merck Manual of Diagnosis and Therapy: 17th edition. Whitehouse Station, NJ. Merck Research Laboratories. 1999; 33.

4. Pauling, L: Orthomolecular psychiatry. Varying the concentrations of substances normally present in the human body may control mental disease. Science, 1968; 160: 265-271.

5. Abbey, LC: Agoraphobia. J Orthomolec Psych, 1982;11:243-259.

6. Prousky, J: Niacinamide's potent role in alleviating anxiety with its benzodiazepine-like properties: a case report. J Orthomol Med, 2004; 19(2): 104-110.

7. Prousky, J: Supplemental niacinamide mitigates anxiety symptoms: report of three cases. J Orthomol Med, 2005; 20(3): 167-178.

8. Prousky, J: Anxiety: Orthomolecular Diagnosis and Treatment. CCNM Press Inc. 2006.

9. Kaplan BJ, Simpson JS, Ferre RC, et al: Effective mood stabilization with a chelated mineral supplement: an open-label trial in bipolar disorder. J Clin Psychiatry, 2001; 62: 936-44.

10. Alpert JE, Mischoulon D, Rubenstein GE, et al: Folinic acid (Leucovorin) as an adjunctive treatment for SSRI-refractory depression. Ann Clin Psychiatry, 2002; 14(1): 33-38.

11. Hoffer, A: Treatment of schizophrenia. In. eds. Williams RJ, Kalita DK. *A Physician's Handbook on Orthomolecular Medicine.* New Canaan, CT. Keats Publishing, Inc. 1977; 83-89.

12. Ames BN, Elson-Schwab I, Silver EA: High-dose vitamin therapy stimulates variant enzymes with decreased coenzyme binding (increased Km): relevance to genetic diseases and polymorphisms. Am J Clin Nutr, 2002; 75: 616-658.

13. Hoffer A, Osmond H: *How to Live with Schizophrenia.* Secaucus, NJ. University Books, Inc. 1974; 174-175.

14. Rudin, DO: The major psychoses and neuroses as omega-3 essential fatty acid deficiency syndrome: substrate pellagra. Biol Psychiatry, 1981; 16: 837-850.

15. Horrobin, D: *The Madness of Adam and Eve.* London, England. Corgi Books. 2001.

16. Stoll, AL: *The Omega-3 Connection.* New York, NY. Simon & Schuster. 2001.

17. Hoffer, A: Vitamin B3 dependency: chronic pellagra. Townsend Lett Doctors Patients, 2000; 207: 66-73.

18. Bender, DA: Pellagra. In. eds. Sadler MJ, Strain JJ, Caballero B. *Encyclopedia of Human Nutrition.* San Diego,CA, Academic Press. 1999:1298-1302.

19. Bicknell F, Prescott F: *Nicotinic acid. The Vitamins in Medicine.* 3rd ed. Milwaukee, WI. Life Foundation for Nutritional Research. 1953;333-389.

20. Bates, CJ: Niacin. In. eds. Sadler MJ, Strain JJ, Caballero B. *Encyclopedia of Human Nutrition.* San Diego, CA, Academic Press. 1999: 1290-1298.

21. Cervantes-Laurean D, McElvaney NG, Moss J: Niacin. In. eds. Shils ME, Olson JA, Shike M, Ross AC. *Modern Nutrition in Health and Disease.* 9th ed. New York, NY, Lippincott Williams & Wilkins. 1999: 401-411.

22. Groff JL, Gropper SS, Hunt SM: The water soluble vitamins. Niacin. *Advanced Nutrition and Human Metabolism.* 2nd ed. St. Paul, MN, West Publishing Company. 1995: 247-252.

23. Hoffer, A: Mechanism of action of nicotinic acid and nicotinamide in the treatment of schizophrenia. In. eds. Hawkins D, Pauling L. *Orthomolecular Psychiatry.* San Francisco, CA, W.H. Freeman and Company. 1973; 202-262.

24. Hoffer A, Osmond H: *How to Live with Schizophrenia.* Secaucus, NJ. University Books, Inc. 1974; 116-132.

25. Miller CL, Llenos IC, Dulay JR, et al: Upregulation of the initiating step of the kynurenine pathway in postmortem anterior cingulate cortex from individuals with schizophrenia and bipolar disorder. Brain Res, 2006; 1073-1074: 25-37.

26. Simopoulos, AP: Genetic variation and nutrition. Nut Rev, 1999; 57: S10-S19.

27. Horrobin, D: *The Madness of Adam and Eve.* London, England. Corgi Books. 2001;253-260.

28. Hoffer, A: Schizophrenia Delenda Est. J Orthomol Med, 2006; 21: 123-139.

Appendix 6. Vitamin Deficiency, Megadoses, and Some Supplemental History

1. See the heading on page B5 "Vitamins Win Support as Potent Agents of Health" and on page B9 "New Support for Vitamins as Agents of Health."

2. Editor's note: Professor Emanuel Cheraskin, MD, DMD, is another one of the persons we can thank for the superior nutrition program at the U. of Alabama at Birmingham.

3. From "Ascorbic Acid in Cancer Prevention," in the book *Nutrition and Cancer Prevention*, New York: CRC Press, 1989. Edited by Thomas E. Moon and Marc S. Micozzi.

Appendix 7. Remembering Dr. William Kaufman

1. Hoffer, A: Treatment of arthritis by nicotinic acid and nicotinamide. Can Med Assoc J, 81: 235–238, 1959.

Appendix 8. Vitamin B$_3$: Niacin and Its Amide

1. Reprinted with the permission of the author: Abram Hoffer, MD, PhD.

2. Horwitt MK: Modern Nutrition in Health and Disease. Fifth Ed. RS Goodhart and ME Shils. Lea & Febiger, Phil. 1974.

3. Canner, PL, Berge KG, Wenger NK, Stamler J, Friedman L, Prineas RJ & Freidewald W: Fifteen year mortality Coronary Drug Project; patients long term benefit with niacin. American Coll Cardiology 8:1245-1255, 1986.

4. Altschul R, Hoffer A & Stephen JD: Influence of Nicotinic Acid on Serum Cholesterol in Man. Arch Biochem Biophys 54:558-559, 1955.

5. Hoffer A: The Schizophrenia, Stress and Adrenochrome Hypothesis. In Press, 1995.

6. Hoffer A: Orthomolecular Medicine for Physicians. Keats Pub, New Canaan, CT, 1989.

7. Hoffer A: The Development of Orthomolecular Medicine. In Press, 1995.

8. Hoffer A: Niacin Therapy in Psychiatry. C. C. Thomas, Springfield, IL, 1962. See also:

Hoffer A & Osmond H: New Hope for Alcoholics, University Books, New York, 1966. Written by Fannie Kahan.

Hoffer A & Walker M: Nutrients to Age Without Senility. Keats Pub Inc, New Canaan, CT, 1980.

Hoffer A & Walker M: Smart Nutrients. A Guide to Nutrients That Can Prevent and Reverse Senility. Avery Publishing Group, Garden City Park, New York, 1994.

9. Wilson B: The Vitamin B-3 Therapy: The First Communication to A.A.'s Physicians and A Second Communication to A.A.'s Physicians, 1967 and 1968.

10. Smith RF: A five-year field trial of massive nicotinic acid therapy of alcoholics in Michigan. Journal of Orthomolecular Psychiatry 3:327-331, 1974. See also:

Smith RF: Status report concerning the use of megadose nicotinic acid in alcoholics. Journal of Orthomolecular Psychiatry 7:52-55, 1978.

11. Kaufman W: Common Forms of Niacinamide Deficiency Disease: Aniacin Amidosis. Yale University Press, New Haven, CT, 1943. See also:

Kaufman W: The Common Form of Joint Dysfunction: Its Incidence and Treatment. E.L. Hildreth and Co., Brattelboro, VT, 1949.

12. Hoffer A: Orthomolecular Medicine For Physicians, Keats Pub, New Canaan, CT, 1989.

13. Jacobson M & Jacobson E: Niacin, nutrition, ADP-ribosylation and cancer. The 8th International Symposium on ADP- Ribosylation, Texas College of Osteopathic Medicine, Fort Worth, TX, 1987. See also:

Titus K: Scientists link niacin and cancer prevention. The D.O. 28:93-97, 1987.

Hostetler D: Jacobsons put broad strokes in the niacin/cancer picture. The D.O. 28:103-104, 1987.

14. Chaplin DJ, Horsman MP & Aoki DS: Nicotinamide, Fluosol DA and Carbogen: a strategy to reoxygenate acutely and chronically hypoxic cells in vivo. British Journal of Cancer 63:109-113, 1990.

15. Nakagawa K, Miyazaka M, Okui K, Kato N, Moriyama Y & Fujimura S: N1-methylnicotinamide level in the blood after nicotinamide loading as further evidence for malignant tumor burden. Jap. J. Cancer Research 82:277-1283, 1991.

16. Gerson M: Dietary considerations in malignant neoplastic disease. A prelimary report. The Review of Gastroenterology 12:419-425, 1945. See also:

Gerson M: Effects of a combined dietary regime on patients with malignant tumors. Experimental Medicine and Surgery 7:299-317, 1949.

17. Hoffer A: Orthomolecular Oncology. In, Adjuvant Nutrition in Cancer Treatment, Ed. P. Quillin & R. M. Williams. 1992 Symposium Proceedings, Sponsored by Cancer Treatment Research Foundation and American College of Nutrition. Cancer Treatment Research Foundation, 3455 Salt Creek Lane, Suite 200, Arlington Heights, IL 60005-1090, 331-362, 1994.

18. Hoffer A: Hong Kong Veterans Study. J Orthomolecular Psychiatry 3:34-36, 1974.

19. Marks J: Vitamin Safety. Vitamin Information Status Paper, F. Hoffman La Roche & Co., Basle, 1989.

20. Mullin GE, Greenson JK & Mitchell MC: Fulminant hepatic failure after ingestion of sustained-release nicotinic acid. Ann Internal Medicine 111:253-255, 1989.

21. Henkin Y, Johnson KC & Segrest JP: Rechallenge with crystalline niacin after drug-induced hepatitis from sustained-release niacin. J. American Medical Assn. 264:241-243, 1990.

22. Hoffer A: Niacin Therapy in Psychiatry. C. C. Thomas, Springfield, IL, 1962. See also:

    Hoffer A: Safety, Side Effects and Relative Lack of Toxicity of Nicotinic acid and Nicotinamide. Schizophrenia 1:78-87, 1969.

    Hoffer A: Vitamin B-3 (Niacin) Update. New Roles for a Key Nutrient in Diabetes, Cancer, Heart Disease and Other Major Health Problems. Keats Pub, Inc., New Canaan, CT, 1990.

For Further Reading

You may receive the *Orthomolecular Medicine News Service* free of charge by email. The subscription link is http://orthomolecular.org/subscribe.html. It is peer-reviewed and contains no advertising. The entire OMNS archive of over 300 articles is at http://www.doctoryourself.com/omns/index.shtml and also at http://orthomolecular.org/resources/omns/index.shtml. All issues are available in English, Spanish, and Portuguese. Many are available in French, Chinese, German, and Norwegian.

American Society for Nutrition. "Symposium: Nutrients and Epigenetic Regulation of Gene Expression." *J Nutr* 139(12) (Dec 2009): 2397–240.

Angell, M. "Is Academic Medicine for Sale?" *N Engl J Med* 342(20) (May 18, 2000): 1516–8.

Benavente, C. A., M. K. Jacobson, E. L. Jacobson. "NAD in Skin: Therapeutic Approaches for Niacin." *Curr Pharm Des* 15(1) (Jan 2009): 29–38.

Benavente, C. A., E. L. Jacobson. "Niacin Restriction Upregulates NADPH Oxidase and Reactive Oxygen Species (ROS) in Human Keratinocytes." *Free Radic Biol Med* 44 (Feb 2008): 527–37.

Berge, K. G., P. L. Canner. "Coronary Drug Project: Experience with Niacin. Coronary Drug Project Research Group." *Eur J Clin Pharmacol* 40 Suppl 1 (1991): S49–51.

Berger, M. M. "Nutrients as Antioxidants—Effect of Antioxidative Trace Elements and Vitamins on Outcome of Critically Ill Burns and Trauma Patients." *Aktuelle Ernaehrungsmedizin* 28(6) (2003): 376–379.

Birkmayer, J. G., C. Vrecko, D. Volc, et al. "Nicotinamide Adenine Dinucleotide (NADH)—A New Therapeutic Approach to Parkinson's Disease. Comparison of Oral and Parenteral Application." *Acta Neurol Scand Suppl* 146 (1993): 32–35.

Boyle, E. "Communication to AA by Bill W." In: *The Vitamin B3 Therapy*. 1967.

Carey, J. "FDA Rejects Merck's Cordaptive." *BusinessWeek*. (April 29, 2008): 11–13.

Challem, J. *Nutrition Reporter* 19 (2008)

Clarkes, R. "Niacin for Nicotine?" *Lancet* 1(8174) (Apr 26, 1980): 936.

Cleave, T. L., G. D. Campbell, N. S. Painter. *Diabetes, Coronary Thrombosis, and the Saccharine Disease.* 2nd. ed. Bristol, ENG: John Wright and Sons, 1969.

DeAngelis, C. D., P. B. Fontanarosa. "Impugning the Integrity of Medical Science: The Adverse Effects of Industry Influence." *J Am Med Assoc* 299(15) (2008): 1833–1835.

El Enein, A., A. M. Hafez, Y.S. Salem, et al. "The Role of Nicotinic Acid and Inositol Hexanicotinate as Anticholesterolemic and Antilipemic Agents." *Nutr Rep Int* 281 (1983): 899–911.

Foster, H. D. "New Strategies For Reversing Vital Pandemics: The Role of Nutrition." *P Int Forum Public Health Shanghai* (2007): 19–23.

Galadari, E., S. Hadi, K. Sabarinathan. "Hartnup Disease." *Int J Dermatol.* 32(12) (Dec 1993): 904.

Graveline, D. "Transient Global Amnesia. A Side Effect of 'Statins' Treatment." *Townsend Letter for Doctors and Patients* 253/254 (Aug/Sept 2004): 85–89.

Hill, K. P., J. S. Ross, D. S. Egilman, et al. "The ADVANTAGE Seeding Trial: A Review of Internal Documents." *Ann Intern Med* 149(4) (Aug 2008): 251–258.

Hoffer, A. *Adventures in Psychiatry.* Toronto, ON: Kos Press, 2005.

Hoffer, A. *Dr. Hoffer's ABC of Natural Nutrition for Children.* Kingston, ON: Quarry Press, 1999. 45.

Hoffer, A. "Epidermolysis Bullosa: A Zinc Dependent Condition?" *J Orthomolecular Med* 7 (1992): 245–246.

Hoffer, A. *Healing Cancer.* Toronto, ON: CCNM Press, 2004.

Hoffer, A. *Hoffer's Laws of Natural Nutrition: A Guide to Eating Well for Pure Health.* Kingston, ON: Quarry Press, 1996.

Hoffer, A. "Hong Kong Veterans Study." *J Orthomolecular Psychiat* 3 (1974): 34–36.

Hoffer, A. "Mechanism of Action of Nicotinic Acid and Nicotinamide in the Treatment of Schizophrenia." In: *Orthomolecular Psychiatry*, R. Hawkins, L. Pauling, eds. San Francisco, CA WH Freeman, 1973.

Hoffer, A. *Niacin Therapy in Psychiatry.* Springfield, IL: CC Thomas, 1962.

Hoffer, A. *Mental Health Regained.* Toronto, ON: International Schizophrenia Foundation, 2007.

Hoffer, A. "An Orthomolecular Look at Obesity." *J Orthomolecular Med* 22(1st Q 2007): 4–7.

Hoffer, A. *Orthomolecular Treatment for Schizophrenia.* A Keats Good Health Guide. Lincolnwood, IL: Keats, 1999.

Hoffer, A. "The Psychophysiology of Cancer." *J Asthma Res* 8 (1970): 61–76.

Hoffer, A. *Treatment Manual.* Toronto, ON: International Schizophrenia Foundation, 2007.

Hoffer, A. *User's Guide to Natural Therapies for Cancer Prevention and Control.* Laguna Beach, CA: Basic Health Publications, 2004.

Hoffer, A. *Vitamin B3 and Schizophrenia: Discovery, Recovery, Controversy.* Kingston, ON: Quarry Press, 2004.

Hoffer, A. *Vitamin B3: Niacin and Its Amide.* http://www.doctoryourself.com/hoffer _niacin.html.

Hoffer, A., H. Osmond. *The Chemical Basis of Clinical Psychiatry.* Springfield, IL: CC Thomas, 1960.

Hoffer, A., H. Osmond. *The Hallucinogens.* Academic Press, New York, 1967.

Hoffer, A., H. Osmond. *How To Live with Schizophrenia.* New York, NY, University Books, 1966. (Also published by Johnson, London, ENG, 1966, written by Fannie Kahan; New revised ed.: Citadel Press, New York, NY, 1992. Revised: Quarry Press, Kingston, ON.)

Hoffer, A., H. Osmond, M. J. Callbeck, I. Kahan. "Treatment of Schizophrenia With Nicotinic Acid and Nicotinamide." *J Clin Exper Psychopathol* 18(2) (1957): 131–158.

Hoffer, A., H. Osmond, J. Smythies. "Schizophrenia: A New Approach. II. Results of a Year's Research." *J Ment Sci* 100 (1954): 29–45.

Hoffer, A., J. Prousky. *Naturopathic Nutrition: A Guide to Nutrient-rich Food & Nutritional Supplements for Optimum Health.* Toronto, ON: CCNM Press, 2006.

Hoffer, A., A. W. Saul. *The Vitamin Cure for Alcoholism.* Laguna Beach, CA: Basic Health Publications, 2008.

Hoffer, A., M. Walker. *Putting It All Together: The New Orthomolecular Nutrition.* New Canaan, CT: Keats Publishing, 1996.

Horton, J. W. et al. "Antioxidant Vitamin Therapy Alters Burn Trauma-mediated Cardiac NF-B Activation and Cardiomyocyte Cytokine Secretion." *J Trauma: Inj Inf Crit Care,* 50(3) (2001): 397–408.

Jacobson, E. L., Jacobson, M. K. "A Biomarker for the Assessment of Niacin Nutriture as a Potential Preventive Factor in Carcinogenesis." *J Intern Med* 233(1) (Jan 1993): 59–62.

Jonas, A. J., I. J. Butler. "Circumvention of Defective Neutral Amino Acid Transport in Hartnup Disease Using Tryptophan Ethyl Ester." *J Clin Invest.* 84(1) (Jul 1989): 200–204.

Jonas, W. B., C. P. Rapoza, W. F. Blair. "The Effect of Niacinamide on Osteoarthritis: A Pilot Study." *Inflamm Res* 45 (1996): 330–4.

Kaufman CS, Saul AW. Niacinamide Therapy Pioneer William Kaufman, MD, PhD, as Remembered by his Wife, Charlotte JOM, Volume 30:1, p ———

Kaufman, W. "Bibliography of Professional Publications." DoctorYourself.com. http://www.doctoryourself.com/biblio_kaufman.html

Kaufman, W. "Collected Papers." University of Michigan, Special Collections Library, 7th Floor, Harlan Hatcher Graduate Library, Ann Arbor, Ml 48109. special.collections @umich.edu Phone: 734-764-9377

Kaufman, W. *Common Forms of Niacinamide Deficiency Disease: Aniacin Amidosis.* New Haven, CT: Yale University Press, 1943.

Kaufman, W. "Niacinamide Improves Mobility in Degenerative Joint Disease." *Am Assoc Adv Sci* Program, Philadelphia, PA: AAAS, May 24–30, 1986. Abstract.

Kaufman. W. "Niacinamide Therapy for Joint Mobility." *Conn. State Med. J* 17 (1953): 584–589.

Kaufman, W. "Vitamin Deficiency, Megadoses, and Some Supplemental History." (1992) Letter. DoctorYourself.com. http://www.doctoryourself.com/kaufman2.html

Kaufman, W. "What Took the FDA So Long to Come Out in Favor of Folic Acid?" Commentary. DoctorYourself.com. http://www.doctoryourself.com/kaufman4.html

Kirkland, J. B. "Niacin Status Impacts Chromatin Structure." *J Nutr* 139(12) (Dec 2009): 2397–2401.

Kunin, R. A. "The Action of Aspirin in Preventing the Niacin Flush and Its Relevance to the Antischizophrenic Action of Megadose Niacin." *J Orthomolecular Psychiat* 5 (1976): 89–100.

Lewis, N. D. C., Z. A. Piotrowski. "Clinical Diagnosis of Manic-depressive Psychosis." In: *Depression*, P. H. Hoch, J. Zubin, eds., New York, NY: Grune & Stratton, 1954. 25–38.

Linus Pauling Institute, Micronutrient Information Center. Oregon State University. J. Higdon 2002; Updated by V. J. Drake 2007. lpi.oregonstate.edu/infocenter /vitamins/niacin

McCarty, M. F. "Co-administration of Equimolar Doses of Betaine May Alleviate the Hepatotoxic Risk Associated With Niacin Therapy." *Med Hypotheses* 55 (2000): 189–194.

McCracken, R. D. *Niacin and Human Health Disorders.* Fort Collins, CO: Hygea Publishing Co., 1994.

McIlroy, A. "A Tip to Get That Monkey off Your Back." *Globe and Mail,* April 7, 2008.

Miller, C. L., I. C. Llenos, J. R. Dulay, et al. "Expression of the Kynurenine Pathway Enzmye Tryptophan 2.3 Dioxygenase is Increased in the Frontal Cortex of Individuals With Schizophrenia." *Neurobiol Dis* 15 (2004): 618–629.

Miller, C. L., I. C. Llenos, J. R. Dulay, et al. "Upregulation of the Initiating Step of the Kynurenine Pathway in Postmortem Anterior Cingulate Cortex from Individuals With Schizophrenia and Bipolar disorders." *Brain Res* 1073–1074 (2006): 25–37.

Morris, M. C., D. A. Evans, J. L. Bienias, et al. "Dietary Intake of Antioxidant Nutrients and the Risk of Incident Alzheimer's Disease in a Biracial Community Study." *J Am Med Assoc* 287(24) (2002): 3230–3237.

Munro, M. "Cholesterol Pill's Side Effects Worry BBC Drug Specialists." Victoria, BC: *Times-Colonist,* September 16, 2003.

Murray, M. F. *Treatment of Retrovirus Induced Derangements With Niacin Compounds.* Cambridge, MA: The Foundation for Innovative Therapies. 9 p.

Murray, M. F., M. Langan, R. R. MacGregor. "Increased Plasma Tryptophan in HIV-infected Patients Treated With Pharmacologic Doses of Nicotinamide." *Nutrition* (*NY*) 17(7/8) (2001): 654–656.

Parsons, W. B., Jr. "The Effect of Nicotinic Acid on the Liver. Evidence Favoring Functional Alteration of Enzymatic Reactions Without Hepatocellular Damage." In: *Niacin in Vascular Disorders and Hyperlipemia.* R Altshul, ed. Springfield, IL: CC Thomas, 1964.

Parsons, W. B., Jr., R. W. P. Achor, K. G. Berge, et al. "Changes in Concentration of Blood Lipids Following Prolonged Administration of Large Doses of Nicotinic Acid to Persons with Hypercholesterolemia: Preliminary Observations." *Proc Staff Meet Mayo Clinic,* 31 (1956): 377–390.

Picard, A. "Beating Cancer: the Good and the Bad." *Globe and Mail,* Toronto, ON: April 10, 2008.

Prousky, J., C. G. Millman, J. J. Kirkland. "Pharmacologic Use of Niacin." *J Evidence-Based Complementary Alt Med* 16(2) (March 24, 2011): 91–101.

Saul, A. "Down Syndrome: The Nutritional Treatment of Henry Turkel, MD" DoctorYourself.com. http://www.doctoryourself.com/turkel.html

Schmidtke, K., W. Endres, A. Roscher, et al. "Hartnup Syndrome, Progressive Encephalopathy and Allo-albuminaemia. A Clinico-pathological Case Study." *Eur J Pediatr* 151(12) (Dec 1992): 899–903.

Silverman, D. H. S. "Altered Brain Function After Chemotherapy." *Neurol Rev* 14(11) (2006).

Silverman, D. H. S. "Changes in Brain Function Persist 10 Years after Chemotherapy, Imaging Study Suggests." *Oncology Times* 28(2225) (November 2006): 50.

Simpson, L. O. "Can the Role of Statins be Discussed Without Recognition of Their Effects on Blood Viscosity? Rapid Response." *BMJ* April 3, 2008.

Spies, T. D., C. D. Aring, J. Gelperin, et al. "The Mental Symptoms of Pellagra: Their Relief with Nicotinic Acid." *Am J Med Sci* 196 (1938): 461.

Spies, T. D., W. B. Bean, R. E. Stone. "The Treatment of Subclinical and Classical Pellagra: Use of Nicotinic Acid, Nicotinic Acid Amide and Sodium Nicotinate, with Special Reference to the Vasodilator Action and Effect on Mental Symptoms." *J Am Med Assoc* 111 (1938): 581.

Stroup, T. S., J. P. McEvoy, M. S. Swartz, et al. "The National Institute of Mental Health Clinical Antipsychotic Trials of Intervention Effectiveness (CATIE) project: Schizophrenia Trial Design and Protocol Development." *Schizophr Bull* 29(1) (2003): 15–31.

Taubes, G. *Good Calories, Bad Calories.* New York, NY: Knopf, 2007.

Titus, K. "Scientists Link Niacin and Cancer Prevention." *The D.O.* 28 (Aug 1987): 93–97.

Taylor, P. "Bad Medicine: Health Care, Under the Influence." *Globe and Mail* April 26, 2008.

Turkel, H. "Medical amelioration of Down syndrome incorporating the orthomolecular approach." *J Orthomolecular Psych 4* (1975):102–115.

Turkel, H. "Medical amelioration of Down syndrome incorporating the orthomolecular approach," in: *Diet Related to Killer Diseases V. Nutrition and Mental Health*. Hearing before the Select Committee on Nutrition and Human Needs of the United States Senate, Washington, DC: U.S. Government Printing Office, 1977: 291–304.

Turkel, H. *Medical treatment of Down syndrome and genetic diseases*, Southfield, MI: Ubiotica, 4th rev. ed., 1985.

Turkel, H. *New hope for the mentally retarded: Stymied by the FDA*. New York, NY: Vantage Press, 1972.

Uneri, O., U. Tural, N. Cakin Memik. "Smoking and Schizophrenia: Where is the Biological Connection." *Turk Psikiyatri Dergisi* 17 (2006): 1–10.

Wald, G., B. Jackson. "Activity and Nutritional Deprivation." *P Natl Acad Sci USA* 30(9) (Sep 15 1944): 255–263.

Wilson, B. *The Vitamin B3 Therapy: The First Communication to A.A.'s Physicians*, Bedford Hills, NY: 1967. Private publication.

Wilson, B. *A second communication to A.A.'s physicians*. Bedford Hills, NY: Private publication. 1968.

Wittenborn, J. R., E. S. P. Weber, M. Brown. "Niacin in the Long-Term Treatment of Schizophrenia." *Arch Gen Psychiat* 28 (1973): 308–315.

Yamada, K., K. Nonaka, T. Hanafusa, et al. "Preventive and Therapeutic Effects of Large-dose Nicotinamide Injections on Diabetes Associated With Insulitis." *Diabetes* 31 (1982): 749–753.

Yang, J., J. D. Adams. "Nicotinamide and Its Pharmacological Properties for Clinical Therapy." *Drug Design Rev* 1 (2004): 43–52.

Yang, J., L. K. Klaidman, J. D. Adams. "Medicinal Chemistry of Nicotinamide in the Treatment of Ischemis and Reperfusion." *Mini-Rev Med Chem* 2 (2002): 125–134.

Yu, B., Zhao, S. "Anti-inflammatory Effect is an Important Property of Niacin on Atherosclerosis Beyond Its Lipid-altering Effects." *Med Hypotheses* 69(1) (2007): 90–94.

Zandi, P. P. "Vitamin C, E in High Dose Combination May Protect Against Alzheimer's Disease." FuturePundit: Future technological trends and their likely effects on human society, politics and evolution. January 20, 2004.

Index

About the Authors

ABRAM HOFFER, MD, PHD (1917–2009)

In the documentary film *Masks of Madness: Science of Healing*, Abram Hoffer says: "Mental illness is usually biochemical illness. Schizophrenia is niacin dependency." Plain-spoken statements such as these have ignited a revolution in psychiatry. The person who would forever change the course of medicine was born on a Saskatchewan farm and educated in a one-room schoolhouse. In 1952, just completing his residency, he demonstrated with the first double-blind, placebo-controlled studies in the history of psychiatry that vitamin B_3 could cure schizophrenia. But in a medical profession that "knows" vitamins do not cure "real" diseases, the young director of psychiatric research was a dissenter. For over half a century Dr. Hoffer would continue to dissent. Harold Foster wrote: "Fathering a new paradigm does not promote popularity. Fortunately, Dr. Hoffer is not just highly intelligent; he has consistently proven to be able to stand up for the truth, regardless of personal cost."

"If patients look up 'schizophrenia' in the old textbooks," said Dr. Hoffer, "they'll die of frustration and fear. That is why I wrote my first book, *How to Live with Schizophrenia*. Linus Pauling was sixty-five and planning to retire. He chanced to see this book on a friend's coffee table. Pauling did not go to bed the first night he read this book. He decided not to retire because of it."

Dr. Hoffer wrote over thirty books and over 600 papers. He is a member of the Orthomolecular Medicine Hall of Fame and received the Dr. Rogers Prize in 2007. He created the *Journal of Orthomolecular Medicine* and was its editor-in-chief for four decades. Having treated thousands of patients, Dr. Hoffer finally retired at age eighty-eight, wryly saying that "Everyone should have a career change every fifty-five years."

Linus Pauling said, "Abram Hoffer has made an important contribution to the health of human beings... through the study of the effects of large doses of vitamins and other nutrients."

ANDREW W. SAUL (B. 1955)

Andrew W. Saul, an orthomolecular medical lecturer for nearly 50 years, is author or coauthor of a dozen books. He is a member of the Japanese College of Intravenous Therapy and the Orthomolecular Medicine Hall of Fame. Saul has taught nutrition, health science, and cell biology at the college level. He is cofounder of the *Orthomolecular Medicine News Service* and has been its editor-in-chief for 19 years. He is the author of the Basic Health Publications books *Doctor Yourself* and *Fire Your Doctor!* and wrote *Orthomolecular Medicine for Everyone, Hospitals and Health*, and *The Vitamin Cure for Alcoholism* with Dr. Abram Hoffer. He is coauthor of five other books: *Vitamin C: The Real Story; The Vitamin Cure for Children's Health Problems; Vegetable Juicing for Everyone; I Have Cancer: What Should I Do?; and The Vitamin Cure for Infant and Toddler Health Problems.* Dr. Saul is on the editorial board of the *Journal of Orthomolecular Medicine* and is featured in the documentary films *Food Matters* and *That Vitamin Movie.* He has twice won New York Empire State Fellowships for teaching, and has published over 200 reviews and editorials in peer-reviewed publications. His internationally famous, noncommercial natural healing website is DoctorYourself.com.

HAROLD D. FOSTER, PHD (1943–2009)

Harold Foster was deeply invested in improving the quality of life for all living things. For more than forty years, Dr. Foster worked as a geomorphologist, professor of medical geography, consultant to the United Nations and NATO in disaster planning, and avid researcher, which culminated in the formation of the Harold Foster Foundation.

A Canadian by choice, Dr. Foster was born in Tunstall, Yorkshire, England, and educated at the Hull Grammar School and University College

London. While at university, he specialized in geology and geography, earning a B.Sc. in 1964 and a PhD in 1968. He was a faculty member in the Department of Geography, University of Victoria, from 1967 to 2008. As a tenured professor, he authored or edited over 300 publications, the majority of which focused on reducing disaster losses or identifying the causes of chronic degenerative and infectious diseases.

His numerous books include *Disaster Planning: The Preservation of Life and Property*; *Health, Disease and the Environment*; and *Reducing Cancer Mortality: A Geographical Perspective*. He also wrote six books in the What Really Causes series, including those on AIDS, Alzheimer's disease, multiple sclerosis, schizophrenia, SIDS, and breast cancer. Dr. Foster made unique contributions in our understanding of health and disease as he explored the complex relationships between genetic inheritance, health and the "nutritional geographies" of the world. He also conducted many groundbreaking studies of selenium in AIDS therapy in Africa.

Dr. Foster served on the editorial board of the *Journal of Orthomolecular Medicine* for fifteen years, and on the board of directors for the International Schizophrenia Foundation for thirteen years. He was inducted into the Orthomolecular Medicine Hall of Fame in 2010. Photos and short biographies of all members of the Orthomolecular Medicine Hall of Fame may be freely accessed at isom.ca/hall-of-fame/.

CPSIA information can be obtained
at www.ICGtesting.com
Printed in the USA
JSHW081722210223
38049JS00001B/1

9 781684 429028